Clinical Applications: Integrated Traditional Chinese Medicine (TCM) and Western Medicine

Volume I

Compiled and Translated by
Scott L. Herbster, OMD, L.Ac.

Edited by
Marc Wasserman, Ph.D, L.Ac.

Copyright © 2017 Scott L. Herbster
All rights reserved.
ISBN: 1979234272
ISBN-13: 978-1979234276

TABLE OF CONTENTS

	Foreword	i
	Preface	iii
	Introduction	vii
1	Cancer	1
2	Head and Cerebrovascular Diseases	94
3	Cardiovascular Disorders	106
4	Vascular Diseases in Other Parts of the Body	116
5	Head and Neck Disorders	124
6	Autoimmune Diseases	130
	Epilogue	174
	Appendix	175

LIST OF CASE STUDIES

I. Cancer

Section 1: Brain Tumors and Brain Pathologies

Case Study #1: Clinical Treatment of Anaplastic Astrocytoma

Case Study #2: Benign Brain Tumor – Postoperative Complications

Case Study #3: Brain Tumors – Impact of Chemotherapy and Radiotherapy on Hematopoiesis

Case Study #4: Postsurgical Radiotherapy Induces Brain Swelling (Edema)

Case Study #5: Advanced Stage Malignant Brain Tumor Necrosis

Case Study #6: Corticosteroids – Firstline Treatment of Brain Swelling (Edema) Following Surgery, Radiotherapy, and Chemotherapy

Case Study #7: Bu Zhong Yi Qi Tang Variant – "Conquers All Pathoconditions"

Case Study #8: Dry Mouth and Eyes Following Radiotherapy – Don't Misuse Glaucoma Drug (Pilocarpine HCl)!
Case Study #9: Hemiparesis Resulting from Cerebral Infarction

Case Study #10: Cerebral Infarction (Stroke) Complicated by Hydrocephalus – Is There Cerebral Atrophy?

Case Study #11: Dizziness Following Cerebellar Infarction

Case Study #12: Non-healing Wound Following Menangioma Resection

Case Study #13: Intracranial (Brain Stem) Lipoma – Is Treatment Necessary?

Section 2: Other Pathogenic Conditions of the Brain

Case Study #1: Head Tremor – Essential Tremor and Cerebellar Atrophy

Case Study #2: Edematous Meninges Affects Vision

Case Study #3: Post-Concussion Syndrome – "Double Vision"

Case Study #4: Head Trauma – Concussion and Hemorrhage

Case Study #5: Concussion – Cold Hands and Feet and Profuse Sweating Following Mannitol Administration

Case Study #6: Post-concussion Complication – Night Sweats

Case Study #7: Post-Concussion Syndrome (PCS) or Neurosis?

Case Study #8: Amnesia and Dysphasia Following Car Accident

Case Study #9: Tuberculous Meningitis

Case Study #10: Multiple Primary Tumors

Section 3: Respiratory System Cancers

Case Study #1: Nasopharyngeal Carcinoma (NPC)

Case Study #2: Lung Cancer: Can TCM Provide Effective Treatment?

Case Study #3: Lung Cancer: TCM Treatment and Medicinal Foods

Case Study #4: Advanced Metastatic Cancer and Malignant Pleural Effusion (PE)

Section 4: Gastric (Stomach) Cancer

Case Study #1: Gastric Cancer Treatment – Xiang Sha Liu Jun Zi Tang

Case Study #2: Gastric Cancer – A Difficult Condition to Treat

Case Study #3: Adenocarcinoma

Case Study #4: Postoperative Vomiting – How Can I Administer TCM Formula Decoction?

Case Study #5: Gastric Tumor Resection – What TCM Formula Should I Prescribe?

Case Study #6: Cerebral Infarction Patient Diagnosed With Gastric Cancer

Case Study #7: Gastric Cancer – Multiple Metastases

Case Study #8: Gastric Cancer – Post-Operative Regional and Distant Lymph Node Metastases

Case Study #9: Do Tumor Markers Correlate With Pulmonary Tuberculosis?

Case Study #10: Gastric Cancer – Colonic and Brain Metastases

Case Study #11: Advanced Stage Gastric Cancer – Peritoneal and Adrenal Metastases

Section 5: Colorectal Cancer

Case Study #1: Granulomatous Polyp Following Surgical Resection

Case Study #2: Recurrence After 7 Years of Remission

Case Study #3: Colorectal Cancer – Liver and Abdominal Cavity Metastases

Case Study #4: Chemotherapy Induced Watery Diarrhea – Wu Ling San Variation

Cast Study #5: Metastatic Colorectal Cancer

Case Study #6: Colorectal Cancer with Fecal Incontinence

Section 6: Pancreatic Cancer

Case Study #1: Vomiting Following Chemotherapy and Radiotherapy

Case Study #2: It's Really Difficult to Treat!

Case Study #3: Advanced Stage Pancreatic Cancer

Section 7: Liver Cancer

Case Study #1: Hepatocellular Carcinoma (HCC)

Case Study #2: Three Formulas for Treating Liver Cancer

Case Study #3: Transcatheter Arterial Embolism (TAE)

Case Study #4: Elevated AFP and Low T-Pro Following Surgery

Case Study #5: Diffuse Hepatocellular Carcinoma (HCC)

Case Study #6: Elevated AFP Levels

Case Study #7: Postoperative Hepatocellular Carcinoma (HCC) Multiple Metastases

Case Study #8: South Korea's Popular "Vegetarian Liver Cancer-Fighting Diet"

Section 8: Breast Cancer

Case Study #1: Frequent Massage for Postoperative Arm Lymphedema

Case Study #2: Intermittent Upper Limb Lymphedema

Case Study #3: Acupuncture and Moxabustion Principles Following Surgery, Radiotherapy, and Chemotherapy

Case Study #4: Postoperative Ileal and Lung Metastases

Case Study #5: Hormonal Therapy

Case Study #6: Lung, Liver, and Lymphatic Metastases

Case Study #7: Vegetarian Diet – Devastating for Chemotherapy and Radiotherapy Patients

Case Study #8: Be Careful of Contracting HPV

Case Study #9: Acupuncture Treats HPV

Case Study #10: Intermittent Plueral Effusion

Case Study #11: Leukopenia Following Radiotherapy

Case Study #12: Is Pregnancy Safe for Breast Cancer Patients Following Treatment?

Case Study #13: Adverse Effects – Long-term Administration of Tamoxifen

Case Study #14: TCM Medicinal Prescriptions Must Flexibly Respond to Patient's Condition

Case Study #15: Increased CA15-3 and Thrombocytopenia

Case Study #16: Lung Metastases – Focus on Increasing WBCs

Case Study #17: Bone Metastases – Add Lu Jiao

Case Study #18: Colorectal Metastases – Nausea and Vomiting Following Chemotherapy and Radiotherapy

Section 9: Other Types of Cancer

Case Study #1: Tonsillar Cancer – Salivary Gland Hypofunction, Xerostomia, and Aguesia Following Chemotherapy and Radiotherapy

Case Study #2: Gastrointestinal Cancer – Pancreatic and Lymph Node Metastases

Case Study #3: Cervical Cancer – Colorectal Metastases

Case Study #4: Prostate Cancer

Case Study #5: Swollen Neck Lymph Nodes

Case Study #6: Non-Hodgkin's Lymphoma (NHL)

Case Study #7: Multiple Spinal Cord Tumors

Case Study #8: Cervical Artery Aneurysm

Case Study #9: Syringoma – TCM Treatment

Section 10: Therapeutic Side Effects and Novel Therapy

Case Study #1: Radiotherapy-induced Salivary Gland and Gustatory Nerve Damage

Case Study #2: Chemotherapy-induced Peripheral Neuropathy of the Upper and Lower Limbs

Case Study #3: Immunotherapy (Biologic Therapy)

II. Head and Cerebrovascular Diseases

Case Study #1: Sexual Headaches (Coital Cephalgia)

Case Study #2: Parkinson's Disease (PD)

Case Study #3: Limb Tremor – Early Sign of Parkinson's Disease?

Case Study #4: Early-Onset Parkinson's Disease

Case Study #5: Hemilateral Edema – It's Not Alzheimer's Disease!

Case Study #6: Parkinson's Disease, CSF Hypovolemia, or Cerebral Atrophy?

Case Study #7: Cerebral Atrophy, Parkinson's Disease, or Atypical Parkinsonism?

Case Study #8: Essential Tremor among the Elderly

Case Study #9: Lower Jaw and Upper Limb Tremor – "Not" Essential Tremor of the Elderly

Case Study #10: Lower Jaw Spasms and Twitching

Case Study #11: Posterior Cerebral Artery "Beating Like a Drum"

Case Study #12: Cerebellar Atrophy and Cerebral Infarction Inducing Dizziness

Case Study #13: Cerebral Infarction Complicated by Hydrocephalus

Case Study #14: TIA – A Type of Cerebral Infarction

Case Study #15: Nocturnal Cramps – Periodic Paralysis "Not" Cerebral Infarction

Case Study #16: Climacteric Hypertension Inducing Headache

III. Cardiovascular Disorders

Case Study #1: Palpitations and Tachycardia – Wolff Parkinson White Syndrome

Case Study #2: What Is Wolff Parkinson White Syndrome?

Case Study #3: Coma Following Cardiac Arrest

Case Study #4: What is Marfan syndrome?

Case Study #5: Angina Pectoris (Stable Angina), Psychosomatic Disorder, or Esophageal Ulcer?

Case Study #6: Arrhythmia Resulting from Anemia

Case Study #7: Sweating from the Chest – One of the Sweating in the Five Hearts

Case Study #8: Coronary Artery Disease (CAD) (aka Ischemic Heart Disease (IHD))

Case Study #9: Lower Limb Edema – Heart Disease or DVT?

Case Study #10: Hyperglycemia Following Coronary Artery Stent Placement

IV. Vascular Diseases in Other Parts of the Body

Case Study #1: Retinal Vascular Occlusion (Ocular Stroke)

Case Study #2: Intermittent Claudication

Case Study #3: Varicose Veins (VV) and Deep Vein Thrombosis (DVT)

Case Study #4: Deep Vein Thrombosis (DVT)

Case Study #5: Hyperlipidemia

Case Study #6: Gangrene – Poor Circulation of the Lower Limbs

V. Head and Neck Disorders

Case Study #1: Foot Tai Yin Phlegm Reversal Headache

Case Study #2: Psychosomatic Disorder, Fibromyalgia, or Foot Tai Yin Phlegm Reversal Headache?

Case Study #3: Intractable Headache, Uterine Fibroids, and Endometrial Hyperplasia

Case Study #4: Swollen Lymph Node in Neck

Case Study #5: Elderly Patient Unable to Rotate Neck

Case Study #6: Nuchal Rigidity

VI. Autoimmune Diseases

Section 1: Rheumatoid Arthritis (RA)

Case Study #1: Five Approaches to Treating RA

Case Study #2: Scan Image Reveals Joint Inflammation

Case Study #3: Differential Diagnosis – Periodic Paralysis (PP), Subacute Combined Degeneration (SCD), Ankylosing Spondylitis (AS), and Rheumatoid Arthritis (RA)

Case Study #4: Ankylosing Spondylitis (AS)

Case Study #5: Zygomatic (Cheek) Bone Swelling – Don't Prescribe Feng Shi Fang

Section 2: Systemic Lupus Erythamatosus (SLE)

Case Study #1: Three Keys to Treating SLE

Case Study #2: SLE – Mediastinal Effusion Indicates Renal and Brain Damage Stage

Case Study #3: SLE – Acupuncture and TCM Medicinals

Case Study #4: SLE and Idiopathic Thrombocytopenic Purpura (ITP)

Case Study #5: Rheumatoid Arthritis (RA) and Systemic Lupus Erythamatosus (SLE)

Section 3: Idiopathic Thrombocytopenic Purpura (ITP)

Case Study #1: It's Probably Purpura

Case Study #2: What Is Idiopathic Thrombocytopenic Purpura (ITP)?

Case Study #3: Gong Zhen Dan – It's Not Sheng Yu Tang!

Case Study #4: Sheng Yu Tang – It's the Best!

Case Study #5: ITP in Menopausal Patient with Vaginal Bleeding

Case Study #6: Why Is the Fluctuation in PLT Count So Extreme?

Case Study #7: Splenectomy – Eliminates Platelet Destruction and Sequestration

Case Study #8: Familial (Inherited) ITP – It's Worth Following Up!

Case Study #9: ITP Prevalence Increasing in South Korea – Patients Seek TCM Treatment

Case Study #10: Other Heat Pattern Conditions Complicated By Idiopathic Thrombocytopenic Purpura (ITP)

Case Study #11: She Also Has Evans Syndrome

Section 4: Behcet's Disease

Case Study #1: My First Behcet's Disease Patient

Case Study #2: Behcet's Requires Long-term Administration of TCM Medicinals

Case Study #3: Once Western Medicine Drugs Have Been Discontinued – (Yu Sheng) Hyperactive Immune Formula

Case Study #4: Painful Oral Ulcerations on the Tongue and Mouth – It Could Be Behcet's Disease

Case Study #5: Sjogren's Syndrome – It's More Than Sicca Syndrome

Case Study #6: Viscous Saliva May Indicate Sjogren's Syndrome

Case Study #7: Exposure to Water Induces Skin Rash (Papules)

Case Study #8: Reversal Cold Inducing Red Rash: Raynaud's Disease

Case Study #9: Irritable Bowel Disease (IBD) – Ulcerative Colitis (UC) and Crohn's disease (CD)

Case Study #10: Aphthous Tongue Ulcers – Heat Pattern of "Fox-Creeper"

Case Study #11: Autoimmune Diseases – Amyloidosis Predisposition

Case Study #12: Adult-onset Still's Disease (AOSD)

ACKNOWLEDGEMENTS

Immeasurable appreciation and gratitude must be afforded to Dr. Lee Chen-Yu (李正育) whose unwavering guidance and dedication to Dr. Juno Yang (梁珠勞), the author and editor of this book, and the thousands of other TCM students he has personally instructed and mentored has made this project possible. Dr. Lee's nearly 40 years of clinical practice; clinical and laboratory research endeavors involving both TCM treatment and integrative TCM and Western medicine; extensive affiliations and cooperation with Western medicine physicians; countless lectures, presentations, and papers; numerous books (both academic and mainstream); and health advocacy radio broadcast programs have reached out to touch the lives of tens of millions of people worldwide. Much gratitude and respect must be given to Dr. Juno Yang whose quest for knowledge and commitment to the clinical practice and research of TCM has made it possible for us to compile and translate this invaluable material.

Further thanks goes out to these fellow students and preceptees of Dr. Lee's: Frank Delaigue (an accomplished TCM practitioner with over 20 years of clinical experience) and Cyril Oswald (an aspiring TCM educator and practitioner) who compiled and translated excerpts of this material for a book they co-authored titled *Les Hommes de l'Art*, which served as a valuable reference for this book; Dan Altschuler, EAMP, PhD (an acclaimed TCM educator and clinical practitioner with over 25 years of experience and currently a faculty member at the Seattle Institute of Oriental Medicine and Bastyr University) whose *Neuropathy: Traditional Chinese Herbal Treatment in a Modern Medical Environment* (English edition) served as reference and inspiration for this book; Chen, Ching-hui (陳環徽), OMD, MSc (aka "Big Brother Hui"), who has studied and served as an assistant of Dr. Lee's for nearly 30 years and has been an inexhaustible source of clarifying details about the clinical application of both TCM and integrated TCM and Western medicine; Paulo Fonte, a talented physiotherapist and TCM practitioner (now practicing at Estoril Wellness Center, Estoril, Portugal) whose professionalism and optimism is always a motivating influence on everyone; and Matthew Stampe (a massage therapist and current TCM student at the Virginia University of Oriental Medicine) for assisting in proofreading and providing critical analysis for this book.

FOREWORD

"The teacher should never be concerned that a student might surpass him in ability, rather the teacher should only worry that he doesn't guide the student well enough." As a pupil of Dr. Lee's, this is something you hear him say often. He doesn't keep secrets and he'll gladly share all of his wisdom with those willing to make a sincere effort.

This book is an extension of his mission to spread knowledge and healing. Readers will face the same challenges as those traveling thousands of miles to study in his clinic. The knowledge available from the case studies in this collection provides limitless opportunity for gaining clinical experience and opens ongoing opportunities for the practical application of integrated traditional Chinese medicine (TCM) and Western medicine in our modern medical environment.

The familiar nature of the correspondences, the focus on difficult cases, the meticulous translation of source text, and the scrupulous compilation of supplemental material all make for an ideal ongoing learning companion. You'll find it challenging, often getting stuck with questions of your own. This is part of the learning process; it allows for exploration of concepts and growth of new ideas. Anyone who has studied and worked with Dr. Lee has gone through it. Be patient, clarify questions in your mind, and continually search for answers both in this text and beyond.

TCM has always been a system that grows and evolves with each generation. This book will give you substantive framework to build upon and find your own ways to innovate. You'll see the way Dr. Lee has updated classical prescription formulas to serve as effective treatments for the severe and intractable diseases of our current times. The balance between classical wisdom and adapting to modern medical trends is his expertise.

If you were to step foot in his clinic, you'd see someone who has mastered his craft. You'd see his ability to diagnose and treat difficult cases. You'd see the comfort and guidance he provides to patients. And you'd see smiles on the faces of patients and staff. The brightness of his work compared to the gloominess of many medical settings speaks for itself.

I'm excited that this book makes a small part of the Yu Sheng Chinese Medicine Clinic available for everyone to experience.

Marc Wasserman Ph.D. L.Ac.
September 2017

i

PREFACE

TCM Applications & Acceptance

Traditional Chinese medicine (TCM) continues resonating with potential, and through a diversity of therapeutic modalities and vast pharmacopeia there are few limitations for its efficacy. The most stark limitations are from the institutional confines of academia and modern medicine in step with the pharmaceutical and insurance industries that seem more than often holding the reins. Of course, cultural factors also play a role in the acceptance of so-called "alternative" therapies, but based on the perpetual exchange of ideas, adaptation of peoples, and acculturation of societies throughout history, the viability and resounding efficacy of TCM has the persuasive power to overcome.

TCM Education and Status in Societies of Chinese (Han) Cultural Heritage

In societies influenced by Chinese culture (such as China, Taiwan, and South Korea) certified TCM (referred to as traditional Korean medicine (TKM) in South Korea) physicians are required to complete formal TCM medical school programs and pass national licensure examinations authorized by the respective nation's education oversight agency. In China, 5- and 7-year bachelor's, master's, and doctoral programs are designed for students to receive a doctor of clinical medicine and doctor of integrated medicine with the option of practicing both Western and TCM and eligibility to take the respective national licensure examinations; in Taiwan, a 5-year post-baccalaureate and an 8-year bachelor's program are designed for students to receive a TCM degree in the former and the option of a dual degree in Western medicine and TCM in the latter and eligibility to take the respective national licensure examinations; and in South Korea, a 4-year post-baccalaureate and a 6-year bachelor's degree program are designed for students to receive a TKM degree and eligibility to take the national licensure examination. The dual Western medicine and TCM degrees in China and Taiwan require students to fulfill all basic coursework in biomedicine and Western medicine specializations along with clinical internships in both Western medicine and TCM. For TCM (TKM) programs in Taiwan and South Korea, two-thirds of the curriculum focuses on coursework in basic biomedicine and specializations, comparative to the requirements for students in dentistry programs, and one-third on TCM along with a clerkship in a Western medicine hospital and a clinical internship in the TCM department of a Western medicine hospital. The relative emphasis on modern biomedicine and Western medicine specializations in the coursework load is balanced out by an intensive TCM curriculum that includes the classics and contemporary texts and their clinical applications. Based on the author's TCM academic pursuits in Taiwan and relationships with a many TCM students, practitioners, and scholars whom have either received TCM educations or are educators themselves in countries such as China, South Korea, the U.S., Australia, New Zealand, Israel, France, England, and Canada, I am confident in saying that the depth and breadth of TCM curriculums in East Asian university TCM programs (at least in Taiwan, China, and South Korea) goes far beyond the that of TCM programs in most other countries. To a large extent this is due to an inherent cultural affinity that accepts this traditional medicine heritage as viable and effective. There is no question the institution of modern medicine is synonymous with Western medicine, but despite the enormous amount of funding and energies devoted to research and development, there are still glaring deficiencies. In Taiwan, China, and South Korea this has opened up the opportunity for TCM to play a role as part of a unified medical system; just as a major hospital may have a dentistry and physiotherapy department, they also have TCM departments. Indeed, this inclusion within the mainstream institution of modern medicine has in ways been a boon ensuring the perpetuation of this form of traditional medicine. However, there has been a price to pay with TCM serving a subservient role recognized as more of a neoadjuvant, adjuvant, complementary, and palliative therapy as opposed to primary and secondary care and first-line treatment. There are still a few TCM physicians with clinical practices outside of the institutional healthcare system who embrace the powers of integrated TCM and Western medicine and have been able to achieve success at providing primary and secondary care and first-line treatment beyond adjuvant, complementary, and palliative therapy roles. Physician's such as Dr. Lee who have dedicated a lifetime of research and clinical practice have gained due respect and elevated status within the medical community. Backed by clinical experience and a thorough understanding of the advantages and disadvantages of various Western medicine drugs and procedures, in certain cases Dr. Lee may advise patients to consult with their Western medicine physician about gradually reducing the dose and eventually discontinuing a given drug or holding off on surgery if the side effects and potential complications outweigh the benefits, particularly if TCM offers a better therapeutic solution. Dr. Lee may also request that patients under hospital admission receive decocted TCM formula through their nasogastric (NG) tube, which requires both the consent of the patient and/or family members and the physician in charge. Obviously, this type of consent and coordination requires a high degree of trust and communication. This poses significant challenges even in East Asian societies with the legal ramifications that may arise if something unexpected happens. There is still a lot of work that needs to be done in establishing protocols and fostering universal acceptance. Evidence-based medicine (EBM) research involving integrated TCM and Western medicine treatment is still sparse. However, based on both the results of evidence-based medicine (EBM) studies and thousands of years of empirical clinical evidence, there is growing impetus towards recognizing the efficacy of TCM and integrated TCM and Western medicine in the treatment of a broad spectrum of diseases.

"Know Your Medicinals" and Define Your Paradigm

There is no single TCM medicinal or formula that must be administered for a specific symptom, pathocondition, or disease pattern (deviation from homeostasis). Classical and contemporary texts and the experience of mentors provide the foundations for the practitioner to clinically apply methodologies, but it is only through experience that dedicated physicians may develop their own paradigm. Medicinals of various natures, flavors, and chemical constituents are grouped together in pairs and combinations – opposing and complementing, restraining and empowering, accentuating and corresponding – to form a formula composition whose overall action will resolve symptoms and promote the return of homeostasis. In addition to personal preference based on clinical experience, a variety of factors may influence a TCM physician's selection of medicinals for a formula composition such as availability, quality, legal regulations, price, storage, and patient preferences (taste, religion, customs, diet, etc.). Medicinal processing plays an integral role in procuring the intended action, storage life, and mitigation of toxicity. If preparation methods are not tightly monitored and controlled, there could be potentially severe side effects (possibly even fatal). In times of antiquity, it was standard practice for TCM physicians to have their own raw medicinal processing facilities (or have a close cooperative relationship with a licensed medicinal dispensary that specializes in preparing and processing medicinals) and herbal dispensaries stocked with decocting pieces (medicinals) of their choice. Nowadays, even in China, Taiwan, South Korea, and other Asian nations where TCM is more prevalent and culturally accepted, the majority of physicians do not have their own processing facilities and most do not even have onsite herbal dispensaries stocked with decocting pieces (medicinals). Their herbal dispensaries are more commonly stocked with extract powders/granules for the sake of convenience and regulatory oversight (in Taiwan this is particularly evident in part due to the National Healthcare Plan (a single-payer system) that provides nominal coverage for TCM)). Dr. Lee is among the remaining TCM physicians who carry on the original spirit of the tradition, believing that you have to really "know your medicinals like the back of your hand" in order to utilize their best qualities, accentuate their weaknesses, temper their volatilities, and harness the extent of their capacity for providing therapeutic efficacy.

Perspectives on the Four Examinations

The **four examinations – inspection, listening and smelling, inquiry**, and **palpation** – was first recorded in the Warring States period (475–221 BC) nearly 2,500 years ago. Patient examinations are conducted to determine the correlation of all **four examinations** and identify the pattern as the basis of treatment. Depending on the type of symptoms, injury, and pathocondition, the four examinations are generally conducted in the following order: **inspection** (includes observing skin, gait, mannerisms, complexion, color of stool and urine, and the tongue) offers an initial "look" at the patient and is the first natural step; **listening and smelling** (includes listening to the sound of speech and breath and smelling the body, breath, and excretions) provides additional information and is the next natural step; **inquiry** (includes patient history, chief complaint, diagnostic images, and lab test results) allows the physician to collect subjective and objective information and data about the patient's condition and may often be the most valuable; and **palpation** (includes touching and feeling the body to determine the presence of heat, tenderness, and accumulations, and also taking the pulse) enables the physician to get a "feel" for the patient's condition and is the last step. As is often the case with experienced physicians, over the years Dr. Lee has developed a refined application of the **four examinations** with a keen sense for observing mannerisms, gait, skin manifestations, speech, temperament, disposition, speech, smells, the nuances of history taking, abdominal palpation, and elucidating the significance of pulse.

Early on in Dr. Lee's clinical practice he would rely on tongue examination much more, but throughout the years this reliance has diminished due to variables such as natural size, color, texture, and fur variations among individuals and the intake of food and beverages that stain the tongue and alter the appearance of fur. In fact, if one observes Dr. Lee's patient interviews during consultations you will notice that he rarely examines the tongue except for those cases in which patients have a pathology of the tongue or mouth proper.

Pulse-taking remains a hallmark of TCM examination and diagnostic protocol, and early on in Dr. Lee's clinical practice he authored a reputable academic book on this topic titled *Illustrated Traditional Chinese Medicine Pulse Reading*. Indeed, in its historical context pulse-taking is a vital source that opens up vistas into the discrete inner workings of the human body and reveals information about the blood flow, volume, and viscosity; the heart rate, cardiac output, and vascular patency; and the organs and physiological systems of the entire body (including endocrine system, autonomic nervous system (ANS), and central nervous system (CNS)). However, since the advent of modern biomedicine's diagnostic imaging and lab tests, offering once unimaginable detail in revealing tangible images and quantitative data, the significance of pulse examination has in many regards been supplanted. This is compounded by the fact that there is not a set, definable and quantifiable standard for interpreting the quality and nature of the pulse with each individual potentially defining the "feeling" of a pulse differently. Though many well-intended TCM pratitioners and devout patients who still cling to the nostalgia may disagree with this assessment, in my opinion pulse-taking is a relatively ambiguous "art" to practice. It is even more difficult to communicate with others; as one pulse-taker's description of a particular pulse may not be the same as another's, even though they may actually be feeling the same pulse! This doesn't entirely relegate its usefulness for the individual practitioner as a reference for conducting pattern identification, but it's subjectivity does limit its function as conveyed to others.

Yet another factor is the widespread administration of Western medicine therapeutic agents for patients with established illnesses and as preventive care. Many of these drugs have a direct affect on the autonomic nervous system and endocrine systems which regulate cardiovascular blood flow and the feedback mechanisms affecting vasoconstriction and vasodilation. The near ubiquitous administration of pharmaceuticals in our modern society makes the "drug pulse" ("藥脈") phenomenon that much more of a challenge to objectively discern the "feeling" of a pulse. That said, just as it was applied traditionally, Dr. Lee takes each patient's pulse and records the reading in the patient's medical record and uses these readings as a baseline for subsequent patient examination. In certain cases where the pulse reading is noticeably inconsistent with the other presenting signs and symptoms, lab tests, and diagnostic imaging findings, then the pulse may play a vital role in pattern identification (e.g., accurately discerning true and false and complex patterns).

TCM Terminology and Usage

Readers familiar with TCM may know that there are several most commonly used terminology 'systems' employed in the description and explanation of TCM concepts. The author began studying the Chinese contemporary and classical texts on subjects such as literature, philosophy, and religion in 1991; and since 2001, I have been focusing energies on studying TCM. These extensive studies have included graduating from a five-year postbaccalaureate program in a prominent Taiwanese medical teaching college with an affiliated hospital, pursuing personal studies of classical and contemporary texts in Chinese and English on my own, and also working professionally translating classical and contemporary TCM texts from Chinese to English. Through these experiences, the author has explored the use of the various 'systems,' mixed and matched various 'systems,' and created my own complementary interpretations. At first, this 'trial and error' approach seemed innocuous enough; after all, the objective is simply to get the idea across, right? Well, the more I began to analyze and realize the seamless congruity and irrefutable underlying logic of Nigel Wiseman's TCM terminology "system," the more I became persuaded to get on board and adopt this lexicon. Wiseman's TCM lexicon is the only comprehensive, standardized "system" to date. It's possible that this particular "system" may appeal to the scholar's bilingual sensibilities, having introspection into the underlying context of the historical usage of a particular character or paired character phrase throughout different eras, I find this "system" most accurately articulates the "original" meaning of the source text. Naturally, there are limitations in any system and the author admits that some of the usage may seem awkward or unorthodox for those not familiar with the "system." But as stated above, the advantages of congruity far outweigh the occasional ambiguity and archaic flavor. It is the comprehensive "system" that I believe is the best format to convey and advance the valuable medical insights and scientific methodology of TCM. It may require a bit of getting used to and looking up some terms at first, but in the end, I am confident you will discover the "rhyme to this reason."

INTRODUCTION

This book comprises the collection of fax and e-mail correspondence between Dr. Lee Chen-Yu (李政育), recognized as one of Taiwan's most accomplished and prominent traditional Chinese medicine (TCM) physicians, and his dedicated student Dr. Juno Yang (梁珠勞) from South Korea. Nearly forty years of clinical experience and insights are made readily available through these clear and concise interactions, offering practical antidotes for the clinical application of integrated TCM and Western medicine.

Dr. Lee Chen-Yu is an acclaimed TCM physician who has been practicing medicine for over 35 years and is renowned as a pioneering innovator at the forefront of integrated TCM and Western medicine. Aside from being the Director of Yu Sheng Chinese Medicine Clinic, which he founded in 1980, he currently serves as the Honorary Chairperson of the R.O.C. Chinese and Western Medicine Neurology Foundation and Honorary Ph.D. Advisor for Liaoning University of Traditional Chinese Medicine among other distinguished positions and accolades. Dr. Lee has authored more than 30 TCM books (and counting!), co-authored numerous others, and has written hundreds of professional papers.

Dr. Juno Yang graduated from the prestigious College of Oriental Medicine (1998) at the Kyung Hee University, and later went on to complete his Master of Science in Pathology (2003), and PhD in Radiation Oncology (2008) from Ajou University. In 2000, Dr. Yang came to study under the mentorship of Dr. Lee Chen-Yu at Yu Sheng Chinese Medicine Clinic in Taipei, Taiwan (ROC). Following this period of immersed clinical study he returned to South Korea where he started his his own TCM clinical practice, gradually honing his capacities over the years until becoming confident and competent in treating patients with serious conditions and intractable diseases. At the onset, Dr. Yang lacked experience and had a lot of questions about how to accurately diagnosis and effectively treat the broad scope of pathological conditions for which patients sought consultation. Thus, the "student" would correspond with his "mentor" by fax or e-mail seeking advice and guidance. Dr. Lee enjoyed sharing the knowledge gained from decades of study, research, and clinical experience, and further imparted the necessity for maintaining a balance between "prudence and confidence" and the importance of continuing education and developing professional capacities to make a positive impact on the lives of those depending on your medical assistance.

This regular correspondence between Dr. Lee ("mentor") and Dr. Yang ("student") took place from 2001 up until 2008, and consequently these interactions formed the content and outline for the conception of this book. Rather than presenting this correspondence in its original chronological order, the author has sorted and collated the material by grouping follow-up of specific patient's cases and associated pathological conditions together as well as modifying some of the letter formatting making the presentation of each case study concise and informative. It contains troves of information on TCM pattern identification as the basis for determining treatment; clinical application of TCM medicinals, formulas, and acupuncture treatment regimens; classical TCM pathological conditions and coinciding Western medicine pathological nomenclature; background information on symptoms, diagnostic tests, and treatment modalities; keys to differential diagnostic; and prognoses.

The sheer breadth and expanse of this material warranted division into a three volume series of which this is the first volume translated into English. Volume I includes chapters on cancer (and benign tumors) of the central nervous, respiratory, gastrointestinal, lymphatic, circulatory systems, and genitourinary systems and breast; cerebrovascular, cerebellar, central nervous system, cardiovascular, and peripheral vascular pathologies; head and neck disorders; and autoimmune diseases.

A full spectra of other pathological conditions will be published in the upcoming Volume II and Volume III of this series. Case studies involving pathologies of the following will be included: respiratory, gastrointestinal, musculoskeletal, and genitourinary systems, neurology, endocrinology, dermatology, renal, metabolic, gynecology and obstetrics, hematology, pediatrics, infectious diseases, ophthalmology, psychiatric, and other conditions such as Tourette's syndrome and autism.

By no means does this book attempt to present a comprehensive analysis of all the pathological conditions TCM is capable of treating, either independently or through Western medicine integration. Its precept stems from the candid correspondence and guidance between a promising TCM physician ("student") and an innovative spirit at the forefront of integrated TCM and Western medicine development ("mentor"). The scope of the pathological conditions and descriptions of the cases presented here are simply derived from the questions a dedicated student has asked seeking guidance from his mentor. The reader should not expect an unabridged, pedagogic explanation of all pathological conditions.

This material will serve as a valuable reference source for practical application – a catalyst that inspires the TCM practitioner to continue applying and integrating the classical traditions within our modern biomedicine environment and an insightful medium for those interested in learning about the vast potential for both the clinical applications of TCM and integrated TCM and Western medicine therapeutic approaches.

1. CANCER

Cancer is among the leading causes of mortality worldwide. Despite the rapid technological advancements in modern medicine and the evolution of new therapeutic modalities, adverse effects and iatrogenic complications remain an overshadowing concern. Many cancer patients experience severe loss of appetite following chemotherapy, resulting in severe malnutrition and cachexia (aka wasting syndrome) and essentially wither away. TCM medicinals have been used in the treatment of cancer for thousands of years and remain an effective choice for supplementing the deficiencies and complementing the overall treatment of modern biomedicine, and in some cases even alleviating the need for toxic pharmaceutical agents and invasive therapies altogether.

Section 1: Brain Tumors and Brain Pathologies

Case Study #1: Clinical Treatment of Anaplastic Astrocytoma

Q: I have asked you many times about the diagnosis and treatment of brain tumors, but have been apprehensive about getting involved in these cases until I was ready. Well, recently a classmate of mine came to me complaining of frequent headaches and blurred vision in the right eye beginning one year ago. A CT scan revealed a 5~6 cm tumor located towards the center of the left cerebral hemisphere below the motor cortex behind the optic nerve. He was diagnosed with anaplastic astrocytoma, and his doctors told him performing surgery would be a difficult task and not curative. Under the advice of his physician, he spent US$2,700/month on the newest U.S. chemotherapy agent, but after taking the drug for several months results have proven ineffective.

Five days ago my classmate felt that the vision in his right eye was blurrier and he had a splitting headache. He went to the hospital where mannitol infusions were administered to relieve increased intracranial pressure (ICP) and also had another CT scan performed, revealing the tumor had enlarged to 7 cm. He made a special visit hoping I could prescribe TCM medicinals that would reduce the tumor size and lower ICP in order to ease the pain. I plan on advising him to undergo surgical resection and then come back to me for follow-up TCM treatment. What do you think I should do?

A: Anaplastic astrocytomas are found towards the middle of the cerebral hemispheres and lower aspect of the motor cortex, which happens to be directly behind the optic nerve. These tumors tend to be deep (infiltrative) and large sized making surgical resection extremely difficult. Your best option is to administer TCM medicinals and advise the patient to receive radiotherapy in order to reduce the tumor size and prevent exacerbation of symptoms, and then go from there.

Temodal (Temozolomide (TMZ)) is currently the first-line chemotherapy agent for the treatment of this type of cancer. Following oral administration or injection of this alkylating agent, it is completely absorbed and broken down into small molecules with the capacity to cross the blood-brain barrier (BBB) directly reaching the tumor where it kills off some of the cancer cells and inhibits proliferation. This is why it is the first-line drug for treating this condition. The problem is that it only provides temporary relief of symptoms with a brief respite in proliferation, but doesn't offer an effective cure. If the ICP continues increasing, the best option is to immediately administer injections of corticosteroids and mannitol.

Radiotheraphy treatment using the LINAC system (X-Knife or CyberKnife) should be performed, while also accompanying the administration of TCM medicinals to enhance therapeutic effectiveness. For larger tumors, proton beam therapy (cyclotron) with the radionuclide cadmium 60 will typically be performed along with administration of corticosteroids.

As for the TCM formula, you should prescribe Ban Xia Tian Ma Bai

Zhu San adding Ren Shen (powder), Chuan Qi (powder), and Wan Ling Dan. If tics, spasms, or seizures present, then add Quan Xie, Wu Gong, and Bai Jiang Can; if there is constipation, then add Da Huang and Pu Huang; and for severe headache add Tian Ma and Wu Zhu Yu. Once the tumor size shrinks change the prescription to Ru Mo Si Wu Tang adding heat-clearing and toxin-resolving and blood-quickening and stasis-resolving medicinals to prevent the tumor cells from proliferating.

If you are still unable to achieve effective control of this patient's condition through this therapeutic regimen, then resulting brain swelling will compress cranial nerves causing abnormalities of vision, hearing, swallowing, breathing, arm and leg motor function, cognitive function, personality, temperament, etc. Severe headache, nausea and vomiting may also present, and eventually severely elevated ICP and extremely high doses of corticosteroids may induce death during sleep.

This is an extremely difficult condition to treat, but you should stand up and face the challenge. Obviously, you need to coordinate treatment with your classmate's attending physicians (e.g., neurologists, oncologists). Solely using TCM medicinals to treat this condition will "not" provide effective treatment. If the ICP continues to increase, it's best to perform decompression surgery and at the least attach a drainage tube to relieve the symptoms. For patients whom have had surgery, an external ventricular drain (EVD) or ventriculoperitoneal shunt (VPS) is commonly inserted. Care should be taken to keep the catheter clean of metabolic waste, and if blockage does occur, then it must be reinserted.

Risky surgery clears away only three-fourths...

Q1: Last week my classmate developed severe brain swelling, and despite the prevailing dangers, surgery was performed in hopes of completely resecting the tumor. The patient's family told me that an MRI was performed prior to surgery revealing an 8 cm tumor; however, during the surgical procedure surgeons found diffuse proliferation of the tumor at a size much larger than 8 cm making clearance impossible. They ended up only clearing away three-fourths of the tumor about "the size of an adult's fist." Initial results following surgery were good as brain swelling and headache resolved; vision improved; and motor, mental status, speech, and personality all returned to relatively normal. However, the attending physician said that the brain tumor had already metastasized and after a period of time would definitely relapse. What can I do to help improve this condition and allow him to maintain a better quality of life?

A1: Happy to hear about the success of your classmate's surgery! At this stage, the focus of TCM treatment is still on treating symptoms and improving the condition. You can prescribe the same TCM prescription as before, Ban Xia Tian Ma Bai Zhu San variation, continuing with this formula until his next MRI. If the tumor has shrunk, then change the prescription to Ru Mo Si Wu Tang adding Huang Lian, "the Three Insects," Tian Ma, Ren Shen (powder), Chuan Qi (powder), Wan Ling Dan and possibly combinations of medicinals such as Xia Ku Cao, Pu Gong Ying, Lian Qiao, and Jin Yin Hua.

Remember! As a general rule, this type of brain tumor's deep infiltration makes it virtually impossible to completely resect regardless of location. A clearance of 80~90% is considered a good result, followed up by adjuvant radiotherapy in attempts to shrink tumor size and eliminate as many of the remaining tumor cells as possible. If ICP presents, then a drainage tube is commonly inserted to drain the fluid that causes swelling. If the cerebral shunt becomes occluded increased ICP will recur, prompting the need for another shunt placement procedure.

Q2: Thank you for clarifying the principles of using TCM medicinals to treat post-operative brain tumor patients. Due to the critical nature of this condition, prior to consulting me the patient had already undergone surgical excision of the tumor with normal motor and congnitive function and absence of secondary bleeding. Thus, I haven't initiated TCM treatment yet and quite honestly I am apprehensive about doing so. According to the information I have found, astrocytomas are extremely difficult to treat, with the outcomes of surgery, chemotherapy, and radiotherapy for all very poor. For glioblastomas, the most malignant type of atrocytoma, the average expected life span after diagnosis is just over 1 year. Following surgical excision, about how long will it be before the tumor recurs? Is there any way to prevent relapse? What TCM medicinals should be prescribed?

A2: Regardless of whether surgery is performed on astrocytoma patients, treatment with corticosteroids must be administered. If chemotherapy and radiotherapy are "not" administered, then in the early stage Ban Xia Tian Ma Bai Zhu San variation can be prescribed, which may induce shrinkage of tumor size. However, it is likely that the tumor may relapse in 3~5 months. At this time, change the TCM formula to Ru Mo Si Wu Tang or Xian Fang Huo Ming Yin variations, adding medicinals that control seizures and convulsions and lower ICP such as Tian Ma, "the Three Insects," Fu Ling, Zhu Ling, Bai Zhu, Cang Zhu, and Ze Xie; or you could consider prescribing Tong Jing Fang or Xue Fu Zhu Yu Tang. If the ICP remains elevated, prescribe Jian Ling Tang, Wu Ling San, or Chai Ling Tang variations. Long-term administration of these TCM treatment regimens may be able to substantially prolong the patient's life. If the tumor does recur, it will be necessary to perform surgery again with follow-up adjuvant treatment as mentioned previously.

Relapse occurs within a year...

Q: My classmate began experiencing headaches and blurred vision last year so he went for an examination. Results revealed an astrocytoma and his doctors performed surgical decompression (decompressive craniectomy) in August. I saw him after the surgery and his condition was good. I wanted to prescribe TCM medicinals as follow-up and preventive treatment, but wasn't confident it would be effective. I read up on this topic and sought your advice about "How long it usually takes for the astrocytoma to recur?" With these thoughts still vivid in my mind, my classmate returned for follow-up consultation revealing a single 1 cm large tumor in his brain and the attending physician told him: "During this last surgery we only excised three-fourths of the tumor tissue so the residual tumor cells will likely grow and proliferate. And since you [my classmate] are still relatively young [37 y/o] and physically fit tumor cell development tends to occur at a faster pace." Thus, the attending physician recommended another surgical resection for my classmate, but this time placing an anticancer agent (capsule) inside his brain. What is your opinion on this case? Is it possible to use TCM medicinals to treat this condition?

A: Despite surgical attempts, the diffuse infiltration of astrocytoma tumerogenesis makes complete resection impossible and the probability of reproliferation highly likely. Chemotherapy, radiotherapy, and 'the American elixir' corticosteroids are administered in full force following surgery to prevent tumor proliferation for as long as possible and hopefully get the cancer under control. As for TCM medicinals, you can use the original formula of Ban Xia Tian Ma Bai Zhu San (including heavy doses of Huang Bo) adding Ru Xiang, Mo Yao, Chuan Qi (powder), Niu Xi, Yu Sheng Wan, and Wan Ling Dan. For some cases involving persistent recurrence, I may recommend prescribing (Yu Sheng) Ru Mo Si Wu Tang adding Tian Ma, "the Three Yellows," "the Three Insects," Chuan Qi (powder), Bai Zhu, Fu Ling, Ze Xie, Yu Sheng Wan, and Wan Ling Dan.

If relapse has already occurred, then in my opinion you should prescribe (Yu Sheng) Ru Mo Si Wu Tang adding large doses of "the Three Yellows" (8 qian each), Bai Zhu, Fu Ling, Ze Xie, "the Three Insects," Tian Ma, Wu Zhu Yu, Ren Shen (powder), Chuan Qi (powder), Yu Sheng Wan, and Wan Ling Dan. If the condition improves initially after taking these TCM medicinals, but then declines again or even further deteriorates, add Gan Jiang, Fu Zi, and Yu Gui. If necessary, you can prescribe Da Huang (incrementally increasing doses to maintain 2~3 stools/day) to loosen the stool and promote excretion. As for Quan Xie, start out with a dose of 3~5 qian adding up to 8 qian, and since Wu Gong is very expensive, start out with 1.5 qian gradually adding up to 3 qian. For the other medicinals such as Bai Jiang Can and Tian Ma you can prescribe up to 8 qian, Wu Zhu Yu (5 qian), and for Wan Ling Dan start out with 8 pills/3x/day gradually increasing as much as threefold over a period of time (the most I have ever prescribed is 28 pill/3x/day). It is possible the patient may experience blurred vision (e.g., 'like looking at an object through a dense fog'), dizziness, and auditory hallucinations, which may resemble a toxic reaction, but it's not! This reaction simply indicates that the potency of the medicinal treatment has reached a level of exhibiting efficacy. All you have to do is gradually reduce the dosage until these 'pseudo-reactions' resolve and then once again gradually return to the doses originally prescribed. The patient's constitution will develop tolerance and the efficacy will remain at peak levels.

Condition deteriorates and efforts abandoned...

Q1: Bad news. Recently my classmates family told me that his condition had deteriorated with a dramatic increase in ICP and left-sided hemiplegia. The attending physician administered mannitol to lower ICP, which was ineffective and also induced repeated vomiting. Another MRI was performed revealing a 20 cm large tumor that could not be resected and his doctors were planning on giving up treatment hopes. My classmate and his family visited me seeking my assistance. I can't just stand by doing nothing. This is why I am seeking your advice.

I am really close to this classmate. We have been friends since our early 20s when we both first came to live in Seoul. We have kept in touch over the years and have gone out for drinks, sharing both the joys and sorrows of life. Three days ago I went to see him. Due to excessive corticosteroid administration his face was severely swollen, he had hemiplegia, and spoke in a slow, slurred manner (dysarthria). The moment he saw me he struggled to mutter: "Brother, I'm about to die, please save me! I know you studied...a famous Chinese medicine doctor in Taiwan...learning advanced approaches...treating complex disease...severe cases. But you're...not willing...try helping me.... Last year...my first surgery...doctors said I...had six months to live. I listened to your advice...following...treatment regimen...have lived fairly well for over a year now. My condition is critical...now, I know,...I believe you can still save me. I'm only 37...old. Please help me."

After listening to my friend all I could do was cry and console him, saying: "Don't worry, everything will be fine." But I knew there was nothing I could do other than rely on your assistance and guidance. Do you think it is possible to save my classmate? Please help me try to save him!

A1: Coming across a severe illness such as your classmate's in the beginning of your medical career will help you formulate your diagnostic and treatment methods and give you direction for future medical research pursuits. There is a great void to fill in developing methods for the treatment of cerebrovasculature and nerve compressing space-occupying lesions. This is in part due to the broad diversity of conditions that affect the brain including infectious, autoimmune, metabolic, and chronic disease along with the simple process of aging. Most pathological conditions of the body start in the brain centers, specifically the brain's functional capacity of regulating and monitoring the endocrine system, hormones, central nervous system (CNS), and autonomic nervous system (ANS). Modern biomedicine still lacks the capacity to sufficiently evaluate and diagnose the subtleties and nuances of brain function. The TCM "five orifices" (sense organs) can be interpreted as a functional blueprint of the brain with exterior pattern infections in the upper, middle, and lower burners almost all deriving from breathing, swallowing, urinary, reproductive, and digestive centers located in and around the brainstem. These centers receive errant signals and transmit false information that leads to intrinsic environmental changes in the respiratory, digestive, and urogenital system, which thus affects or alters adaptation to various bacteria, virus, and microorganisms. As stated in the *The Yellow Emperor's Inner Canon*: "Evil will encroach when the qi is vacuous." The term "qi" used here may very well refer to brain centers receiving errant signals and thus transmitting false information that suppresses chelonianin (a protective secretion in the mucous membrane of the oral cavity that secretes leukocyte protein enzyme inhibitors) and thus makes the body susceptible to contraction of external evil.

Based on the information you have provided, it sounds like there is still some hope. Don't allow yourself to become so disheartened and discouraged that you lose confidence. If he wants to take TCM medicinals, then by all means you should prescribe treatment for him. You can prescribe Ru Mo Si Wu Tang adding large doses of "the Three Yellows" and "the Three Insects" (8 qian each), Qi Cao (5 qian), Ren Shen (powder) and Chuan Qi (powder) (3 qian each), Da Huang (adding incremental doses of 0.5 g until the patient maintains 2~3 stools per day), "the Four Ling's," Huang Qi, Yin Xing Ye, Yu Sheng Wan, and Wan Ling Dan (adding incrementally up to as much as 28 pills/3x/day (for maximum total of 84 pills/day)). These relatively large doses will ensure optimal therapeutic results. You must have confidence! By carefully monitoring your friend's condition and choosing the appropriate medicinals and doses, you will be doing everything you can to take care of him. Keep me updated on how the treatment progresses and contact me if you have any questions or observations.

Q2: Thank you professor! The TCM formula you prescribed really did help revive my friend from critical condition. After taking these medicinals not only was he able to make it through the crisis, it seems the tumor has plateaued, maintaining the same size without enlarging. However, he still suffers from hemiplegia, which you explained was a result of "brain tissue damage" caused by radiotherapy and chemotherapy. The attending physician thinks the reduction in tumor size (down to 6 x 17 cm) and the revitalization of the patient is due to the "effects of chemotherapy." Thus, his oncologists have decided go on the offensive when the cancer cells appear to be on the defensive by performing another tumor resection next week followed by a regimen of radiotherapy and chemotherapy. Since this will induce further brain tissue damage, what preemptive TCM medicinals should I prescribe? How can I prevent the tumor from enlarging?

A2: It's great to hear that the patient's tumor shrunk following administration of TCM medicinals and so far his condition is being kept under control. After surgery, you can continue prescribing Ru Mo Si Wu Tang adding "the Three Yellows," "the Four Ling's," "the Three Insects," Chuan Qi (powder), Ren Shen (powder), Da Huang, Yu Sheng Wan, and Wan Ling Dan along with small doses of Gan Jiang, Fu Zi, and Yu Gui. This approach should promote further progress.

3 cm large tumor appears again with the sensation of ants crawling...

Q: The patient's condition has been stabilized following the most recent surgery and administration of TCM medicinals. On March 6, another MRI was performed revealing an astrocytoma 3 cm in size and the sensation of ants crawling (formication) on the left side of his body. Western medical physicians believed this to be a sign that the tumor was undergoing abnormal differentiation and thus administered additional antitumor agents. Unexpectedly, the tumor grew in size to 7 cm within a one-month period of time, and the WBC count decreased dramatically. I was worried he might pass away if things continued to regress, so I prescribed Ru Mo Si Wu Tang variant increasing the amount of Huang Qin from 4 qian to 1.5 liang. The patient's CBC and liver function tests improved and I felt relieved.

About two weeks ago the patient felt numbness and tingling on his left side again, but not complete paralysis and imaging tests revealed brain edema. I was concerned that the tumor had already begun to proliferate once again. What I couldn't figure out was why there would be brain edema if the tumor had remained the same size (7 cm). His father wanted to have another procedure performed to reduce ICP, but the attending physician deemed the the patient's chance of survival dismal (0.01%) and thus advised against going ahead with decompression surgery. I felt that surgery to lower ICP would give my friend a chance to survive. At worst, dying on the operating table seemed a better option than lying there suffering on an ICU bed, so I strongly recommended performing another surgery.

Surprisingly, the surgeons discovered that 90% of the brain tumor had shrunk and undergone necrosis and there was extensive cerebral edema. It seemed that the vicious cycle of relapse and proliferation had somehow been altered and now the treatment objective was simply to remedy the brain swelling. The physician in charge was shocked by these findings; over his nearly 20 years of practicing medicine he had never witnessed a neoplasm undergo necrosis and shrinkage like this. I knew TCM treatment was the reason for these results and was so happy that I couldn't sleep the whole night, thinking about the exceptional efficacy and potential of TCM medicinals. I felt like I was floating on clouds and almost started crying from joy!

Soon after, my classmate was moved to a general ward room. He cried and thanked me for saving his life, saying that when he is able to leave the hospital he wants to write a book entitled *How I Overcame Astrocytoma!* and planned to spread the news through the media. Myself, I was thinking about conducting further research and presenting the results that would undoubtedly draw a lot of attention.

The experiment would use your (Yu Sheng) Ru Mo Si Wu Tang variant adding Huang Qin 1.5 liang, Fu Ling 8 qian, Ze Xie 8 qian, Huang Bo 1 liang, Chuan Qi (powder) 3 qian, and Wan Ling Dan. What do you think about this idea?

A: I am also excited about the results of (Yu Sheng) Ru Mo Si Wu Tang variant in the treatment of brain tumors. Over the past year, I have been using this formula primarily on brain tumor patients with normal (or slightly raised) ICP whose corticosteroid administration has already been fully metabolized and those whom have undergone surgery and radiotherapy with ensuing tumor relapse. This formula can also improve brain function and stabilize the condition of patients with iatrogenic brain tissue damage (e.g., hypoxia, scarring, vascuslar injury, necrosis, swelling) resulting from chemotherapy and radiotherapy.

Currently, the Western medicine treatment regimen focuses on improving symptoms with surgery, radiotherapy, and chemotherapy. The problem is there really aren't any effective chemotherapeutic agents that can treat this pathocondition. Human trials have shown that surgery and radiotherapy can only reduce tumor size, but not completely eradicate it, leaving neoplastic cells behind that rapidly reseed and relapse. The newest

LINAC systems (e.g., CyberKnife) that rotate around the lesion at multiple angles are capable of achieving better results. However, regardless of the regimen, to achieve the best results it is essential to use TCM medicinals such as Ru Mo Si Wu Tang variant. Regarding your interest in conducting a study and presenting the research report, I think it would be best to wait for a while to further assess your classmates condition and then we can talk about it later.

Moved to general ward and is able to walk...

Q: Yesterday I went to check up on my classmate. His vision (left eye) was impaired (unable to depict objects) and he had rigidity in his left arm with better mobility in his left leg. Basically, he was still afflicted with left-sided hemiparesis. His radiologist is also my former professor, a very experienced professional whom had worked in the U.S. for nearly 15 years, and has used 3D-CRT extensively. But since this was a very large and deep astrocytoma, he couldn't use Gamma Knife; instead he recommended corticosteroid administration to control the condition. This treatment resulted in the patient developing a red, swollen face.

A: The treatment of astrocytomas can lead to irreversible loss of peripheral vision. A case like this occurred not long ago in a major hospital here in Taiwan. The accumulated effects of repeated, long-term radiotherapy regimens may induce brain swelling and epileptic seizures. If the positioning and wavelength of the radiotherapy are not strictly controlled, normal cells will be damaged and necrosis may occur. Thus, I recommend administering TCM medicinals during the radiotherapy regimen as a means of mitigating these potentially severe iatrogenic complications.

Generally, for large tumors that compress nerves, resection is the best approach because radiotherapy is not very effective regardless of the type (i.e., Gamma Knife, X-knife (photon knife), Cyberknife). TCM medicinals should be administered in the treatment of this condition regardless if corticosteroids are administered or not; it's just a matter of altering the formula composition. If corticosteroids are being administered, a commonly used formula is Ban Xia Tian Ma Bai Zhu San combining Bu Yang Huan Wu Tang, which is essentially (Yu Sheng) Ban Xia Tian Ma Bai Zhu San adding Chuan Qiong, Chi Shao, Yin Xing Ye, Ren Shen (powder), and Chuan Qi (powder). Once corticosteroid administration has been discontinued wait about 3~5 months up until the side effects have resolved and then change formulas to Ru Mu Si Wu Tang variant.

Q2: Can malignant brain tumors be cured? My classmate can walk on his own now, but he always worries about the possibility of relapse. This kind of malignant tumor is really a nightmare; it attacks out of nowhere turning a perfectly healthy young man into an invalid virtually overnight. I remember the first time my classmate's brain tumor relapsed, causing hemiplegia. He received treatment for a time, narrowly avoiding the grasp of death before progressing to recovery. You never know when it will relapse next or what effects it will have on the patient.

Now, my classmate has regained mobility and can get around but is still weak. I continue prescribing Ru Mo Si Wu Tang adding Huang Qi (1 liang), Huang Qin, Ze Xie, Chuan Qi (powder), Bai Jiang Can (8 qian each), Chuan Qiong, Chi Shao, Yin Xing Ye (4 qian each), and Wan Ling Dan (8 pills/3x/day). Do you think this is a good prescription?

A2: My treatment principle for malignant brain tumors is really quite simple. For patients who have undergone surgery and corticosteroid administration, and two years have elapsed without relapse, then prescribe Ban Xia Tian Ma Bai Zhu San variant; and if the tumor has shrunk to the point it is virtually indiscernible from the MRI, PET and CT scan images, then change the formula to Ru Mo Si Wu Tang variant adding "the Three Yellows" (similar to Wen Qing Yin variant). If relapse does occur, you can still prescribe Ru Mo Si Wu Tang variant adding "the Three Yellows" which offers tumor-suppressing action. This is what I have learned from my clinical experience so far. If you have any further discoveries or insights share them with me and we can learn from one another!

The anticancer agent Timodol has shown some efficacy in 70% of the subjects in trial studies, but up to now, only animal experiments have been conducted. I am still gathering information on this drug and cooperating with Western medical doctors on experimental studies. If I find out anything new, I will contact you about it.

Q3: Since our last correspondence, in addition to 1/3 of his left eye having visual impairment, my classmate currently presents with slight edema in his left lower leg and a slight gait abnormality, but his mobility is improving and, most significantly, the tumor has not relapsed. I am considering adding Ren Shen (powder) into his current formula – Ru Mo Si Wu Tang adding Fu Ling, Ze Xie, "the Three Yellows," Yin Xing Ye, Dan Shen, Chuan Qi (powder), Da Huang, Pu Gong Ying, and Wan Ling Dan. Do you think this is a good idea? Will it induce tumor proliferation? [2007/04/09]

A3: Ren Shen (powder) will not induce proliferation and growth of brain tumors. You don't need to be concerned about that. Ren Shen is an adaptogen that complements as opposed to assuming a predominating role in the overall formula composition. Depending on the dosage and formula it is in, it can be used as a sovereign medicinal and also serve the role of minister, assistant, or envoy. For instance, adding Ren Shen to cold and bitter heat-abating medicinals accelerates the heat-abating, swelling-dispersing, and antitumor actions; added to yang-supplementing medicinals, it assumes a great yang-supplementing action; added to blood-quickening and stasis-transforming medicinals, it promotes quickening of blood and transformation of stasis; and added to other antitumor (especially for brain tumors) medicinals, it serves to suppress proliferation of cancer cells. In the case of brain tumors, corticosteroids is the first-line treatment administered, regardless if surgery, chemotherapy, and radiotherapy are part of the treatment regimen. The administration of corticosteroids inevitably causes side effects of edema and swelling (fluid retention) and fat deposition (especially the face and neck). Adding Ren Shen (powder) into your TCM formula actually helps prevent brain swelling, atrophy, and marrow failure. You don't have to worry about using it!

Tumor shrinks with no signs of relapse...

Q1: An MRI performed on 04/12 confirmed that the postsurgical tumor remnants had shrunk. The attending physician said: "Very odd, usually the tumor will relapse about 3 months after surgical excision. This patient's neoplasm has not spread; on the contrary, it has incurred a marked reduction in size." The patient's parents were grateful and his father was drinking liquor and singing overwhelmed with tearful joy. My friend is still young and should be able to look forward to a bright future. Originally, he thought there was no hope and couldn't imagine ever recovering; and now he is ecstatic. I want to change formula to Ru Mo Si Wu Tang adding Yin Xing Ye and Dan Shen (8 qian each). What do you think about his idea? [04/19/2007]

A1: Yes, this might be a good idea, and actually you could add a small amount of Huang Qi as well. But remember! You only need to use a small dose. Once the tumor has been suppressed, TCM medicinals can be used to promote nerve conduction and functional compensation. This is why I always say that TCM medicinals also have a rehabilitative action. You don't want to inundate the body with supplementing medicinals, prescribe just enough to activate this process and let the body's natural capacity to restore itself take effect. Completely depending on medicinals or other agents will have the deleterious effect of accelerating degeneration of the brain's functional capacities and possibly even result in dementia.

Q2: My classmate has gone two years without malignant brain tumor relapse. This is great, but the problem he faces now is being badly overweight (verging on obesity) due to long-term administration of the tumor cell suppressor drug Tamoxifen and a host of digestants. He has experienced a dramatic weight gain now tipping the scale at 120kg (height: 182 cm). This is troubling, what can I do? [04/17/2008]

A2: The main side effect involving the long-term administration of the tumor cell suppressant Tamoxifen is "water amassment." If not carefully monitored, the patient will inevtiably gain weight. I suggest you prescribe either Zhi Bo Di Huang Tang; Ru Mo Si Wu Tang adding "the Three Yellows"; Wen Dan Tang combining Huang Lian Jie Du Tang; or Xian Fan Huo Ming Yin variant (these formulas will inhibit estrogen receptors and prevent rapid weight gain). If water amassment presents, then add Bai Zhu, Fu Ling, and Ze Xie; for mild seizures add Tian Ma, Wu Zhu Yu, "the Three Insects," and Zhu Ru.

Q3: An MRI performed in July 2009 revealed the presence of a heart-shaped polyp at the site of the original brain tumor lesion. It doesn't appear to be cancerous. Left-side arm and leg mobility, function, and strength has improved and the patient can now easily raise his arm and lift his leg, but the tips of fingers and toes severely ache and tingle. Is this a good or bad sign? I hope it isn't a neoplasm. [07/16/2009]

A3: From what you've described it sounds like the fortuitous signs of brain cell regeneration. I have seen this before during experiments on animals and in patients here in my clinic. There is no doubt TCM medicinals can induce stem cell regeneration and inhibit neoplastic stem cells. You should compile these results and present them as research paper. The title could be something like "Traditional Korean Medicine (TKM) regenerates normal brain stem cells in astrocytoma patient." You can show the images before and after and explain the recovery process of limb and facial function. I am confident these results will attract international attention and acclaim. Don't forget to mention my name in the report!

Q4: On a related topic, a senior traditional Korean medicine doctor says that the administration of Dao Tan Tang will reduce tumor size within 2 months. Is this possible?

A4: Dao Tan Tang can definitely reduce tumor size, but it depends on the size and type of tumor. If the tumor is large causing severe compression, patients with increased ICP must first have surgical decompression and then resection with adjuvant radiotherapy. Oral administration of formulas such as Er Chen Tang, Wen Dan Tang, Di Tan Tang, and Dao Tan Tang variants; or Meng Shi Gun Tan Wan, Xiang Sha

Liu Jun Zi Tang, Ren Shen Gan Jiang Ban Xia Wan, and Ban Xia Tian Ma Bai Zhu San variants can be prescribed at this time. First, you must accurately identify the pattern; and if it is indeed phlegm heat pattern or cold phlegm (rheum) pattern, then these types of formulas will be effective.

I remember telling you about my animal experiments and how the most effective formulas were Ban Xia Tian Ma Bai Zhu San, Da Chai Hu Tang, Long Dan Xie Gan Tang, Huang Lian Jie Du Tang, Wen Dan Tang, and Qing Xin Niu Huang Wan variants addingYu Sheng Wan and Wan Ling Dan. However, in cases involving iatrogenic brain tissue damage (e.g., hypoxia, scarring, vascuslar injury, necrosis, swelling); or if chemotherapy and/or radiotherapy are a part of the treatment regimen with initial tumor shrinkage or resolution but then grows back again, then this can be identified as repletion heat pattern or stasis heat pattern. For this pattern, it is best to prescribe Ru Mo Si Wu Tang, Da Chai Hu Tang, or Chai Ling Tang variants adding large doses of "the Three Yellows" (Huang Qin, Huang Lian, and Huang Bo), "the Three Insects," Da Huang, Chuan Qi (powder), Tian Ma, Yu Sheng Wan, and Wan Ling Dan.

Obviously, I am still in the exploratory stages of treating brain tumors myself. I wish there were some "golden elixir" that I could share with you, and if there is, I haven't found it yet. This is an intensely involved and multifaceted condition that offers great challenge, but also promise. Next year, I will be collaborating with Dr. Ma Hsing-yi, Director of the Division of Neuro-Oncology, Department of Neurological Surgery at Tri-General Services Hospital, on an integrated TCM and Western medicine national cancer research project. The project involves CTS, MRI, and PET diagnosis, surgical procedures, biopsies for conducting gene research, and treatment using radiotherapy and Timodol accompanied by administration of TCM medicinals. This research is very expensive requiring the acquisition of national project funding and assistance from the pharmaceutical manufacturer of Timodol. I hope this research will propel my clinical work into the international spotlight, advancing the administration of TCM medicinals as a part of the conventional treatment regimen for brain tumors. The good news is that we have already applied for and are currently in the patent pending phase for patents on 9 TCM formulas for the treatment of brain tumors; and if accepted, patent licensing will be issued in three months. Plans are also being made for conducting further research in the future.

Case Study #2: Benign Brain Tumor – Postoperative Complications

Q: Thanks for your encouragement and support. Since you gave me the confidence and guidance to treat my classmate's malignant brain tumor, I have gone on to treat several other brain tumor cases. However, I know this is just the beginning and there are so many things for me to learn. I look forward to your continued support, guidance, and instruction.

Now, I have a 39 y/o male patient whom on February 14 underwent surgical excision of a brain tumor (right-side). Following the surgery he presented with right-sided facial paralysis and had difficulty rotating his head. The diagnosis was postsurgical complications of benign brain tumor. I also gave the patient acupuncture for over a month without any noticeable effect. He is still taking drugs to lower ICP. What do you think the best course of action is from here?

A: Most surgeries for brain tumors induce postsurgical complications. Facial paralysis is one of these and is similar to the complications of cerebrovascular accident (CVA). First, if the tumor enlarges it will occupy space and compress nearby stroma and parenchyma causing nerve damage and impairment; second, iatrogenic nerve damage from the surgical procedure may occur; and third, the toxins secreted from the tumor itself may cause nerve damage as well. Regardless of the cause, TCM medicinals should be prescribed. Admittedly, efficacy manifests slowly, but the sooner treatment is started the greater the potential for nerve regeneration and functional recovery. As for acupuncture, only corresponding "distal points" should be selected: local points on the affected side will not provide efficacy due to the nerve conduction block deep in the parenchyma.

Case Study #3: Brain Tumors – Impact of Chemotherapy and Radiotherapy on Hematopoiesis

Q: A brain tumor patient was first administered chemotherapy and then underwent more than 10 cranial surgeries. This resulted in decreased CBC counts: WBC 1,000, Hb 7, and PLT 6,000. After being administered emergency blood transfusions (whole blood 1x and Hb 6 packs), amounts increased to WBC 2,200, PLT 60,000, and Hb 10.2. As you advised, I prescribed (Yu Sheng) You Gui Yin (including Gan Jiang, Fu Zi, Yu Gui (5 qian each)) adding Ren Shen (powder) and Chuan Qi (powder). Two weeks later levels had increased to WBC 3,800 and Hb 15,000. The entire medical staff couldn't believe this had happened.

The first time the patient received a Procarbazine injection CBC counts dropped: WBC 2,400 and PLT 64,000. After administering the (Yu Sheng) You Gui Yin variant above, his CBC counts increased: WBC 3,800 and PLT 15,000. This time following injections of anticancer chemotherapeutic agents WBC levels remained at pretty much normal levels, but the PLT dropped to 48,000, and a week later hit a low of 32,000. Do you think I should add large doses of Gan Jiang, Fu Zi, Yu Gui, and Ren Shen (powder)? Or should I add Lu Rong and Zhu Jie?

I once prescribed (Yu Sheng) You Gui Yin adding Ren Shen (powder) to a patient undergoing chemotherapy, and the tumor shrunk by 1/3. It appears that it was effective!

A: Hematopoietic function will inevitably be inhibited following chemotherapy and radiotherapy for the treatment of brain tumors. (Yu Sheng) You Gui Yin adding Ren Shen (powder) and Chuan Qi (powder) will improve hematopoietic function and relieve symptoms; so yes, I would continue prescribing this formula. However, if chemotherapy and radiotherapy are no longer being administered, then you could consider changing the original formula to Ban Xia Tian Ma Bai Zhu San or (Yu Sheng) Ru Mo Si Wu Tang adding Huang Qin, Huang Lian, Huang Bo, Bai Zhu, Fu Ling, Ze Xie, Tian Ma, Wu Zhu Yu, Chuan Qi (powder),Yu Sheng Wan, Wan Ling Dan, and possibly small doses of Gan Jiang, Fu Zi, and Yu Gui. Remember! Administration of these TCM medicinals may not always produce noticeable effects right away, but don't get deterred, it's best to stay the course.

Generally, inhibition of hematopoietic function is most marked during the second week following anticancer agent infusions. In addition to blood transfusions and injections of EPO or G-CSF, oncologists commonly administer corticosteroids or autologous stem cell transplantation (ASCT) to improve hematopoietic function. However, adverse effects are severe, because the proliferation of both good and bad cells is greatly increased. This method does kill cancer cells (hematologic and imaging tests verify), but after a period of time these neoplastic cells will proliferate again, and once they do these renegade cells run rampant. TCM medicinals can promote renal secretion of hematopoietic factors and the secretion of hematopoietic stem cells in the bone marrow without the adverse effects of Western medicine drugs. It's best to begin TCM medicinal treatment soon after (about 1 week) administration of chemotherapy to ensure optimal results at preserving hematopoietic function.

Note: For the treatment of chemotherapy side effects in brain tumor patients, there is no need to begin promoting hematopoietic function right away, because complete blood count (CBC) tests will remain normal. Typically, about two weeks after treatment, signs of decreased hematopoietic function present. With this in mind, it is best to begin prescribing TCM medicinal treatment 1 week after administration of chemotherapy. You could consider prescribing Ban Xia Tian Ma Bai Zhu San adding qi-supplementing, blood-supplementing, and yang-supplementing medicinals; or You Gui Yin adding Tian Ma, Gu Sui Bu, Xu Duan, Mu Dan Pi, Chi Shao, Huang Qin, Wu Zhu Yu, and "the Three Insects." The administration of TCM medicinals will dramatically shorten the period of time hematopoietic function is inhibited. Of course, it would be even better to coordinate efforts with the hematology-oncology specialist, ensuring that chemotherapy be administered in smaller doses (say 80% or even 50% of the normal dose) spread out over several times. That way the adverse effects can be minimized. (Anitcancer agents are developed in Western countries with people of European descent the primary focus of research studies and clinical trials. The dosage standards are based on this focus group. For the majority of Asians, who tend to be smaller in physical stature, this dosage is too heavy; it's no wonder there are so many adverse effects!)

You are starting to get the hang of the integrated TCM and Western medicine approach to treating brain tumors. I can tell by the formulas you are prescribing and the questions you are asking. Just remember! 2~3 weeks (at the absolute uppermost limit 2~3 months) after the completion of chemotherapy you need to change formulas. Yang-supplementing medicinals improve low blood protein concentrations and BUN and Cr levels, thus remedying the side effects of Western medicine drugs, and also prevent tumor growth. However, administration of yang-supplementing medicinals over too long a period of time (upper limit of 3~6 months) has the potential of inducing rapid proliferation of the brain tumor. At this time, the condition can be identified as repletion heat pattern. The formula should be changed to either Ru Mo Si Wu Tang, Wen Dan Tang, or Ban Xia Tian Ma Ban Zhu San variants adding Gan Jiang and Fu Zi as channel conductors directing the medicinals to the lesion site.

Case Study #4: Postsurgical Radiotherapy Induces Brain Swelling (Edema)

Q: The patient is a 46 y/o male with a brain tumor located near Broca's area presenting with symptoms of speech impairment, gait disturbance, limb weakness, and poor appetite. A brief history is as follows:

He underwent his first surgery in April 2007 and following radiotherapy he incurred massive brain swelling. After receiving chemotherapy his WBC and PLT counts severely decreased and he was admitted into ICU three times. In March of the next year (2008) his condition worsened and his doctors said they couldn't do anything for him. On June 30, he came to my clinic by referral for consultation. First, I prescribed Ban Xia Tian Ma Bai Zhu San adding Chi Shao, Dan Pi, Gu Sui Bu, Xu Duan (1 liang of each), and Wan Ling Dan (6 pills/3x/day), which proved effective in improving strength. By the end of July, the patient's condition had deteriorated presenting with symptoms of heightened dysphasia, gait disturbance, and severe headache; thus, the attending physician decided to perform the second surgery on August 20 (2008). The strange thing is on August 15 the patient awoke from sleep without a headache and the dysphasia and gait disturbance also gradually resolved, so his doctor decided to cancel the second surgery. How could this have happened?

A: Treatment of brain tumors involves reducing brain swelling, lowering ICP, inhibiting angiogenesis, preventing seizures, averting tumor exacerbation, and stabilizing the overall condition. If there is no improvement after receiving surgery, chemotherapy, and radiotherapy, the administration of TCM medicinals will usually stabilize the patient's condition, even to the extent where the tumor is not visible on an MRI image. This is when you must change back to using the "essential state" formula, otherwise the yang-supplementing medicinals may induce relapse. I have mentioned this many times now— you must remember this!

Case Study #5: Advanced Stage Malignant Brain Tumor Necrosis

Q: I am currently treating an advanced stage malignant brain tumor patient whom has already received the full regimen of Western medicine cancer therapies prior to seeking my consultation. I prescribed Ru Mo Si Wu Tang, and after taking the formula for 2 months an MRI image revealed tumor contrast enhancement along with right-side motor dysfunction and visual disturbance. Concerned that sections of the tumor had undergone necrosis, his doctors have decided to perform another craniectomy.

A: This could be a sign of liquefactive necrosis in an advanced stage brain tumor. To quickly resolve these symptoms you can simply add large doses of "the Three Yellows," Bai Zhu, Fu Ling, Ze Xie, and Da Huang to your original formula, which will accelerate the clearance of metabolic waste and resolve the toxins. Your patient's doctors may alos decide to insert a drainage tube, which will also promote resolution of the lesion. For brain tumors there are three possible results of treatment: tumor apoptosis, calcification, and necrosis. Your treatment approach has accurately identified the pattern and thus has produced effective results. The contrast enhancement in your patient's MRI simply indicates that the tumor has necrosed, releasing profuse amounts of blood and lymph fluids that accumulate due to inadequate resorption. You should advise the patient to have follow-up CT scan and MRI performed to evaluate the amount of fluid and adjust your TCM formula prescription accordingly.

Case Study #6: Corticosteroids – Firstline Treatment of Brain Swelling (Edema) Following Surgery, Radiotherapy, and Chemotherapy

Q: A 50 y/o male patient was administered an injection of vincristine, cyclophosphamide, and procarbazine (PCB and CCVV) to treat a brain tumor. He suffered severe adverse effects from chemotherapy and came to my clinic seeking consultation. First, I prescribed You Gui Yin variant to remedy the side effects, but it turns out, in addition to improving energy level and strength, this formula also had an anitcancer action inducing shrinkage of the patient's tumor. The patient's children were grateful, telling me that I had brought their father back to life and given their family renewed hope. Actually, the credit really goes to my mentor whose guidance and instruction walked me through this process. For both the family and me, we thank you so much!

I remember you asked me at the time, "Has the patient been administered corticosteroids?" Without verifying to make sure I told you that he hadn't. It wasn't until later that I found out he had taken corticosteroids for a period of time. I admit, I wasn't detailed enough while conducting the patient interview and must be more attentive in the future. Now, I also have another question: Does You Gui Yin really have an anticancer action?

A: When I talked to you on the telephone you said that this patient had "not" taken corticosteroids, but the patient's medical records that you faxed me clearly indicated corticosteroid administration. Remember! Every brain tumor patient who undergoes surgery and follow-up radiotherapy and chemotherapy will incur brain swelling (edema), and to alleviate the damaging effects on brain cells caused by increased ICP, general protocol calls for the administration of corticosteroids. Once corticosteroids have been either injected or taken orally, the patient's condition is identified as kidney yang deficiency pattern. At this time, regardless of the formula prescribed you must add Gan Jiang, Fu Zi, Rou Gui, and Ren Shen (powder). If severe swelling and elevated ICP present, mannitol or glycerin will be administered to reduce ICP levels. At this time, the TCM physician must add Bai Zhu, Fu Ling, Zhu Ling, Ze Xie, Tian Ma, Wu Zhu Yu, "the

Three Insects," and Yu Sheng Wan to prevent aberrant electrical discharges that might induce seizures. If the patient's condition exacerbates and becomes difficult to control, add Wan Ling Dan.

Chemotherapy inhibits hematopoietic function in the bone marrow as well as hematopoietic function and growth factor pathways in the kidneys. You Gui Yin improves this condition and promotes hormone secretion and pathway function. Since the administration of corticosteroids puts the patient in a kidney yang deficiency pattern state and the brain (sea of marrow) belongs to the kidney, prescribing You Gui Yin effectively treats this condition, preventing the brain tumor from proliferating and possibly even shrinking or completely eradicating the tumor.

But you must remember! Once corticosteroids have been discontinued you should change the formula to (Yu Sheng) Ban Xia Tian Ma Bai Zhu San variant. After 2~3 months of administering this formula, you should then change to either Ru Mo Si Wu Tang adding Fu Ling, Bai Zhu, Ze Xie, "the Three Yellows," Tian Ma, Wu Zhu Yu, "the Three Insects," Chuan Qi (powder), Yu Sheng Wan, and Wan Ling Dan; or Chai Ling Tang adding Da Huang, Tian Ma, "the Three Yellows," Wu Zhu Yu, "the Three Insects," Dan Pi, Chi Shao, Qing Hao, Di Gu Pi, Yu Sheng Wan, and Wan Ling Dan. The principle here is that you want to bring the patient's condition back to the "essential state" of repletion heat pattern, which is the state it was at the onset of disease before the patient received chemotherapy and radiotherapy. The problem with administering yang-supplementing medicinals over too long a period of time is that it could induce neoplastic differentiation in stem cells peripheral to the tumor, thus accelerating proliferation and deterioration of the patient's condition.

If the patient receives chemotherapy and radiotherapy without administration of corticosteroids, then you should prescribe Da Chai Tang, Chai Ling Tang, or Ru Mo Si Wu Tang variants from the onset. Do "not" administer yang-supplementing formulas such as (Yu Sheng) Ban Xia Tian Ma Bai Zhu San and (Yu Sheng) You Gui Yin. If you feel it is necessary to add Gan Jiang, Fu Zi, and Yu Gui, then only use small doses adding corresponding amounts of "the Three Yellows" and large doses of, Qing Hao, Zhi Mu, Di Gu Pi, and Dan Pi, which combine to counterbalance the heat and protect the yin aspect. You could also consider prescribing Wen Dan Tang or Zhi Bo Di Huang Tang variants instead. Clearly understanding this basis of reasoning and applying this approach in clinical practice is fundamental to the integrated Chinese and Western medicine treatment of disease.

Case Study #7: Bu Zhong Yi Qi Tang Variant – "Conquers All Pathoconditions"

Q: Recently, I was invited to the Department of Radiation Oncology at the affiliated hospital of Ajou University to treat patients and also asked to collaborate with Kyung Hee University on a research project. We plan to design several TCM formula compositions within three years to provide the Western medical community with reference sources. The focus of our research is to improve the adverse effects of dry mouth following radiotherapy to the head and neck in cancer patients and the symptoms that mimic menopause syndrome such as tidal heat and facial sweating following chemotherapy in breast cancer patients.

The treatment for improving symptoms of dry mouth simply entailed acupuncture treatment (no moxa nor TCM medicinal formulas) needling Ting Gong (SJ19), Yi Feng (SJ17), and He Gu (LI4) (1x/week for 1 month (total of 4 treatments)). This 4-treatment regimen proved effective in improving symptoms (patients were able to naturally secrete saliva on their own). Similarly, I needled acupoints San Yin Jiao (SP6), Shui Quan (K5), and Xue Hai (SP10) 1x/week for 1 month (total of 4 treatments), which proved effective in improving the symptoms that mimic menopause syndrome such as tidal heat and facial sweating in breast cancer patients. We are presently conducting further studies on animals and humans, essentially using your three main formulas: Xiao Chai Hu Tang combining Sheng Yu Tang, Shi Quan Da Bu Tang, and You Gui Yin. Additionally, I want to slightly modify these formulas adding blood-activating and stasis transforming and heat-clearing and toxin-resolving medicinals due to the climate and environmental differences here in South Korea. What do you think about this project? Any suggestions or advice?

A: Acupuncture is very effective at treating "early stage" salivary gland atrophy, but if there is lymphatic obstruction or swollen and sclerosed glands and the muscle tissues of the head, face and neck have undergone fibrosis, then warm needling (moxa cubes on the needle) will offer better results. As for treating menopause symptoms with yin-nourishing and heat-abating acupoints and TCM medicinals, these modalities offer excellent efficacy in the treatment of psychosomatic symptoms and autonomic nervous system disorders arising during menopause. Based on my experience, they are also effective at treating the tidal fever and facial sweating induced by chemotherapy in breast cancer patients. Keep up the good work and publish your results. The only way to ensure your efforts make an "enduring" impact is getting these results down in "print." Let's go!

Bu Zhong Yi Qi Tang variant is a good TCM formula for treating the adverse effects of chemotherapy and radiotherapy in cancer patients. Adding medicinals such as Huang Qin, Yuan Hu, Mu Xiang, Dan Shen, Ren Shen (powder), and Chuan Qi (powder) to this formula promotes wound healing from surgery and the initial liver damage caused by chemotherapy. Large doses of Huang Qi may also be included (anywere from 1.5~2 liang) for its center-supplementing and blood and flesh-engendering actions. If hematopoietic dysfunction presents add Gan Jiang, Fu Zi, Yu Gui, and Lu Rong; if low total protein (TP) levels present with edema (i.e., sternocostal, abdominal, lower leg regions) add Bai Zhu, Fu Ling, and Ze Xie; and for increased BUN and Cr add Ren Dong Teng, Ding Shu Xiu, and Pu Gong Ying. If I had to make a choice of one formula that could "conquer all conditions," an elixir if you will, it would be Bu Zhong Yi Qi Tang variant.

Case Study #8: Dry Mouth and Eyes Following Radiotherapy – Don't Misuse Glaucoma Drug (Pilocarpine HCl)!

Q: A 24 y/o male received radiotherapy for a brain tumor with increased β-HCG levels. Following radiotherapy the patient suffered from adverse effects of severe dry mouth, dry eyes, insomnia, and irritability, and came to my clinic for consultation. The patient said that he was using pilocarpine hydrochloride (prescribed by an ophthalmologist), which provided relief for dry eyes within minutes of application and also improved dry mouth symptoms, but induced side effects of profuse, generalized (entire body) sweating and the relief lasted for only a short time. Is TCM effective at treating this condition?

A: Pilocarpine hydrochloride is an externally applied cholinergic agonist used for treating glaucoma and doesn't contain any active properties that can improve dry eye syndrome (DES). In fact, long-term application of this drug can lead to even drier eyes, a "burning" sensation in the eyes, unstable blood pressure, cataracts, and glaucoma. Elevated β-HCG levels are present in endometrial cancer in women and testicular, prostate, and adrenal gland pathologies in men. For brain cancer patients with elevated β-HCG levels, TCM medicinals that clear kidney and liver heat should be administered. In cases of severe dryness, the treatment regimen for Sjogren's syndrome can be followed, prescribing Hyperactive Immune Formula variant; and if insomnia presents add Dai Zhe Shi or Long Gu and Mu Li. Also, bleed Zan Zhu (UB2), Si Zhu Kong (SJ23), and Da Zhui (DU14); and needle the acupoints Feng Chi (GB20), Wan Gu (GB12), He

Gu (LI4), San Yin Jiao (SP6), Yin Ling Quan (SP9), Tai Chong (LV3), Shen Men (HT7), Nei Guan (PC6), Xin Shu (UB15) and Shen Shu (UB23).

Administration of cholinergic agonists may induce profuse sweating, and if severe, then you can change the formula to Jian Ling Tang (including Gan Cao) adding "the Three Yellows," Qing Hao, Zhi Mu, and Di Gu Pi.

Case Study #9: Hemiparesis Resulting from Cerebral Infarction

Q: I have a male patient who suffers from hemiparesis resulting from cerebral infarction and has a history of chronic, bleeding hemorrhoids. One day last year he overstrained while on the toilet leading to a stroke that caused left-sided hemiparesis manifesting as stiffness in the left arm and leg. The patient's doctor diagnosed him with cerebral infarction. How do you treat cerebral infarction? Using TCM medicinals, how long do you think it will take to recover function of the stiff appendages (able to move about freely and autonomously carry out basic daily activities)? At least one year, right?

A: Overstraining while on the stool (e.g., holding the breath and straining at the same time) in people with constipation, bleeding hemorrhoids, or anal prolapse can most certainly cause cerebral ischemia (hypoxia), cerebral infarction, and cerebral hemorrhage, resulting in hemiparesis (sensory and motor deficits) and in severe cases hemiplegia. In fact, overstraining while on the toilet is the most common cause of anal prolapse with incidence rates on the rise.

There are increasing numbers of people with anal prolapse and anal fissures. People of today eat a lot of rich foods, not enough fruits and vegetables, and don't get enough exercise – dietary and lifestyle habits that lead to constipation problems. Additionally, sit-down toilets are now in virtually every modern household. These toilets offer the benefit of convenience for those physically unable to squat; alleviate the discomfort of soreness, numbness, and pain for those who have to wait for their bowels to move; and even provide a leisurely gettaway for those in the habit of reading periodicals or browsing on their smartphone while "doing their business." The problem is these toilets were invented by people of European descent with designs standardized to accommodate the physical stature of Europeans and Americans not the relatively smaller statures of Asians whose legs are often left hanging in the air or straining in flexion to reach the floor below. People with constipation sit on the toilet for long periods of time exerting themselves unsuccessfully and not getting everything evacuated. Since sitting there is a relatively comfortable endeavor, constipated people tend to spend excessive amounts of time straining away. This puts too much pressure on the anal orifice, constricting the canal instead of opening it, and making it difficult to defecate and more likely to induce anal fissures and anal prolapse. In severe cases, this overstraining may lead to cerebral hypoxia and ischemia (especially for those with anal fissures or anal prolapse who sit on the toilet and bleed) and possibly may even induce cerebral infarction (ischemic stroke) that results in hemiparesis or hemiplegia.

For cerebral infarction patients, it's best to administer both TCM medicinals and acupuncture (with moxa). Prescribe Bu Yang Huan Wu Tang adding Gan Jiang, Fu Zi, Yu Gui, Huang Qin, Ren Shen (powder), and Chuan Qi (powder). This formula's sovereign medicinal is Huang Qi, and you can start out prescribing 2 liang incrementally increasing up to 2.5 liang and then 3 liang to strengthen the qi-supplementing action. These are all effective in treating hemiparesis and hemiplegia caused by cerebral infarction (ischemic stroke), improving motor function and strengthening the limbs. As for acupuncture, to treat hemiparesis (or hemiplegia) you can consider needling (with moxa) acupoints such as He Gu (LI4), Shou San Li (LI10), Wai Guan (SJ5), Zhong Zhu (SJ3), Zu San Li (ST36), Yang Ling Quan (GB34), Xuan Zhong (GB39), San Yin Jiao (SP6), Tai Chong (LV3), Di Wu Hui (GB42), Feng Chi (GB20), Tian Zhu (UB10), Bai Hui (DU20), Guan Yuan Shu (UB26), Wei Zhong (UB40), and Kun Lun (UB60). Naturally, if the patient actively engages in rehabilitation the outlook for functional recovery (especially the arms) is even better. For remedying hemorrhoids, anal fissures, and anal prolapse, you can needle He Gu (LI4), Shou San Li (LI10), Chi Ze (LU5), Xia Bai (LU4), Bai Hui (DU20), and the "four anal perimeter acupoints"; and bleed Shang Yang (LI1), Er Jian (LI2), and San Jian (LI3).

Remember! The duration of treatment for hemiparesis and hemiplegia varies greatly with each patient. Sometimes it is a quick process and other times it can be very slow. It depends on the extent of brain damage, both the size and location of the lesion, and also on how motivated the patient is to achieve recovery along with the level of family support. Patients with mild hemiparesis who retain motor function capacity and mental clarity should stay actively involved in hobbies and interaction in social settings. For example, getting together with friends for "therapeutic mahjong" sessions is a great way to combine an interest that stimulates the brain, encourages social interaction, and provides rehabilitation for upper limb motor function.

Case Study #10: Cerebral Infarction (Stroke) Complicated by

Hemorrhage and Hydrocephalus – Is There Cerebral Atrophy?

Q: A 62 y/o male patient had incurred cerebral infarction and received treatment that successfully stabilized his condition; and about 6 months later hydrocephalus developed followed by another cerebral infarction and hemorrhage. After this episode, the patient and his family sought my consultation. I prescribed Bu Yang Huan Wu Tang variant for 3 months, which dramatically improved his symptoms of malaise, heaviness over the entire body, and cognitive dysfunction. The patient said he felt almost like a normal, healthy person again. And then yesterday, I received a call from his daughter saying that her father had once again presented with cognitive and motor dysfunction starting about 1 month ago. Recently, the patient had an MRI performed revealing the recurrence of hydrocephalus, but ICP was normal and there was no fever. Is there cerebral atrophy? What's the best way to treat this condition?

A: In patients with cerebral infarction, a loss of cerebral tissue occurs and the ventricular system enlarges to compensate for this loss, resulting in a secondary (normal-pressure or communicating) hydrocephalus. For this condition, you can consider prescribing either Wu Ling San (Nephritis Formula) adding Da Huang, Ren Shen (powder), and Chuan Qi (powder); or Ban Xia Tian Ma Bai Zhu San variant. If constipation presents, add Da Huang to promote the stool, and if heavy doses of up to 8 qian still prove ineffective, then add Pu Xiao starting at 5 fen adding incremental doses until the patient maintains 1 stool/day. Remember! If the hydrocephalus is caused by a cyst or tumor that blocks CSF circulation (i.e., obstructive (noncommunicating) hydrocephalus), the patient will present with increased ICP, requiring the prescription of a different formula. You should also advise the patient to avoid rigorous activities and situations that might injure the already compromised brain tissue (cells).

Case Study #11: Dizziness Following Cerebellar Infarction

Q: This patient is male with robust stature who likes to drink alcohol and has a history of high blood pressure. Recently, he went to the hospital to examine the cause of his severe dizziness and get treatment. An MRI revealed left-sided cerebellar infarction. The patient's urine output and stool are normal. What's the best approach for treating this patient?

A: There are many causes of dizziness, and cerebellar infarction is one of them. You must carefully identify the pattern and then decide on the right treatment. Here are three formulas you may consider prescribing: 1) Bu Yang Huan Wu Tang adding Gan Jiang, Fu Zi, Yu Gui, Tian Ma, Huang Qin, Chuan Qi (powder), and Ren Shen (powder); 2) Ban Xia Tian Ma Bai Zhu San adding heavy doses of Tian Ma, Huang Qi, Chuan Qi (powder), Chi Shao, and Yin Xing Ye; and 3) for visceral agitation, prescribe Ban Xia Tian Ma Bai Zhu San adding Gan Cao and Long Yan Gan (or Hong Zao).

Case Study #12: Non-healing Wound Following Meningioma Resection

Q: Recently, a female patient diagnosed with meningioma sought my consultation. She has already undergone brain surgery 5 times (including Gamma Knife and CyberKnife) and also received several regimens of radiotherapy. At the time, she presented with right-sided hemiplegia and I prescribed Ru Mo Si Wu Tang variant for 1 month. After her symptoms improved a bit she never returned for consultation and treatment (I heard that she had had a stroke and was consulting another TCM doctor closer to her home). Well, the meningioma grew back, requiring another surgical resection. After surgery, the wound would not heal and the skin graft didn't take well either. The patient's husband was worried sick about her condition and wanted her to come back to visit me, but she declined, saying, "I want to use the little time I have left to go see things and have fun." Infection set in and she ended up dying. When I heard the news, I was very sad and wondered why a person would not cherish their own life. If this were your patient, what would you have done?

A: Meningioma relapse following resection could induce stroke-like symptoms such as hemiparesis, asthenia, seizures, and hallucinations (aural, visual, spatial, olfactory, and gustatory). If the TCM physician is inexperienced and treats this hemiparesis as a stroke (mistakenly administering TCM supplementing medicinals), the tumor will again likely relapse and grow back at a faster rate and develop into a "space-occupying lesion," which requires cranial surgery to "reduce the intracranial pressure" (decompressive craniectomy). Following surgery, adjuvant radiotherapy is typically administered with the skin and tissue that has been exposed to radiotherapy susceptible to damage and necrosis. Failure of the granulation tissue to grow makes it difficult for the wound to heal; and even if skin grafts are performed, success rates are low and infection prevalent.

In cases where infection spreads to the brain, rapid tumor proliferation and expansion readily occurs in the presence of a compromised immune system (from the invasive surgical procedure) often developing into a space-occupying lesion. At this time, corticosteroids must be administered to prevent cerebral swelling (edema) and inflammation. The problem is that long-term administration of corticosteroids will also end up suppressing the immune system, leaving the patient susceptible to infection and resulting in tumerogenesis. On the surface, it appears that the decompressive surgery was successful (decreased ICP levels), but the patient's condition may rapidly deteriorate and eventually result in death due to secondary pathologies.

So remember! You must explain to patients and their families how vital it is to comply with TCM treatment. Even when symptoms improve and the patient appears to be on the path to recovery patients must continue with this treatment regimen for at least 3~5 months longer up until the image scans indicate no sign of relapse, then you can begin to gradually reduce the dosage. And in the future, the patient must be vigilant for any signs and symptoms of common cold (external contraction) and immediately seek treatment (preferably TCM); otherwise, the patient is highly susceptible to subsequent infection and brain swelling (edema).

Case Study #13: Intracranial Lipoma – Is Treatment Necessary?

Q: I have a 42 y/o male patient with an 8 cm lipoma on the left side of his brain stem. He has no presenting symptoms or signs of impairment or discomfort. Is it necessary to treat this condition?

A: Although this patient with the brainstem lipoma doesn't have any presenting signs or symptoms right now, the tumor will continue growing slowly over time. If its growth isn't inhibited, then it could compress breathing and swallowing nerve centers resulting in airway obstruction and aspiration pneumonia, possibly resulting in death. I recommend prescribing Ru Mo Si Wu Tang adding "the Three Yellows," Tian Ma, "the Three Insects," Bai Zhu, Fu Ling, Ze Xie, Chuan Qi (powder), Ma Huang, Xing Ren, Di Long, Yu Sheng Wan, and Wan Ling Dan. This formula will effectively shrink the size of the lipoma and possibly even achieve complete resolution.

Section 2: Other Pathogenic Conditions of the Brain

Case Study #1: Head Tremor – Essential Tremor and Cerebellar Atrophy

Q: A 50 y/o male patient began having head tremors about 3 years ago. When he is nervous or angry his tongue will even tremble, and the only time he doesn't experience these tremors is during sleep. The patient went through a full range of tests to rule out dopamine, blood sugar, or blood pressure abnormalities. His diet and sleep habits are healthy, but he is impatient and loses his temper easily. I diagnosed his condition as "head tremor" (essential tremor) and prescribed Bu Yang Huan Wu Tang adding Gan Jiang, Fu Zi, Yu Gui, Huang Qin, "the Three Insects," Ren Shen (powder), and Chuan Qi (powder). Is there anything in particular about this condition that I should look out for?

A: When head tremor presents (especially in males), you can't overlook the possibility of Parkinson's disease or brain stem pathology. Now let's take a look at what the cause of your patient's head tremor could be. Generally, if head tremor presents when a person is calm and at rest (e.g., sitting down talking, watching television) this is called "quiet" tremor, which is strongly suggestive of Parkinson's disease. If the head tremor is brought on by action (e.g., walking, working with hands) this is called "intention" tremor, which is suggestive of essential tremor, cerebellar atrophy, or pathologies of the nerves or vasculature in sub-cerebellar regions. One sign in particular that verifies the diagnosis of cerebellar atrophy is when the patient cannot walk down the stairs even when accompanied by someone alongside (oftentimes even the slightest degree of slope will cause reluctance and apprehension). For all of these conditions you can prescribe Bu Yang Huan Wu Tang variant.

In cases of elevated ICP, the patient will present with neck flaccidity and weakness and a gait like someone with poliomyelitis, lurching forward one step at a time. For these patients, it is best to prescribe (Yu Sheng) Ban Xia Tian Ma Bai Zhu San combining (Yu Sheng) Bu Yang Huan Wu Tang along with the supplementing medicinals you prescribed above. Overall, for any type of brain atrophy, degeneration, or dementia caused by vascular disease, long-term administration of Bu Yang Huan Wu Tang variant will prove very effective.

Case Study #2: Edematous Meninges Affects Vision

Q: I have a 28 y/o male patient who is overweight. He came to see me for a consultation because of difficulty passing stool and urinating and loss of vision in his left eye. The patient explained that he had been this way for over a year. He had an MRI performed at a hospital revealing edematous meninges in the turchean region. The swelling was approx. 1 cm x 1.5 cm large. He doesn't want to follow the advice of Western medical doctors recommending that he have surgery so he came to visit me instead. Do you think this is a case I should take on?

A: Overweight people tend to have poor metabolism and are inherently susceptible to metabolic disorders. Difficulty passing stool and urinating and loss of vision in his left eye due to edematous meninges indicate that the condition is very serious. If he isn't willing to receive Western medical treatment, then you can consider prescribing either Da Chai Hu Tang variant or Ru Mo Si Wu Tang variant adding Bai Zhu, Fu Ling, Ze Xie, Tian Ma, and Chuan Qi (powder). These formulas will gradually promote the absorption of the edematous fluid by the body. As long as the edema resolves and doesn't compress on the optic nerve, vision can usually be restored.

Case Study #3: Post-Concussion Syndrome – "Double Vision"

Q: On the afternoon of August 16, a 9 y/o boy accidentally fell off his bed while playing and hit his head on the floor (head trauma) and there was concern he may have a concussion. Sure enough that evening he developed symptoms of headache and nausea and was immediately sent to ER and admitted into the hospital where he received mannitol infusions. The next day he still had a severe headache. The MRI revealed a small hemorrhagic lesion in his brain and he had "double vision" (diplopia). The attending physician planned to give the patient drugs to promote the absorption of the hemorrhage, but his mother came to me first to ask my opinion. To tell you the truth I am not sure myself about the prognosis of solely relying on Western medicine treatment for this condition. I hope you can give me advice and direction on this case. Your input and instruction is greatly appreciated!

A: Post-concussion "double vision" can be caused by damage to the visual center at the back of the head or the oculomotor nerve and optic chiasma in the brain stem. Persistence of cerebral edema and headache despite administration of mannitol suggests that the brain injury has produced a large amount of exudate with brain tissue (cell) swelling. Also, the MRI also shows hemorrhage. Taking these factors into consideration, this condition can clearly be identified as stasis heat with water amassment pattern headache. As for TCM treatment, you can prescribe (Yu Sheng) Ru Mo Si Wu Tang adding "the Four Ling's," Tian Ma, Huang Qin, Huang Lian, and Chuan Qi (powder) to expedite stabilization of ICP, minimize the area damaged, and reduce the extent and severity of the ensuing adverse effects and complications. Once ICP has stabilized, you can add Gan Jiang, Fu Zi, and Yu Gui (gradually increasing the dose up to 5 qian each) to the original formula. Administer this treatment for a period of time until the symptoms have stabilized, then change the prescription to either Bu Yang Huan Wu Tang, Sheng Yu Tang, or Ban Xia Tian Ma Bai Zhu San variants adding Chuan Qi (powder), Chuan Qiong, Chi Shao, and Yin Xin Ye. The patient should continue taking this formula for a minimum of 6 months~1 year. There will be noticeable improvement in the patients condition. If the patient has epileptic seizures, then the formula should be adjusted according to the presenting symptoms.

Presently, the treatment of cerebral hemorrhage in most hospitals involves promoting spontaneous resorption by administering the anticoagulants aspirin and warfarin (Coumadin), which merely function to lower blood viscosity. There aren't any pharmaceuticals specifically targeted at treating this condition. TCM medicinals, on the other hand, have proven efficacy in facilitating spontaneous resorption and can also prevent other sites from hemorrhaging. You can definitely prescribe TCM formulas for this patient!

Case Study #4: Head Trauma – Concussion and Hemorrhage

Q: A patient of mine suffered a concussion causing hemorrhage and edema. The patient was admitted into the hospital for treatment and management of his condition, and his family sought my consultation for TCM treatment. After administering TCM medicinals, an MRI revealed that 2/3 of the hemorrhagic lesion had already been resorbed. The patient's doctor prescribed antiepileptic drugs and processed the patient for discharge.

A: Naturally, in cases of concussion resulting in epidural, subdural, or subarachnoid hemorrhage, the sooner resorption occurs the better. This will minimize the amount of brain cells damaged from compression and the ensuing swelling and lysis (necrosis), dramatically reducing the potential for causing behavioral changes, cognitive impairment, and progressive brain atrophy. You must be vigilant about these potential outcomes. Brain hemorrhage will usually spontaneously resolve within 2 weeks. If spontaneous hemorrhage does not occur within 2 weeks, TCM identifies this as cold stasis pattern. As is the case for many types of brain disorders antiepileptic medication must be administered to prevent epileptic seizures. If severe (e.g., grand mal) epileptic seizures may lead to cerebral vasospasm, cerebral infarction, or cerebral infarction secondary to cerebral hemorrhage, resulting in enlargement of the necrosed area and an increased severity and frequency of epileptic attacks (a viscous cycle!). My belief is that antiepileptic medication should be prescribed and combined with the administration of TCM medicinals that regulate the constitution. This integrated approach provides the best method of both accelerating the resorption of blood and protecting the patient's brain tissue (cells).

Case Study #5: Concussion – Cold Hands and Feet and Profuse Sweating Following Mannitol Administration

Q: A patient suffered a concussion and was admitted into the hospital where he was administered a mannitol injection. Afterwards, the patient developed cold hands and feet and profuse sweating. Why would this happen?

A: Once the condition of a patient with concussion stabilizes, the patient will be susceptible to a host of autonomic nervous system and neuropsychiatric symptoms, such as spontaneous sweating, night sweats, aversion to cold (phantom cold), aversion to heat (phantom heat), fear, fright palpitations, circadian rhythm disturbance, late afternoon tidal heat, etc. These symptoms will resolve as brain circulation improves and returns to normal.

Case Study #6: Post-Concussion Complication – Night Sweats

Q: I am treating a 41 y/o male patient whom suffered a head trauma injury (hemorrhage). He never underwent cranial surgery, but stayed in the hospital for 6 months following the accident receiving medication until recovery. What is strange about this case is that since the accident occurred every night for the past 3 years just about 5 minutes after falling asleep he has profuse sweating "flowing like water" on the neck and upper back. The patient has received both TCM and Western medicine treatment, but none has provided any significant efficacy. How would you treat this condition?

A: Patients suffering from a concussion resulting in intracranial hemorrhage and leading to the complication of night sweats can be identified as Yang Ming channel with Shao Yang enduring heat pattern. You can consider prescribing (Yu Sheng) Jian Ling Tang (including Gan Cao) adding Hong Zao (or Long Yan), Huang Bo, Qing Hao, Zhi Mu, Di Gu Pi, and Ma Huang Gen. You should add up to 8 qian of Huang Bo and if necessary add Chuan Qi (powder). Following the administration of these medicinals his symptoms should rapidly improve. But remember! In the future, if the patient catches a cold (external contraction), you should "not" prescribe Ma Huang or substances with ephedra (TCM or Western medicine). If cough presents, then you can add extra amounts of Xing Ren, Gui Zhi, and Hou Po to avoid hyperstimulation of the patient's perspiration centers. You can also administer acupuncture treatment selecting the acupoints Feng Chi (GB20), Feng Fu (DU16), Bai Hui (DU20), San Yin Jiao (SP6), Tai Xi (KD3), Xuan Zhong (GB39), Tai Chong (LV3), and Shen Men (HT7).

Case Study #7: Post-Concussion Syndrome (PCS) or Neurosis?

Q: A 50 y/o female patient suffers from post-concussion complications of blurred vision in her left eye explaining that "it feels like it's swollen" (but actually it's not) along with mental fogginess, limb weakness, dizziness, nausea, sensation of heat on the vertex, heaviness in the chest, and slight edema of the arms and legs. In March of this year, she was standing at the doorway of a bank when the metal security door dropped down on her forehead. The MRI revealed nothing abnormal with her neck and head, and her blood pressure is normal, but the patient continues to worry about the concussion and insists she is suffering from post-concussion syndrome (PCS). What do you think I should do?

A: This doesn't sound like post-concussion complications to me; it sounds more like neurosis. People with neurotic disorders have an uncanny way of finding "points of attack" to blame for all of their discomforts (either real or perceived). If they have been injured, hit by something, contracted an infection, been irritated, felt pressured in some way, etc., they just can't get over it, mired and overcome by a cascade of travails. You can prescribe Wen Dan Tang or Ban Xia Tian Ma Bai Zhu San adding Gan Cao, Hong Zao, Qing Hao, Zhi Mu, Di Gu Pi, and Yu Sheng Wan. Make sure to verify if the patient really does have edema of the arms and legs or it just "feels like heaviness and swelling." If there really is edema, then add large doses of Bai Zhu, Fu Ling, and Ze Xie; and if there is just the "feeling of heaviness and swelling," then simply add Yu Sheng Wan and either Hong Zao, Long Yan Gan, or Hei Tang (dark, unrefined, cane sugar); and if pitting edema presents, then add Gan Jiang, Fu Zi, and Yu Gui.

Case Study #8: Amnesia and Dysphasia Following Car Accident

Q: I have a 35 y/o male patient who suffers from amnesia (trouble remembering complex ideas and concepts) and dysphasia (speaks like a young child) following a car accident. Motor function is normal. How would you treat this patient?

A: It is very common to suffer amnesia following a concussion. The first thing I would do is determine whether he has undergone surgery and/or been administered large amounts of corticosteroids. If not, then prescribe Ru Mo Si Wu Tang adding Dan Shen, Chuan Qi (powder), Yin Xing Ye, Huang Qi, and a small dose of Da Huang. This formula will activate the blood, break stasis, and promote circulation; thus resolving the static blood (thrombosis) in the prefrontal and temporal lobes which is causing this patient's condition.

Case Study #9: Tuberculous Meningitis

Q: I have a 61 y/o female patient with tuberculous meningitis. Two months ago she began presenting with exterior pattern symptoms of headache, mild fever, body aches, and dry cough. One week ago she suddenly began vomiting and suffered from a severe, splitting headache. After hospital admission, examination revealed tuberculous meningitis. Now, after taking a regimen of antibiotics the headache and vomiting have resolved, but the nausea remains. Her doctors told her that she needs to continue treatment for at least 1 year. What's the best way to treat this condition?

A: Tuberculous meningitis can be identified as Shao Yang heat pattern. You can prescribe Xiao Chai Hu Tang adding Qing Hao, Zhi Mu, Di Gu Pi, and Tian Ma. If increased ICP and abscesses present, but a shunt has "not" been surgically implanted, then you should add Bai Zhu, Fu Ling, and Ze Xie to promote resolution. An integrated regimen of TCM medicinals and Western medicine drugs should be administered concomitantly. After about 3 months, ask the patient to get another blood, mucus, and CSF culture performed. If these results show no sign of the mycobacterium, then continue administering the treatment regimen for 3 more months changing the formula to Zuo Gui Yin adding Tian Ma, Qing Hao, Zhi Mu, Di Gu Pi, Chai Hu, and Qin Jiao.

Case Study #10: Multiple Primary Tumors

Q: Not long ago a 56 y/o female patient weighing 60kg came to my clinic seeking consultation and treatment for multiple primary tumors. The earliest detection of this condition came during a routine physical examination when a malignant thyroid tumor was discovered. Surgical resection was performed upon the recommendation of her physician. Two years later, tumor cells were discovered in her brain, and ever since then it seems as if malignant tumors have been "popping up like bamboo shoots after a rain." Tumors have grown in all parts of her body, such as her right thigh and right upper arm (deltoid muscle) among other places, and the patient and her family are very worried. After taking TCM medicinals for 2 months, she began to feel improvement; for instance, before she couldn't even walk on her own without someone supporting her and now she can take short hikes on her own. However, the tumors in her right thigh and upper arm continue to enlarge and she was considering having another surgical resection. Recently, she went for a routine examination at the hospital, revealing metastatic spread to the ovaries and uterus. That's when I really started having reservations about this case. Am I providing the right treatment? What advice should I give her? Please, as always, offer your invaluable advice and guidance on this case. Thank you for your help!

A: This patient suffers from post-illness depression and dual blood and qi deficiency resulting from chemotherapy and radiotherapy. In addition to prescribing qi-supplementing, yang-supplementing, and dual qi- and blood-supplementing medicinals, you must also be attentive to caring for the patient's emotional well-being and mental health. Prescribing Yu Sheng Wan (starting out at doses of 1 pill and gradually adding up to 3 pills) should help resolve some of the anxiety and depression.

Section 3: Respiratory System Cancers

This section encompasses pathological conditions extending from the nasal cavity to the lungs– the respiratory system. In TCM theory the lung governs the skin, but since there are so few cases relating to skin cancer compiled here and the types of skin conditions are so variegated, skin conditions will be presented in another volume of this series. This section will primarily present cases concerning nasopharyngeal carcinoma and lung cancer.

Case Study #1: Nasopharyngeal Carcinoma (NPC)

Q: Recently, I treated a patient with nasal lymphoma. Following radiotherapy the patient experienced side effects of dry mouth and tongue, middle ear effusion, and loss of olfactory sense. He wanted to try acupuncture for treating these symptoms, but in my opinion TCM medicinals have the capacity to offer much better results. Please explain your approach for treating this condition.

A: Atrophy of the salivary glands, olfactory nerve, and auditory nerve are all common side effects of radiotherapy treatment for nasopharyngeal carcinoma (NPC). Some patients may present with obstruction of the Eustachian tube and middle ear effusion (purulent discharge) that causes dizziness and vertigo, and others may incur lymphatic swelling, which when severe may result in the patient looking "like a toad with eyes swollen shut." This condition requires patience and compliance from the patient with the administration of both TCM medicinals and acupuncture necessary to achieve the quickest and best efficacy. For patients with lymphatic swelling that resembles 'elephantiasis,' prescribe (Yu Sheng) Wu Ling San (Nephritis Formula) adding heavy doses of Huang qi, Gan Jiang, and Yu Gui along with Yin Xing Ye (8 qiang~1 liang), Ren Shen (powder), and Chuan Qi (powder). At the onset of taking this prescription the affected area will soften and become even more swollen; and after taking the formula for 1~2 months, the swelling will begin to disperse with the condition showing marked improvement and resolution in roughly 6 months~1 year.

If there is no lymphatic swelling, then simply follow the principles of my *Integrated TCM and Western Medicine Treatment of Cancer* using Xiao Chai Hu Tang combining Sheng Yu Tang adding Ma Huang, Xi Xin, Bai Zhi, and Xin Yi (pounded). For Ma Huang start out in small doses gradually adding up to 5~6 qian (or even more if the patient's sleep isn't affected);

for Xi Xin start out in small doses gradually adding up to 3 qian; and for the remaining medicinals you can prescribe doses of up to 8 qian. Once the middle ear effusion has gradually been resorbed you can begin adding Gan Jiang, Fu Zi, and Yu Gui. If after adding these yang-supplementing medicinals hematopoiesis is still insufficient, then you should change the prescription to either Shi Quan Da Bu Tang or You Gui Yin adding Ma Huang, Bai Zhi, Xin Yi, and Xi Xin.

For acupuncture you can needle the "trigeminal nerve special points" corresponding with the pathways of the trigeminal nerves (CNV) and facial nerves (CNVII) (starting at point about 1 cun out from Ting Gong (SI19) below the zygomatic arch transversely insert 3 needles joining Si Zhu Kong (SJ23), Quan Liao (SI18), and Jia Che (ST6) respectively), Feng Chi (GB20), Feng Fu (DU16), He Gu (LI4), Zu San Li (ST36), Bai Hui (DU20), Da Zhui (DU14); or needle Ying Xiang (LI20) joining Qing Ming (UB1), San Yin Jiao (SP6), Yin Ling Quan (SP9), and Xue Hai (SP10). Of course, you could choose Fei Shu (UB13), Ya Men (DU15), and Jing Chuan Dian (aka Bai Lao (EX-HN15)) as well, but due to their anatomical location be very careful when needling these points, only inserting at shallow depths. Warm needling (and also electroacunpuncture, though I don't use this method myself) generally offers better results compared to needling without moxa.

Case Study #2: Lung Cancer – Can TCM Provide Effective Treatment?

Q: Recently, a 59 y/o male with lung cancer visited my clinic accompanied by his wife. Two years ago he was diagnosed with Stage III lung cancer and over the past three months he has experienced shortness of breath, persistent cough, dysphagia, often feels heat sensation, and has lost weight. While conducting the patient interview, I found out that he has a brother with lung cancer who went through 8 years of Western medical treatment with what he described as a very unpleasant process and not very effective results. His brother's experience made him want to give TCM a try. Please advise me on the best approach for treating lung cancer.

A: For lung cancer patients already presenting with neoplastic fever, I recommend prescribing Chai Ling Tang adding Qing Hao, Zhi Mu, Di Gu Pi, Ren Shen (powder), Chuan Qi (powder), Fu Ling and Ze Xie (large doses each), Ting Li Zi, Ma Huang, Xing Ren, Fang Ji, Xian Zha and Ji Nei Jin (to aid digestion), and Yu Sheng Wan. This prescription should effectively provide relief for these symptoms. Once symptoms have been relieved, then subtract Qing Hao, Zhi Mu, and Di Gu Pi. If the above symptoms return once again, then consider adding combinations of the following medicinals: Gan Jiang, Fu Zi, and Yu Gui; Zi Yuan, Kuan Dong Hua, and Wu Wei Zi; or Xu Duan, Gu Sui Bu, Qian Cao, and Huai Niu Xi. The guiding principle is to apply pattern identification as the basis for determining treatment and adjusting your formula accordingly based on the presenting signs and symptoms.

Case Study #3: Lung Cancer – TCM Treatment and Medicinal Foods

Q: I have a 60 y/o male patient with advanced lung cancer who drinks three bottles of soju (Korean rice wine) and smokes three packs of cigarettes every day. Recently, he had been feeling tired and lacked energy so he decided to stop smoking cigarettes. Two days after he quit smoking, he started coughing so he went to a Western medical doctor who prescribed some medicine for the cough. One week later, he began coughing blood (hemoptysis). He went to get it checked out at a hospital and discovered widespread proliferation of cancer cells in his lungs. The patient did not want to take TCM medicinals because "it tastes bad," but he did want to try eating medicinal foods. What kind of food is good for patients with lung cancer?

A: Unfortunately, at this stage medicinal foods are going to be enough to prevent lung cancer from proliferating and spreading. Medicinal foods, though beneficial, are not the most important part of the treatment regimen. Right now, it is critical that you have a serious discussion with him and his family, clearly explaining the need to take TCM medicinals and potentially be open to Western medical intervention – that is if he "really values life." If the patient incessantly shuns your compassionate attempts of concern, then you could resort to a more prodding approach by saying something like this: "Can't eat this, don't want to take that...if you are no longer living then we won't even need to have this conversation."

TCM medicinals is an essential part of the treatment regimen for lung cancer patients, either administered as a first-line therapy or accompanying Western medicine intervention. I recommend prescribing either Chai Ling Tang or Tong Jing Fang variants. For patients presenting with qi vacuity, you can continue prescribing Chai Ling Tang adding Ren Shen (powder), Chuan Qi (powder), Huang Qi, Gan Jiang, Fu Zi, and Yu Gui; or change the formula to Bu Zhong Yi Qi Tang variant. These are formulas with proven efficacy. I have used this approach to treat innumerable lung cancer patients over the years and all have shown improvement in their conditions with some going into sustained remission. Sometimes the institution of modern Western (orthodox or biomedicine) medicine simply gives up and isn't willing to treat these types of patients, not even with radiotherapy or chemotherapy. Time and again, I have successfully administered Chai Ling Tang variant to improve their condition and remedy troubling symptoms, thus dramatically prolonging and increasing their quality of life. One 80 y/o patient was told by doctors that he wouldn't make it 3 more months, but he began taking TCM medicinals and it's already been over 1 1/2 years now and the patient is still going strong and feels healthy!

If the patient insists on just eating medicinal foods and not taking TCM medicinals, then you can advise him to stew some of the "ingredients" (aka TCM medicinals) prescribed in the formulas above adding his choice of fish or meat. This is the best kind of medicinal food. It will help his body maintain the physical strength and stamina to overcome the trials and travails of this chronic condition.

Case Study #4: Advanced Metastatic Cancer and Malignant Pleural Effusion (PE)

Q: I have a 34 y/o male patient with advanced lung cancer. Just 6 months after getting married, he discovered that he had non-small cell lung cancer (NSCLC) with pleural invasion. What I don't understand is that despite currently undergoing chemotherapy (the anticancer agents Gemzar and Cisplatin) there have not been any adverse effects arising, not even dry cough. Please share your advice and guidance on this condition.

A: Typically, lung cancer isn't discovered until the later stages of disease. Prior to clinical diagnosis the majority of these patients have healthy appetites and lead normal, active lives. But after diagnosis...bam!...everything changes. This is in fact one of the major topics of debate going on in "medical ethics": Lung cancer is "discovered" (diagnosed) during a random physical examination (e.g., annual employee health checkup) and metastases has occurred, but the patient has a healthy appetite and no symptoms nor any discomfort whatsoever – Should the patient be "informed" about his or her illness, and should "treatment" be obligatory? Nowadays, Western medical physicians in many advanced nations are advocating that the best approach is to "monitor" the patient's condition taking a "wait and see" approach, instead of telling the patient about the diagnosis. I agree with this approach, because being diagnosed with cancer more often than not leads to a traumatic psychological impact with many losing confidence and the will to survive.

The main formula I prescribe for metastatic lung cancer is still Chai Ling Tang variant, making the appropriate modifications based on the degree and extent of hematopoietic, hepatic, and renal function impairment that has been caused by chemotherapy. Once the patient has weathered the storm of chemotherapy's adverse effects, then you can change back to the original formula variant consisting of either Chai Ling Tang, Shen Ling Bai Zhu San, Xiang Sha Liu Jun Zi Tang, Wu Wei Yi Gong San, or Si Shen Tang variants adjusting the formula based on pattern identification and presenting signs and symptoms.

Section 4: Gastric (Stomach) Cancer

There are four main types of gastric (stomach) cancer – adenocarcinoma (90%), lymphoma, stromal, and carcinoid. Gastric cancer has a relatively high incidence rate in East Asia, and this section will introduces those cases that "student" (Dr. Yang) has sought advice and direction from his "mentor" (Dr. Lee). Additionally, cases involving the diagnosis and treatment of regional and distant metastases are also presented.

Case Study #1: Gastric Cancer Treatment – Xiang Sha Liu Jun Zi Tang

Q: A 34 y/o male patient visited his doctor 3 months ago due to poor appetite and further examination with gastroscopy revealed gastric cancer. The hospital advised him to immediately undergo laparoscopic exploratory surgery, which revealed widespread proliferation of neoplastic cells (end-stage). Thus, they decided it would be best to go ahead and resect as much of the tumor as possible and administer adjuvant chemotherapy and radiotherapy to prevent the continued proliferation of the cancer cells. However, this approach would inherently have its limitations. Eventually, the patient developed pyloric stenosis and ascites along the left hypochondrium, but his doctors said it was a mild case. The patient also had constipation, loss of appetite, weight loss, acid regurgitation, and belching. This is when he sought my consultation and treatment. Since there was nothing abnormal about his CBC and other lab test results, I prescribed Xiang Sha Liu Jun Zi Tang. Do you think this is the correct approach for this case?

A: Yes, that is a good formula, but it would be best to also add Gan Jiang, Fu Zi, Da Huang, Lai Fu Zi, Ze Xie, Ren Shen (powder), Chuan Qi (powder), Yi Ren, and Wan Ling Dan. For Da Huang, you should gradually add incremental doses (up to as much as 7~8 qian) until the patient is able to pass 2~3 stools/day. If the patient still cannot pass stool, then you can try adding larger amounts of Gan Jiang, Fu Zi, and Yu Gui; and if the patient still cannot pass stool, then add Pu Xiao to soften hardness, or even consider changing the formula to Tong Jing Fang adding combinations of the above medicinals.

Case Study #2: Gastric Cancer – A Difficult Condition to Treat

Q: A 37 y/o male patient whom was recently married just two months ago explained that he used to have bad eating habits (usually only taking 1 or 2 meals a day and drinking alcohol almost every evening) along with gastrointestinal discomfort for many years. After getting married, his wife convinced him to get a check up at the hospital where he could have an endoscopy performed. The endoscopic image showed that he had a grain size lump growing in the submucosa of his stomach, and the biopsy confirmed it to be malignant. Not long after, he underwent a follow-up examination revealing that the cancer cells had spread rapidly and extensively throughout to the lymph nodes and distant areas of the body. His physicians deemed his condition so dire that they informed him he may only have about 6 months to live. In his disappointment and despair, he decided to try novel "natural healing" methods and immunotherapy (biologic therapy), which are very popular in Japan. But his condition didn't improve and he lost even more weight. That's when he decided to try TCM treatment instead and came to see me. This is the most serious case of gastric cancer I have attempted to treat, and if I understand correctly, gastric cancer with submucosal invasion is very difficult to treat! Once it has been discovered it typically has already proliferated to the advanced stages. Please provide me with your invaluable insight. Is there any chance of improving this patient's condition, or at least relieving his symptoms?

A: Gastric cancer is so difficult to treat because of the broad scope of symptoms and complex patterns types. According to TCM theory, gastric tumors can be classified into 4 main patterns: 1) Yang Ming exterior with stomach heat pattern; 2) stasis heat, static blood, and stasis obstruction pattern; 3) spleen qi and yang vacuity pattern; and 4) spleen qi and yang vacuity with cold stasis pattern. Remember! This is just a generalization for the purpose of categorization and simplification, but in actual clinical practice these stages and patterns blend together into complex and overlapping patterns.

1) The early stage of gastric cancer can be identified as Yang Ming exterior with stomach heat pattern, requiring the administration of formula variants such as Ge Gen Qin Lian Tang or Xian Fang Huo Ming Yin. For instance, if endoscopic examination reveals a tumor growing on the surface of the stomach lining (aka stromal tumor) with a bright, fleshy color of cinnabar (vermilion), then this can be identified as Yang Ming exterior with stomach heat pattern heat, requiring the administration a formula such as Ge Gen Qin Lian Tang adding Pu Gong Ying, Lian Zhao, Jin Yin Hua, Da Huang Wan Ling Dan, and Yu Sheng Wan.

2) The stomach is continually exposed to the external environment via solid foods and liquids, bringing legions of bacteria and viruses (evil qi) along for the ride. Continual bombardment by this "evil qi" may induce stasis heat, static blood, and stasis obstruction pattern. For this pattern you can prescribe either Tong Jing Fang, Ru Mo Si Wu Tang, or Xuan Fu Dai Zhe Shi Tang adding combinations of medicinals such as Huang Qin, Chuan Qi (powder), Pu Huang (if heat presents), Shan Dou Gen, Liang Jiang, San Leng, E Zhu, Yan Hu Suo, San Nai, Yu Jin, Yu Sheng Wan, and Wan Ling Dan.

3) This stasis heat, static blood, and stasis obstruction taxes the stomach and spleen's functional capacity leading to spleen qi and yang yang vacuity pattern. For these patients you should prescribe formula variants such as Xiang Sha Liu Jun Zi Tang, Bu Zhong Yi Qi Tang, Shen Ling Bai Zhu Tang, or Dang Gui Shao Yao San adding combinations of medicinals such as Shan Dou Gen, Liang Jiang, Chuan Qi (powder), Ru Xiang, Mo Yao, and Gu Sui Bu.

4) In the later stages of this pathocondition, spleen qi and yang vacuity may evolve into spleen qi and yang vacuity with cold stasis pattern, requiring the administration of a formula such as Xiang Sha Liu Jun Zi Tang combining Shen Ling Bai Zhu Tang adding adding Liang Jiang, Fu Zi, and Yu Gui.

If you are treating a gastric tumor in its early stages when the true heat pattern still predominates and there has been no Western medicine intervention, then you should prescribe Xian Fang Huo Ming Yin variant. Nowadays, in my clinical practice more and more patients are presenting with static blood and stasis obstruction pattern types.

Case Study #3: Adenocarcinoma

Q: The spouse of an acquaintance of mine, Professor Cui, visited me a couple of days ago explaining that she had just gotten back results from a physical examination at the university affiliated hospital revealing a gastric tumor. A biopsy confirmed it as gastric carcinoma, and though the tumor is very small, doctors recommended that she undergo surgical resection. What's the best TCM formula I can prescribe for treating this condition?

A: Based on TCM pattern identification, adenocarcinoma can be identified as stomach heat with Yang Ming exterior pattern in the early stages of disease. You can consider prescribing Ge Gen Qin Lian Tang adding Ban Xia, Shan Dou Gen, Gao Liang Jiang, Hai Piao Xiao, Zhe Bei Mu, Chuan Qi (powder), Yu Sheng Wan, and Wan Ling Dan.

Case Study #4: Postoperative Vomiting – How Can I Administer TCM Formula Decoction?

Q: A 49 y/o female patient experienced discomfort in the stomach and went for an examination. Her doctors diagnosed her with early stage gastric cancer (not even at T0), but they advised her to undergo total gastrectomy to "cure her once and for all." About 3 hours after surgery, the patient vomited continuously for 10 minutes, and these vomiting attacks continued occurring at about the same interval (every 3 hours) and duration (lasted for 10 minutes). Administration of Western medicine drugs was ineffective and her doctors didn't know what to do, telling her, "We've never seen this type of complication before." This is when the patient's family came to see me hoping I could prescribe TCM medicinals to remedy the patient's condition. Initially, I prescribed Ban Xia and Fu Ling 1 liang each, but it wasn't effective either. What do you think about adding Ding Xiang, Shi Di, Dai Zhe Shi, and Yu Sheng Wan?

A: Vomiting 3 hours after eating is usually caused by either duodenal stenosis or obstruction. Since the patient is able to pass stool, we know that food is being digested, which thus suggests either duodenal stenosis or partial obstruction. It can't be complete obstruction, because the patient wouldn't be able to absorb nutrients and defecate, and possibly would have passed away by now.

Generally, when total gastrectomy is performed the patient would "not" be allowed to eat or drink right away. So if vomiting presents at regular intervals (e.g., vomiting every 3 hours), I suspect the condition is psychosomatic. With this in mind, I would try prescribing Gan Mai Da Zao

Tang combining Ban Xia Hou Po Tang adding Yu Sheng Wan (3 pills/day; taking 1 pill after every meal or eating the pill with meals). You can instruct the patient to casually sip or drink this decoction like a beverage throughout the course of the day. This prescription will serve the dual function of remedying the physical symptoms and calming the spirit on the psychological level.

Case Study #5: Gastric Tumor Resection – What TCM Formula Should I Prescribe?

Q: A 31 y/o male patient was diagnosed with advanced stage gastric cancer and has already undergone surgical resection and received chemotherapy. Now, the tumor is virtually imperceptible. What TCM medicinals should I prescribe for this patient? He is happily married with a 2-month old newborn and really has a strong will to survive. What formula should I prescribe to boost appetite and promote digestion? Or should I just wait until symptoms present and prescribe medicinals accordingly based on pattern identification?

A: Regardless of the device (e.g., endoscopy, laparoscopy) used for examination, type of surgery (e.g., endoscopic resection, subtotal or total gastrectomy), or if imaging scans reveal the presence of a tumor or not, all gastric cancer patients should be administered TCM medicinals as soon as possible following surgery. The main purpose is to regulate the function of the stomach and a wide selection of formulas can achieve this goal such as Xiang Sha Liu Jun Zi Tang, Si Jun Zi Tang, Si Shen Tang, Yue Ju Wan, and Bao He Wan variants. You should also add selected combinations of the following medicinals based on presenting symptoms and pattern identification: Yi Ren, Gao Liang Jiang, and Shan Dou Gen; Yuan Hu, Mu Xiang, San Leng, E Zhu, and Chuan Qi (powder); Gu Ya, Mai Ya, Nei Jin, and Xian Zha (these food-dispersing and stomach qi-supplementing medicinals are very important!); "the Three Yellows" and Mu Dan Pi; and Bei Mu (Tu Bei Mu or Zhe Bei Mu) and Hai Piao Xiao. Remember! Yu Sheng Wan and Wan Ling Dan are essential medicinals for the treatment of cancer and should be included as a part of your therapeutic regimen regardless of which formula you choose to prescribe. As a part of a formula composition, these spleen and stomach qi-supplementing, blood quickening and stasis transforming, heat-abating and toxin resolving, and acid-controlling medicinals offer exceptional anticancer efficacy.

For gastric cancer patients 75 y/o and above Western medicine standard protocol does not advocate surgery, and in many cases doctors are not willing to aggressively treat the condition. In these situations you can prescribe Shen Ling Bai Zhu San variant, which will help remedy symptoms. If heat presents, you can add "the Three Yellows" and Mu Dan Pi; and if anemia presents, then add yang-supplementing medicinals. Remember! You must understand that Cu Lu Rong offers greater efficacy for treating tumors and Xi Lu Rong offers greater efficacy for promoting hematopoiesis. Thus, for de novo neoplasms and in younger patients, unless there is severe malnutrition or if chemotherapy and radiotherapy has induced hematopoietic dysfunction, then Cu Lu Rong should be administered and "not" Xi Lu Rong. If Xi Lu Rong is administered, it could lead to the acceleration of tumerogenesis, and we obviously don't want that.

Case Study #6: Cerebral Infarction Patient Diagnosed With Gastric Cancer

Q: A 63 y/o male patient explained that one day 4 years ago he suddenly began salivating profusely and continuously. Upon examination an MRI revealed signs of a cerebral infarct in the upper left hemisphere, but he did not aggressively treat this condition and simply began taking antihypertensive medication. About 2 years ago, he was diagnosed with gastric cancer, underwent a complete gastrectomy, and has suffered from dysphagia since the procedure; meanwhile, complications caused by the cerebral infarct have worsened. During his last visit he presented with dysphagia, weakness in his right leg, and normal stool and urine. Do you think it is a good idea to prescribe Bu Yang Huan Wu Tang combining Huang Lian Jie Du Tang?

A: Cerebral infarction patients commonly incur progressive cerebral atrophy. Once degeneration begins there is an even greater possibility for another infarct and hemorrhage causing more complications for the patient. Since the patient has already had a total gastrectomy to remove the gastric tumor, you can go ahead and prescribe Bu Yang Huan Wu Tang combining Huang Lian Jie Du Tang, but also add Gao Liang Jiang, Sha Ren, Shan Dou Gen, Ban Xia, San Leng, E Zhu, Ren Shen (powder), Chuan Qi (powder), Yu Sheng Wan, and Wan Ling Dan for better results.

Case Study #7: Gastric Cancer – Multiple Metastases

Q: Recently, I have been treating a 59 y/o male patient with gastric cancer. About 3 years ago he was diagnosed with gastric cancer and in October of that year he underwent gastrectomy and colectomy (patient previously underwent several less-invasive surgeries). In February of the following year, metastatic spread to the lymph nodes below the pancreas was discovered with resection immediately performed and 10 sessions of chemotherapy administered. Three months later (mid May), inguinal lymph nodes on both sides were resected; and in August, malignancies were resected in the abdomen and left lung. In January of the following year (third year), abdominal lymph node metastases had occurred but with subsequent shrinkage in size, while the left lung tumor had gradually enlarged. Now, I am treating him with Chai Ling Tang adding Gan Jiang, Fu Zi, and Yu Gui (1 qian each) to control WBC levels; and also Bai Zhu, Fu Ling, Ze Xie, Huang Qin (8 qian each), and Wan Ling Dan (4 pills/3x/day). Do you think this is a good approach? Should I advise him to discontinue chemotherapy?

A: Yes, this formula should be effective. The patient must be a very strong-willed person to continue pushing on in the face of adversity. He will have even better results under your care receiving integrated TCM and Western medical treatment. The only thing I would suggest is to consider adding larger doses of Wan Ling Dan, along with Ma Huang, Ting Li Zi, Fang Ji, and Bai Bu to help relieve the complications arising from the lung and lymph node tumors. You can also consider adding Ren Shen (powder) and Chuan Qi (powder). As for chemotherapy, if the cancer has already reached the advanced stage, the most important aspect is for the patient to maintain a relatively high quality of life and enjoy themselves as much as possible during this final period. Though ultimately it is the patient's decision (in consultation with his oncologist), in my opinion it may be the best choice to forego chemotherapy.

Case Study #8: Gastric Cancer – Post-Operative Regional and Distant Lymph Node Metastases

Q: A 51 y/o male patient was diagnosed with gastric cancer in 1993 and underwent a complete gastrectomy. In 2006, he went to have a swelling on his right arm examined revealing relapse of cancer. His doctors suspected regional and distant lymph node metastases from gastric cancer and the patient received chemotherapy, which was not very effective and dramatically weakened the patient's physical condition. Now, the patient presents as follows: lymphoma in the right arm and both legs, mild ascites, and normal CBC. What formula do you think would be most effective?

A: Patients are consistently seeking your consultation and treatment for relapse of gastric cancer and lymph node metastases. This proves that you have gained some notoriety and the trust of South Korean patients. Keep up the good work! For this condition you can prescribe Chai Ling Tang adding Qing Hao, Zhi Mu, Di Gu Pi, Shan Dou Gen, Gao Liang Jiang; Huang Qin and Huang Lian (large doses); Chuan Qi (powder), Yu Sheng Wan, and Wan Ling Dan; Ma Huang and Xing Ren (small doses); and also Cang Zhu, Fu Ling, Ze Xie, Ting Li Zi, and Fang Ji for ascites, pleural effusion, and lung metastases.

Just remember! Most adenocarcinomas (and lymphomas) can be identified as Shao Yang pattern. If the above formula doesn't effectively reduce ascites, then you can add Ren Shen (powder). If the blood tests show normal levels of HB, PLT, LDH, and CPK with only CA72-4, CEA, and CA19-9 elevated, then you should continue monitoring the condition; and if necessary, add larger doses of Huang Qin, Huang Lian, and Wan Ling Dan. If the tumor markers are normal, but T-PRO and ALB are low, then add Yi Ren, Shan Yao, Qian Shi, and Bai Guo; Gan Jiang and Fu Zi (small doses); or consider adding Sha Ren and Cao Dou Kou (Rou Dou Kou or Hong Dou Kou).

Case Study #9: Do Tumor Markers Correlate With Pulmonary Tuberculosis?

Q: I have a gastric cancer patient (female) with regional metastatic spread to the lymph nodes in the abdomen. The patient had undergone treatment for 2 years at a major hospital receiving several regimens of chemotherapy prior to seeking my consultation. To regulate and strengthen her physical constitution, I started out by prescribing Chun Ze Tang adding Bai Zhu, Fu Ling, Ze Xie, Huang Bo, Chi Shao, Mu Dan Pi, Chuan Qi (powder) (large dose), and Wan Ling Dan (large dose). I also advised her to temporarily discontinue taking Western medicine drugs. Western medical doctors were still prescribing the anticancer agent fluoroucil (5-FU) via rapid injection and slow infusion, and after completion of the second cycle, the secondary cancer in the lymph nodes virtually disappeared. However, a follow-up examination revealed a 1 cm opacity in the right lung with an elevated CA19-9 (100), and there was concern the patient may have pulmonary tuberculosis as well. Thus, doctors decided to go ahead with 2 doses of chemotherapy, which resulted in a mild reduction of the opacity size and CA19-9 dropped to 50. Do tumor markers correlate with pulmonary tuberculosis? What are the best TCM medicinals to treat this condition?

A: High CA19-9 tumor marker levels may have correlations with gastrointestinal cancers and hence lymph node malignancies, but not with pulmonary tuberculosis. I have a liver cancer patient who had percutaneous ethanol injection (PEI) performed 3 times. Follow-up examinations showed CA19-9 tumor marker levels at 69, confirming the presence of metastatic spread to the lymph nodes with a high degree of probability. The administration of 5-FU to treat lymph node malignancy may be effective in reducing the size of the tumor or even making it disappear; however, if TCM medicinals aren't a part of the treatment regimen, then the anticancer agent 5-FU will inhibit hematopoiesis resulting in low PLT count, prolonged PT, and activated APTT that likely will lead to cancer progression and accelerated mortality.

If it is determined that the increase in tumor marker levels reflects the tumor growth, proliferation, or further spread to the lymph nodes (identified as Shao Yang heat pattern) and the diagnosis of pulmonary tuberculosis is confirmed (identified as steaming bone taxation heat pattern), then you can simply prescribe either Xiao Chai Hu Tang, Di Gu Pi Yin, or (Yu Sheng) Hyperactive Immune Formula variants adding Yuan Shen, Sha Shen, Bai He, Bai Bu, Tian Men Dong, and Mai Men Dong.

Case Study #10: Gastric Cancer – Colonic and Brain Metastases

Q: A 34 y/o male patient with gastric cancer and metastatic spread to the brain suffered from dysphagia and underwent exploratory laparoscopy, discovering a 3 cm tumor in his stomach and the presence of regional lymph node metastases. Following surgery, he received a regimen of Leucovorin, Oxaliplatin, and 5-FU, and after 1 cycle the tumor shrunk from 3 cm to 2 cm while the lymph node metastases remained the same. The patient then decided to discontinue chemotherapy and took Jie Geng extract instead. Two months later, an emergency surgery was performed on an acute intestinal obstruction and then another regimen of chemotherapy was administered (5-FU and Cisplatin) with dissatisfactory results. Now, he has 1 bowel movement every 1~2 days with variable consistency (sometimes loose), and his blood tests are normal. What formula would you use to treat this condition?

A: In gastric cancer patients with metastatic spread to the small intestine causing obstruction you can consider prescribing Xiang Sha Liu Jun Zi

Tang adding Yi Ren, Liang Jiang, Shan Dou Gen, Huang Qin, Huang Lian, Tian Ma, Ze Xie, Fu Ling, Da Huang (wine-steeped) (gradually increasing dose until the patient passes stool 2~3x/day), Chuan Qi (powder), Yu Sheng Wan, and Wan Ling Dan. This formula will improve the patient's condition over time.

Case Study #11: Advanced Stage Gastric Cancer – Peritoneal and Adrenal Metastases

Q: A 35 y/o male advanced stage gastric cancer patient had a stent inserted to relieve intestinal obstruction and not long after suffered from nephritis and scrotal edema (both gonads). Recently, examination revealed metastatic spread to the stomach, peritoneum, and adrenal gland (right), along with severe ascites (daily drainage of 2.1 liters). He still has difficulty passing stool (1 stool every 2~3 days). I prescribed Ban Xia, Mang Xiao, Fu Ling, and Shi Gao, but his condition did not improve (still unable to pass stool daily). Western medical doctors informed his family "to be prepared," but the patient is strong-willed and won't give up hope. What's the best way going forward?

A: Caring for an advanced stage cancer patient is most certainly a difficult endeavor. That's why so many hospitals admit these patients into hospice care units. The purpose is to allow the conditions of terminally ill patients to decline gradually with as little pain as possible until they peacefully pass away. This approach is essentially described in the following excerpt of a TCM classical text: "Disperse accumulations and gatherings as much as possible (70~80%) and rely on food and drink for the rest." However, there is still a rift right now between TCM and Western medicine about what type of diet is best for advanced cancer patients.

Many hospitals in Taiwan and South Korea serve a Western (European/U.S.) style diet (the entire meal including the relatively large portions) without any consideration of the patient's body type, weight, and customary dietary habits. There is a lot of food on the plate that the patient doesn't have a palate for and thus doesn't eat, leading to a lack of nutrients and poor physical condition. For example, most South Koreans have eaten kimchi all their lives and have grown so accustomed to the chili peppers that their bodies actually become physically reliant on the capsicum to function properly. Once the patient is diagnosed with cancer, the doctors and dieticians may claim that eating spicy foods had something to do with it and specifically advise advanced stage cancer patients "not" to eat chili peppers. Instead, the amount of animal proteins and dairy products (e.g., milk, cheese) are increased. They don't realize that chili peppers are vital for stimulating these patients gastrointestinal system. Of course they don't have an appetite! If the appetite control center in the brain is not stimulated, digestive secretions are not produced. This leads to a "poor appetite" and also compromised gastrointestinal immune function, and is the main reason advanced stage cancer patients lack physical strength and energy. Just like Taiwanese (people throughout East and southeast Asia as well) have the habit of eating steamed rice, taro, and steamed buns, and all of a sudden you want them to change their diet to leavened bread. Naturally, it wouldn't feel right so they don't want to eat.

TCM emphasizes the concept of "local foods" with the "local" having the connotation of most "suitable." This means meal schedules and the kinds of food should be based on local eating customs in order to maintain the healthiest diet. This includes those popular overseas dietary supplements (especially those claiming to have medicinal effects) sold on the local market. The individual's digestive system (e.g., microbiome) has already grown accustomed to a specific style of diet and the GI tract must have these types of foods in order to effectively absorb nutrients and receive sustenance that will boost the immune system's natural disease fighting mechanisms.

TCM emphasizes the patient's physical constitution and severity of the pathocondition (degree of imbalance or deviation from homeostasis). Prescribing "mild medicinals to treat serious conditions" offers no beneficial value, while prescribing "potent medicinals to treat mild conditions" may inadvertently harm the constitution (further compromising homeostasis) and lead to the manifestation of other diseases. This premise is evident in the TCM materia medica classic *In The Essential Herb Foundation*, where under the template for Chuan Qiong this quote from the *The Yellow Emperor's Inner Cannon* cautions: "frequently taking large doses and for long durations [of Chuan Qiong] will cause overabundance of one organ, leading to sudden collapse and death."

The approach Western medical hospitals commonly take to treat disease typically transpires like this: The patient feels ill or has discomfort, then goes to the hospital where the patient is most likely immediately administered high-dose infusions or intravenous injections (IV), resulting in edema for those patients with poor metabolic function. Once malignancy is confirmed in patients with tumors, they will inevitably be advised to "first have surgery to resect the lesion, then follow-up with adjuvant radiotherapy and/or chemotherapy" or possibly use "targeted drugs and therapies" in attempts to eradicate all of the cancer cells. This is tantamount to "clearing the fields and leaving nothing behind" and "killing off the bad along with the good" since chemotherapy eradicates both cancer cells and healthy cells in the process. During treatment patients mainly eat a diet recommended by a dietician. Though this diet "technically" meets the nutritional needs of the patient, patients often find these foods unappealing, lose their appetites, and just don't eat enough. After the completion of several chemotherapy cycles, this vicious cycle spirals out of control with patients continuing to lose more and more weight; and in the end, they just get "burnt out" and die.

TCM advocates the approach: "Disperse accumulations and gatherings as much as possible (70~80%) and rely on food and drink for the rest." For advanced stage cancer patients whose physical conditions are already extremely compromised and weak, you should start out prescribing small doses of relatively mild TCM medicinals and then assess the patient's condition to determine if incrementally larger doses of more potent medicinals should be prescribed. Remember! Trying to expedite the process with large doses is fundamentally contraindicated. For treating accumulations, gatherings, concretions, and conglomerations (nomenclature that includes both benign and malignant tumors) you only need to eliminate about 70~80% of the cancer cells and tumor mass; it isn't necessary to achieve complete clearance (in fact, technically, it is impossible to completely eliminate all of the cancer cells!). The rest of the treatment involves maintaining a healthy diet, which will open the stomach and spleen so that the remaining pathogenic qi can be eliminated, allowing the patient to "live a long life in harmony with the condition."

Thus, it's a good idea to prescribe advanced stage cancer patients small doses of Gu Ya, Mai Ya, and Ji Nei Jin along with Shan Yao and Ou Jie (powder) to open the stomach and spleen (promote appetite). If the patient has a craving for their favorite foods, it would fine to go ahead and eat small amounts; and even if they wanted to drink a few classes of Jinro soju that's ok too! Advanced stage gastric cancer patients lead exceedingly bland lives "dried up like dead wood." In this stage of their condition, there is no decisive evidence that a healthy diet will have anything but a marginal effect at best, so let the patient eat the foods they like and feel a sense of joy and satisfaction. It may not be very long until they pass away, and they won't have any regrets about it. In fact, these savory foods just might increase their appetites, like "dried up twigs and wilted leaves" on a tree receiving nourishment and moisture to once again flourish and become vibrant. Taking TCM medicinals will only be effective if the patient has a good appetite, moderate physical strength, and adequate hematopoietic function. This is a quintessential principle you must always remember as you treat patients.

Before, you told me of a patient you prescribed large doses of Huang Lian Jie Du Tang for the treatment of chronic active hepatitis, which conversely led to an increase in AST (GOT) and ALT (GPT). At that time, I thought you should have prescribed Zhi Zi Bo Pi Tang (pulverized powder) instead (with each medicinal at 2~3 qian) adding Xian Zha, Mai Ya, and Ji Nei Jin. This is an example of the principle I just mentioned above.

Remember! For patients with chronic illness, serious disease, or advanced stage cancer, you must prescribe small doses of TCM medicinals, otherwise you may "outsmart yourself" making matters worse instead of better. Just remember the principle: "Disperse accumulations and gatherings as much as possible (70~80%) and rely on food and drink for the rest." You must first "moisten" and "nourish" the intestines and stomach and then prescribe TCM medicinals to treat the condition. This is the most effective approach.

Section 5: Colorectal Cancer

Colorectal cancer is among the most common types of cancer in Taiwan (ROC) and South Korea with postsurgical metastases frequently occurring. This section is devoted to these cases.

Case Study #1: Granulomatous Polyp Following Surgical Resection

Q1: A 64 y/o male colorectal cancer patient visited me with a history of undergoing 3 partial colectomies and 1 right-sided nephrectomy during the past ten years, and now a recent periodic examination revealed the presence of a granulomatous polyp. The patient's physician told him that since he had already undergone colectomy there wasn't much left to remove so the best option was to perform endoscopic laser therapy. Feeling disappointed and frustrated, the patient sought my consultation for TCM treatment. I prescribed Ru Mo Si Wu Tang variant. Please offer your guidance on this case.

A1: Colorectal cancer patients with metastatic spread to the kidneys and recurring polyps and granulomas following surgical resection can be identified as damp heat and stasis heat pattern. Prescribing Ru Mo Si Wu Tang variant should be effective or you could also consider Tong Jing Fang variant as well. However, make sure to add Huang Qin, Huang Lian, Huai Hua, Di Yu, Bai Zhi, Chuan Qi (powder), and Wan Ling Dan to your formula. If the patient is physically weak, then consider prescribing Bu Zhong Yi Qi Tang adding the aforementioned medicinals (equivalent to Ti Gang San variant).

After taking the above formula for 1~2 months, the patient should have another endoscopy and CT scan performed to determine if the granulomatous polyp has disappeared. Even if the polyp has disappeared, the patient should still continue taking TCM medicinals for 2~3 more months.

Q2: The colorectal cancer patient said he had another endoscopy performed about 3 weeks after starting TCM treatment confirming the granulomatous polyp had indeed disappeared. Thank you so much for your guidance. Could you please further elaboborate on your approach to treating colorectal cancer?

A2: The physical constitutions of Asian's make it less likely for colorectal polyps to manifest into cancer. So the presence of granulomatous polyps on inspection shouldn't cause too much alarm and there is no rush to immediatley peform biopsy or undergo surgical resection. In some patients these polyps are simply the swelling and distention arising from stasis, depression, dampness, or heat in the large intestine channel; and their condition will improve after taking TCM medicinals. If the polyp does turn out to be colorectal cancer, then at the onset you should prescribe Xian Fang Huo Ming Yin adding Huai Hua, Di Yu, Da Huang, Chuan Qi (powder), and Wan Ling Dan. Doses of Da Huang should be incrementally increased until the patient maintains 3 or more bowel movements per day. Even if the patient presents with loose stools, slightly bloody stool, or even anorectal mucosal prolapse and lymphocytic-rich exudates, there is still no need to be too worried. Simply change the formula to Xue Ku Fang adding yin-supplementing medicinals such as Bai Zhi (channel-conducting medicinal), Fang Feng (intestinal wind bleeding) Tian Men Dong, Mai Men Dong, Dang Shen, Huang Qin, Huai Hua, Chuan Qi (powder), Ren Shen (powder), and Wan Ling Dan.

Case Study #2: Recurrence After 7 Years of Remission

Q: A 63 y/o female was diagnosed with colorectal cancer 7 years ago and received radiotherapy and chemotherapy, but surgical resection was not performed. Recently, there was recurrence and the patient followed the advice of her doctor receiving targeted therapy with EGFR inhibitor. During follow-up examination elevated CEA was discovered, but she didn't present with any other noticeable signs or symptoms. What should I make of this?

A: As long as hematopoietic function is not compromised then it's all right. This condition is identified as blood heat and blood-aspect stasis heat pattern. So you should prescribe formulas that contain heat-abating with cold and bitter, blood-activating and stasis-transforming, and blood-cooling medicinals, and also add Huang Qin, Chuan Qi (powder), Cang Zhu, Fu Ling, Ze Xie, Bai Zhi, Fang Feng, and Wan Ling Dan. Remember! Huang Qin enters the large intestine channel so make sure to include this medicinal.

Case Study #3: Colorectal Cancer – Liver and Abdominal Cavity Metastases

Q1: This case is similar to another patient of mine [Case Study #2]. A female patient was diagnosed with colorectal cancer 7 years ago and received radiotherapy, chemotherapy, and targeted therapy with EGFR inhibitor. Recently, she had felt distension and discomfort in her right flank with occasional dull pain, occasional sharp pain in the left lower abdomen, and pain in the left inguinal region upon walking. I prescribed Ru Mo Si Wu Tang adding Huang Qin and Huang Lian (8 qian each), Fu Ling and Ze Xie (5 qian each), Yu Sheng Wan, and Wan Ling Dan. After taking this formula for 1 1/2 months (though not fully in compliance with the prescribed dosage), one day she suddenly incurred a small amount of anal bleeding (only 1 time). She immediately went to the hospital for examination, which revealed CEA over 100 and a PET-CT scan confirmed the presence of metastatic spread to the liver and abdominal cavity. However, the 2 tumors in the abominal cavity 5 cm and 3 cm in size shrank to 4 cm and 2 cm respectively; and the liver tumor remained the same size, but there were also numerous small cystic growths of varying sizes (no larger than 1 cm). Liver function tests (i.e., AST, ALT, BIL) were normal, and the flank distension and pain in her abdomen and inguinal region has resolved.

What kinds of cystic growths are precancerous? Do you think the unspecified growths (no larger than 1 cm) revealed on the PET-CT scan is neoplastic growth from the existing colorectal cancer? Or do you think the liver cancer is spreading?

One week ago the patient visited me again explaining that she had followed the advice of her oncologist and received chemotherapy, but the treatment hasn't been effective. Now, she plans on receiving radiotherapy on the large intestine, liver, and cervix. What is your opinion about this?

A1: CEA over 100 does not necessarily indicate cancer progression; elevated levels most likely arose from tumor cell necrosis and release of metabolic enzymes during the breakdown process. The cystic growth likely is a blood-filled cyst resulting from the process of tumor necrosis, which first liquifies, then forms a cyst, and will eventually be resorbed. A PET-CT scan will be able to confirm if the growth is malignant or benign. Typically, metastases involving the celiac artery (trunk) is identified as stasis heat, so you can simply add Xu Duan, Gu Sui Bu, and Chuan Qi (powder) to your Ru Mo Si Wu Tang variant prescription.

Overall, administration of radiotherapy and chemotherapy to treat patients with colorectal cancer metastases to the liver rarely, if ever, offers effective results. The types of radiotherapy currently used are CyberKnife, photon knife, or Gamma Knife. Radiotherapy treatment of liver cancer with any of these systems will lead to complications of liver stasis and swelling, sudden onset of hepatitis, cirrhosis, and liver failure (though these complications are usually less severe compared to the adverse effects of conventional cobalt 60 irradiation!). If these complications present, then prescribe either Chai Ling Tang, Tong Jing Fang, or Ru Mo Si Wu Tang variants, and monitor for any changes in GOT/GPT, T-Pro, A/G, T/D-Bil, Hb, PLT, BUN/Cr, and ammonia.

Q2: Cancer has spread to the patient's lungs and she presents with cough (dry cough or with very little phlegm), constipation, pain in the left inguinal region, and sore back. I suspect that the lung metastases was a result of radiotherapy, but since the hepatic cancer enlarged, she planned on receiving radiotherapy again.

As adjuvant TCM treatment, I prescribed Ru Mo Si Wu Tang adding "the Three Yellows," Da Huang, Fu Ling, Ze Xie (8 qian each), and Yu Sheng Wan (2 pills/day). What is your perspective on this case?

A2: There is no doubt about it, patients with colorectal cancer that has metastasized to the liver, lung, spine, and pelvis really deserve a lot of sympathy! The 'good' thing is that the administration of TCM medicinals still offers effectiveness and hope. I would prescribe Ru Mo Si Wu Tang adding "the Three Yellows," Da Huang, Fu Ling, and Ze Xie (8 qian each); Cang Zhu, Qing Hao, Di Gu Pi, and Ting Li Zi (8 qian each); Fang Ji, Ma Huang, Xing Ren, and Chuan Qi (powder) (3 qian each); Xu Duan, Gu Sui Bu, and Niu Xi, Gou Ji, Zhi Mu, and Di Long (5~8 qian); Sheng Du Zhong (4 qian); Lu Jiao (1 liang); Wan Ling Dan (incrementally increase the amount week-by-week starting out with 12 pills/3x/day adding up to 26~30 pills/3x/day); and Yu Sheng Wan (up to 6~9 pills/day). If the patient has dry mouth following radiotherapy and doesn't drink enough water, you can advise the patient to regularly drink fresh vegetable and fruit juices (carrot, pear, apple, etc.) or drink Kudzu (Ge Gen) root juice. Keep working hard and making headway!

Case Study #4: Chemotherapy Induced Watery Diarrhea – Wu Ling San Variation

Q: I have a colorectal cancer patient whom has suffered from watery diarrhea ever since starting chemotherapy. How should I treat this and how long will it take to remedy? If the patient doesn't have a lot of faith in TCM treatment, what can I do to convince the patient? (Unfortunately, this is the situation with most cancer patients in South Korea.)

A: Following chemotherapy colorectal cancer patients may incur side effects such as burns and edema of the intestinal mucus membrane that causes iatrogenic mucositis (resembling Behcet's syndrome and Stephens-Johnson syndrome) and most commonly manifests in watery diarrhea. When treating these patients, you must determine the extent of the mucositis with the first priority being to check diarrhea.

In the TCM classic *Essential Prescriptions of the Golden Coffer* diarrhea is treated with Ge Gen Qin Lian Tang and Bai Tou Weng Tang. If these formulas are unable to check diarrhea (heat dysentery), and you're certain the patient hasn't eaten contaminated food or contracted an infection (putrid-smelling stool), then the condition can be diagnosed as "unable to astringe the intestines" watery diarrhea, requiring the administration of Chi Shi Zhi Yu Yu Liang Tang variant. And if this is ineffective, then prescribe Wu Ling San variant, utilizing its separation of the clear and turbid action to restore the absorption capacity of the large intestine so it can regulate water flow from the cecum to the kidney and bladder and thus promote excretion. This approach is quite simple, just prescribe Wu Ling San (Cang Zhu, Fu Ling, and Ze Xie as the sovereign medicinals) and add Huang Qin and Huang Lian.

Cast Study #5: Metastatic Colorectal Cancer

Q: A 58 y/o male patient had surgical resection performed on metastatic colorectal cancer and he also presented with inflammation of the cecum (it turned out to be metastatic spread to the cecum). Two years later, the cancer spread to the rectum and he underwent partial surgical resection; but only 3 years later, it recurred resulting in another partial resection with adjuvant chemotherapy (anticancer agent Xeloda and Oxaliplatin). The treatment was ineffective and 1 year later it spread to the lymph nodes near the abdominal aorta and pelvis, resulting in another surgical resection and chemotherapy (this time changing to Xeloda and Irinotecan, and then Erbitux). One year later, the patient's condition deteriorated once again, and the family insisted upon changing hospitals where a different chemotherapy regimen (5-FU, Oxaliplatin, and Leucovorin) was administered. Up to now, the patient's condition has remained stable without additional metastases, but he is very weak, and if metastases occurs again there aren't any other drugs available. This is when he came to me seeking TCM treatment. I prescribed Chai Ling Tang variant. What's your opinion on treatment from here on out?

A: This case offers a prime example of the difference in approach between TCM and Western medicine. We can see in this case that the Western medicine protocol is still to "eliminate the lesion" as the only option. TCM prioritizes its treatment approach in this way: 1) Treat and prevent iatrogenic vasculitis, circulatory system disorders, and myocardial disease; and 2) Prevent iatrogenic hepatitis and nephritis and hypertrophy, and iatrogenic cerebral and peripheral nerve damage.

For this patient, as long as the hematopoietic function and serum protein levels are normal, the treatment principle is to open the spleen and stomach (promote appetite) and increase the absorption of nutrients. Doing so will help the patient regain strength, activate immune response, and stablize the condition, thus fostering a physiological environment that enables the patient to go into remission. As for the TCM principle: "Disperse accumulations and gatherings as much as possible (70~80%) and rely on food and drink for the rest." This "...food and drink for the rest" refers to nutrient supply and includes the absorption of nutrients by the small intestine (receptor sensitivity and responsiveness), the liver's storage and conversion function, and the kidney's capacity of producing essence (essential physiological substances). As for TCM treatment, I would start out by prescribing variants of Chai Ling Tang; Xiang Sha Liu Jun Zi Tang, Shen Ling Bai Zhu San or Bao He Wan; or Bu Zhong Yi Qi Tang or Gui Pi Tang adding medicinals accordingly based on pattern identification and presenting signs and symptoms.

For instance, if water amassment presents, then add Bai Zhu, Fu Ling, Ze Xie, Ting Li Zi, and Fang Ji. If serum protein levels are low, then add combinations of medicinals such as "the Four Ling's," Shan Yao, Lian Zi, Qian Shi, Yi Yi Ren, Bai Guo, Da Jin Ying, Huang Qi, and Ren Shen (powder). If iatrogenic hepatitis presents, for the acute stage prescribe "the

Three Yellows" and Mu Dan Pi; and for the chronic and remission stages, prescribe Qi Bao Mei Ran Dan or Xue Ku Fang adding Wu Wei Zi and Nu Zhen Zi. If hematopoietic bone marrow function is suppressed, then add Tu Si Zi, Rou Cong Rong, Du Zhong, and Niu Xi along with Gan Jiang, Fu Zi, Yu Gui, Xi Lu Rong, and Huang Bo. If there is nerve damage, then prescribe Bu Yang Huan Wu Tang adding Ma Huang, Di Long, and Tian Ma. If tidal fever presents, then add Qing Hao, Zhi Mu, and Di Gu Pi.

Metastatic spread to the lympatic system can be identified as Shao Yang heat pattern and is similar to the Shao Yang heat pattern of osteomyelitis, nephritis, and neuritis. These types of "steaming bone" and drug-induced (iatrogenic) fever symptoms (unless there is low WBC count and/or hematopoiesis dysfunction) can all be identified as Shao Yang heat. Treatment involves first supplementing the spleen and stomach, and if the cancer relapses, then add "the Three Yellows," Mu Dan Pi, Chuan Qi (powder), Yu Sheng Wan, and Wan Ling Dan. The main channel-conducting medicinals for colorectal cancer are Bai Zhi and Sheng Ma; Fang Feng is an essential medicinal for intestinal wind bleeding; and Huai Hua and Di Yu are both essential blood-cooling and blood-stanching medicinals for the large intestine channel.

Case Study #6: Colorectal Cancer with Fecal Incontinence

Q: Following a partial colectomy a 64 y/o male patient with colorectal cancer and metastatic spread to the liver visited me complaining of poor appetite and inhibited defecation. I prescribed Xiang Sha Liu Jun Zi Tang variant. After taking this formula, he said the symptoms had improved a bit and that he had gained a little weight. Recently, he came back for another visit, this time complaining of fecal incontinence (examination by a gastroenterologist discovered muscular hyperplasia in the rectum near the anus). His doctors said this was a very difficult condition to treat, and the only thing the patient could do is wear adult diapers or change his underwear "frequently" (about 10 times/day). I am thinking this might be caused by yang vacuity pattern (similar to crab's-foot swelling (keloid)). How would you treat this patient?

A: Colorectal cancer with fecal incontinence can be identified as qi vacuity with stasis obstruction pattern, requiring administration of Bu Zhong Yi Qi Tang variant. If the patient hasn't received radiotherapy or chemotherapy, then you can add Ru Xiang, Mo Yao, Huang Qin, and Ze Xie. If he has received RT and CT, then add Gan Jiang and Fu Zi instead.

Section 6: Pancreatic Cancer

Case Study #1: Vomiting Following Chemotherapy and Radiotherapy

Q: A 61 y/o female patient with pancreatic cancer has recently suffered from vomiting following chemotherapy and radiotherapy. She also has poor intestinal motility and has lost a lot of weight (down to 33kg). If this were your patient, what formula would you prescribe?

A: For pancreatic cancer patients you can prescribe either Da Chai Hu Tang or Chai Ling Tang; Xiang Sha Liu Jun Zi Tang or Xie Xin Tang; or Wen Dan Tang or Ban Xia Tian Ma Bai Zhu San variants adding Shan Dou Gen, Liang Jiang, and Da Hui Xiang. If persistently increased CEA and CA19-9 levels present, add large doses of "the Three Yellows," Yu Sheng Wan, and Wan Ling Dan. TCM (Kampo) practitioners in Japan often prescribe Yan Nian Ban Xia Tang adding Ren Shen (powder) and Chuan Qi (powder) for this condition, and you could consider this formula as well.

Case Study #2: It's Really Difficult to Treat!

Q1: I have a 62 y/o female patient with a pancreatic tumor near an artery at the center of the pancreas. Radiotherapy was performed on one occasion and results of recent lab tests are as follows: blood– BUN 5.1 (normal 8-25), T.P. 5.6 (normal 6-8.5), and S-Alb 3.1 (normal 3.5-5.3); and liver function– GOT 18 (0-40) and GPT 6 (1-30). Results of a CT scan reveal the tumor has shrunk and there is mild ascites. Later on, metastatic spread to the peritoneum was discovered and the oncologist at the hospital said: "Now, it will be tough to administer aggressive treatment." They couldn't prescribe diuretics nor could they perform aspiration of ascites. Please help me understand this condition better: Is ascites a result of low s-Alb? Or is it caused by peritoneal metastases? Is it possible for her condition to improve? How should I treat this patient?

A1: The way I see it is that ascites is caused by low s-Alb along with low

BUN/Cr. Therefore, you can consider prescribing large doses of Ren Shen (powder), Bai Guo, Huai Shan, Da Jin Ying, Fu Ling, Ze Xie, Qian Shi, and Yi Ren. If T-Pro and A/G levels don't increase, then add Tu Si Zi; and if levels still don't rise, then add small doses of Gan Jiang, Fu Zi, and Huang Qin.

Remember! You cannot prescribe Gan Jiang and Fu Zi too early in the treatment regimen for this condition, but Gao Liang Jiang and Xiang Fu are ok. Second, if peritoneal metastases has already occurred, then the ascites will usually be rapid and profuse, and it can't be resolved regardless of the method employed (e.g., paracentesis, automated pump system). The sooner you administer the TCM medicinals mentioned above the better; this will help relieve symptoms and improve the patient's condition.

Typically, unless it is repletion heat pattern ascites (e.g., acute fulminant heptatitis complicated by liver failure with the administration of too much IV fluid), then you should prescribe Chai Ling Tang variant adding incremental doses of medicinals that address the presenting signs and symptoms. If T-Pro, A/G, Hb, and C3/C4 levels are low and BUN/Cr high, then prescribe Chai Ling Tang adding Gan Jiang, Fu Zi, Yu Gui, Ren Shen (powder), and Huang Qi. For all of these medicinals start out with small doses and gradually increase as needed: Don't overdo it all at once! Even in the case of acute ascites, you can still prescribe Chai Ling Tang combined with either Da Xian Xiong Tang, Shi Zao Tang, Dan Dong Shen You Wan, or Shu Zuo Yin Zi variants. In cases of low T-Pro and A/G, then add Bai Guo, Huai Shan, Qian Shi, Yi Yi Ren, Lian Zi, Da Jin Ying, and Xiao Jin Ying.

Typically, after pancreatic cancer has been treated and calcification occurs, the symptoms will improve. But remember! Even if CA19-9, amylase, lipase, and GLU all test out at normal levels, the patient should continue taking TCM medicinals for a minimum of 6 months~1 year with periodic lab tests being monitored. You must be vigilant!

Q2: Unfortunately, this pancreatic cancer patient has passed away. At the onset of administering TCM medicinals her symptoms did improve, but towards the end it didn't seem to matter how strong of dose I prescribed, it still wasn't enough to prevent the progression of cancer and ascites. Do you think it would have been helpful for the patient to continue with CT and RT when her condition was in remission? For cases like this, what do you think is the best approach for treatment?

A2: Pancreatic cancer is always difficult to treat. Once a diagnosis has been confirmed, many doctors will tell the patient's family: "The patient can do whatever she (he) wants to do." This infers that the hope for a cure is dismal. Administering TCM medicinals for this condition and having the patient survive for 6 months is in itself a commendable accomplishment. Only TCM physicians with exceptional skills can achieve results of having patients survive for more than 1 year. So if you have a similar patient in the future, I would stick to the same treatment approach. Don't feel discouraged and lose confidence in yourself. After all, doctors are only human; the capacity of the medicinals we use and the institution of modern medicine as a whole has inherent limitations. Through thick and thin we as doctors must continue striving for development and progress. The day you are able to cure a severe illness such as pancreatic cancer is when you will be acknowledged as a "master physician," a luminary respected throughout the medical community.

Case Study #3: Advanced Stage Pancreatic Cancer

Q: There is a 74 y/o male patient with pancreatic cancer. Since the diagnosis was confirmed he has been administered anticancer agents in attempts to control the condition, but results have been poor. The patient has a sallow complexion and often feels nauseated with occasional dry heaving. He has been diagnosed with cirrhosis and maintains 1 stool per day. The family decided to give TCM a try since all their options with Western medicine have been exhausted. Can you give me any advice on this case?

A: The pancreas is anatomically located at the back of the abdominal cavity behind the stomach. It is among the body's silent organs, and thus when afflicted with disease (e.g., cancer), detection and diagnosis remains difficult in the early stages. This condition isn't usually discovered until the tumor has already enlarged to the point where it presses down on the bile duct obstructing the bile flow and subsequently enters the bloodstream causing hyperbilirubinemia, sallow facial complexion, and light-colored stools. Some patients will have nausea, vomiting, poor appetite, tidal fever, fatigue, weight loss, constipation, and severe hemilateral pain between the nipples and diaphragm (these symptoms are most pronounced after eating deep-fried foods or drinking hard liquor.) Once the diagnosis of pancreatic cancer has been confirmed, it is usually already in the advanced stages. Really a tough situation!

The most common causes of mortality from this condition are from hyperbilirubinemia and hepatic coma. However, poor nutrition, and low levels of T-Pro, ALB, and Hb will induce generalized edema, cerebral hypoxia, and cerebral edema, which may also lead to mortality.

My formula of choice for treating this condition is either Chai Ling

Tang or Da Chai Hu Tang adding Da Huang, Liang Jiang, and Shan Dou Gen. However, you could also consider the Xie Xin Tang series, Yan Nian Ban Xia Tang, or Gui Pi Tang. If T-Bil levels drop then rise again, you should add Gan Jiang, Fu Zi, and Yu Gui (starting out in small doses adding incrementally).

Section 7: Liver Cancer

Case Study #1: Hepatocellular Carcinoma (HCC)

Q: I have a 73 y/o male hepatocellular carcinoma patient whose lab test results are as follows – T/D Bil: 0.6 / 0.2, AST: 86, ALT: 42, ALP: 805 (normal range 102-333), r-GT: 162 (normal range 11-78), PT: 11.9 (normal range 11-14), R-Feto protein: 159.73 (normal range 0-13.4), CA19-9: 49.5 (normal range below 33), CEA: 1.49, PLT: 148 (normal range 150-350), CYFRA 21-1: 2.72 (normal range < 3.3ng/ml), HbsAg (+), and HBV (-).

Results of the most recent CT scan reveal:

1. Slight increases in size and number of multiple, variable sized, conglomerated hepatic masses involving the entire liver, especially Lt hepatic lobe, and focal adjacent IHBD dilatation.

Slight increase in size and number of multiple intrahepatic metastatic nodules in the Rt hepatic lobe.

Little interval change of possible focal Lt portal vein invasion, and some cavernous transformation of the portal vein.

2. No ascites, no varices, no splenomegaly.

3. About 1.5 cm, Bosniak 1 cyst, Lt kidney.

A: From the CT scan we know that there are multiple HCC tumors. This means Western medicine won't be able to perform percutaneous ethanol injection (PEI) or TAE (TACE), so their only option is administering chemotherapy. The problem is that the available HCC chemotherapy agents aren't very effective. For now, the most important thing to do is make sure the patient is getting enough nutrients. I suggest you tell the patient: "Eat whatever you like, but just make sure it isn't too hot." Remember! This is important because liver cancer patients will often have esophageal varices or gastric ulcers and ingesting scalding hot foods (or liquids) could exacerbate an already precarious condition.

As for TCM medicinals, I would still prescribe Chai Ling Tang variant adding Fu Ling and Ze Xie (large doses), Ma Huang (small dose), Xing Ren, Da Huang (adding incrementally to maintain 2~3 stools per day), and of course Ren Shen (powder) and Chuan Qi (powder). If chemotherapy has not been administered, then add "the Three Yellows" (large doses), Ru Xiang, Mo Yao, San Leng, E Zhu, and Wan Ling Dan. Patients who have received chemotherapy will have suppressed hematopoietic function so it is beneficial to add large doses of Gan Jiang, Fu Zi, and Yu Gui.

For patients just completing a chemotherapy regimen, as long as their liver function indices (GOT/GPT) remain elevated, then continue prescribing Chai Ling Tang variant, but the dose of Huang Qin can be reduced to 3 qian each (down from 5~8 qian). For patients who incur drug-induced hepatitis, doses of Huang Qin can be increased, while concomitantly lowering the dosage of or "temporarily" discontinuing chemotherapy altogether until the drug-induced hepatitis has resolved.

For HCC patients with elevated AFP (tumor marker) levels following chemotherapy, you should prescribe the above TCM formula adding large doses of "the Three Yellows"; and if this is still not effective, then add Gan Jiang, Fu Zi, and Yu Gui.

Applying an integrated TCM and Western medicine approach (concomitantly administering TCM medicinals throughout the chemotherapy regimen) offers excellent efficacy. Even when the condition has stabilized and the CT scan, MRI, and PET scan reveal no signs of tumor, the patient must still take TCM medicinals for at least 6 months up to 1 year. Remember! For patients who have been administered Gan Jiang, Fu Zi, and Yu Gui continously for 3 months or longer, you must subtract these medicinals at this time to alleviate the potential for inducing relapse of the tumor. If AFP rises again, then simply add large doses of "the Three Yellows"; and if doses of 8~10 qian fail to bring down AFP, then add large doses of Gan Jiang, Fu Zi, and Yu Gui along with San Leng, E Zhu, and Yu Sheng Wan.

In the event none of these approaches offers efficacy, then change formulas to Ru Mo Si Wu Tang adding "the Three Yellows", Cang Zhu, Fu Ling, Ze Xie, Ren Shen (powder), Chuan Qi (powder), San Leng, E Zhu, Pu Gong Ying, Da Huang, Yu Sheng Wan, and Wan Ling Dan; and if this still is ineffective, then once again add Gan Jiang, Fu Zi, and Yu Gui.

Currently, regardless of the treatment approach (i.e., TCM, Western medicine, or integrated TCM and Western medicine), for advanced cancer typically the best prognosis that can be hoped for is to extend survival for 6 months (at most up to 1 year). My hope is that we can all work toghether (TCM and Western medicine) striving for breakthroughs that will result in survival rates of 3~5 years with a good quality of life. This would be a rewarding consolation for the entire field of medicine.

Case Study #2: Three Formulas for Treating Liver Cancer

Q1: I have a 73 y/o male patient with multiple (more than 20) tumors whose liver function tests (including T/D-bil levels) are normal. I prescribed Chai Ling Tang (including Fu Ling and Ze Xie 5 qian each) adding Da Huang (5 fen); San Leng and E Zhu (3 qian each); "the Three Yellows" (8 qian each); and Pu Gong Ying (1 liang). He has taken this formula for 1 week, and I don't have any information about his AFP test results yet. Please offer your advice on this case.

A1: For this type of liver cancer with multiple liver masses you can consider prescribing several formula options:
1) Chai Ling Tang adding large doses of "the Three Yellows" (at least 8~10 qian each), San Leng, E Zhu, Shan Nai, Yu Jin, and Chuan Qi (powder).
2) Ru Mo Si Wu Tang adding large doses of "the Three Yellows" (at least 8~10 qian each), Cang Zhu, Fu Ling, Ze Xie, "the Three Insects," Chuan Qi (powder), San Leng, E Zhu, Shan Nai, and Yu Jin.
3) Tong Jing Fang adding "the Four Ling's" and large doses of "the Three Yellows" (at least 8~10 qian each).

Also, Yu Shen Wang and Wan Ling Dan should be added to each of these three formulas, and the patient should be advised to maintain a well-balanced diet with plenty of nutrients to prevent ascites. It is also optimal to maintain 2~3 stools/day in order to avoid the formation of hyperdynamic circulation arising from portal hypertension, ascites, and esophageal varices.

If liver function indices and AFP levels happen to increase or T-Pro and GPT decrease, then you should add Gan Jiang, Fu Zi, Yu Gui, Ren Shen (powder), Si Shen Tang (Huai Shan, Qian Shi, Lian Zi, Yi Ren, and Fu Ling), Bai Guo, Da Jin Ying, and Xiao Jin Ying. Remember! If the patient presents with repletion heat pattern, then you should "not" add Ren Shen (powder), Gan Jiang, Fu Zi, Yu Gui, Si Wu Tang, or Huang Qi, because these supplementing medicinals may induce accelerated proliferation and tumerogenesis. During this repletion heat pattern stage, you should prescribe heat-clearing and toxin-resolving medicinals. Yes, you can also select heat-clearing, toxin-vanquishing, and swelling-dispersing and bind-dissipating "anticancer" medicinals such as Pu Gong Ying, Lian Qiao, Jin Yin Hua, Ban Zhi Lian, and Bai Hua She Ku Cao. But quite frankly, you may just as well use the most common and broadly available broad-spectrum heat-clearing and toxin-resolving medicinals Huang Qin, Huang Lian, and Huang Bo (aka "the Three Yellows"). In my clinical experience, I have found that the anticancer efficacy of "the Three Yellows" is comprable to, if not better, especially if prescribed in large doses in combination with other essential medicinals.

Once the patient's condition has stabilized and enters the chronic stage, then you can also add warm and acrid medicinals such as Jiang Huang, Bai Jie Zi, Hua Jiao, Hu Jiao, Bin Lang, Lao Ye, Bi Bo, Liang Jiang, and Sha Ren Gen.

Q2: I didn't realize the survival expectancy for HCC was so short. I have a question about why you would add "the Three Insects" to formula 2) (Ru Mo Si Wu Tang) in your previous response?

A2: Right now, if only Western medicine treatment is administered, liver cancer will typically relapse in 3~5 months and possibly manifest as proliferation of diffuse pinpoint lesions. Integrating TCM treatment will overcome the insufficiencies of Western medicine treatment and can achieve remission periods of up to 2 years (as documented in some of my patients). As for adding "the Three Insects," the use of toxic proteins and chitin in TCM medicinal insects is aimed at suppressing tumor proliferation. The combination of these insect medicinals with heat-clearing and toxin-resolving medicinals produces the dual action of suppressing tumor proliferation and also inhibiting hyperstimulation of the central nervous system and thus preventing the recurrence of cancer cell proliferation signals.

Q3: After receiving treatment, the patient's liver function test results remained normal, he gained 1kg, and AFP dropped to 600 (down from a high of 890). Now he feels pretty much back to normal and the distending pain in the right hypochondrium has mostly resolved. A CT scan didn't show any signs of ascites, but did reveal that the tumor was still there. The patient's attending physician was surprised to find there were no signs of jaundice. T-Bil has dropped to 0.8 and the pain in the right hypochondrium has resolved so the patient doesn't need to apply lidocaine patches. The patient occasionally feels nausea but there is no ascites. The patient and I are genuinely grateful for your advice and guidance.

A3: Congratulations you are starting to see results! Even though the tumor has not disappeared, it hasn't enlarged or spread. Now, we can anticipate the tumor will gradually become "calcified" and inactive. Remember! The patient must continue to take TCM medicine.

Case Study #3: Transcatheter Arterial Embolism (TAE)

Q: I have a 43 y/o female patient with chronic HBV infection whose condition deteriorated with progression to hepatocellular carcinoma. She has already undergone transcatheter arterial embolism (TAE) several times, yet regional metastases to the abdominal lymph nodes still occurred. The patient has no ascites, 1 stool/day, and the CT scan images show numerous diffusely distributed HCC lesions. Liver function tests are as follows – GOT/GPT: 150/113, AFP: 192, and T/D Bil: 3.4/1.6. How would you treat this patient?

A: Chai Ling Tang variant is still the best option adding large doses of Fu Ling, Ze Xie, Huang Qin, and Mu Dan Pi along with Ma Huang, Ren Shen (powder), Chuan Qi (powder), Yu Sheng Wan, and Wan Ling Dan. This approach should be able to prevent tumor enlargement and promote dissolution. If you feel it is necessary to include other medicinals you could add San Leng and E Zhu or Yuan Hu, Yu Jin, and Jiang Huang. You can also consider adding a tablespoon of white vinegar (distilled vinegar) into the pot with the other medicinals, soaking for at least 30 minutes up to 12 hours, and then decocting the formula until there is 2 1/2 or 3 rice bowls (200ml) of liquid remaining. Instruct the patient to drink this decoction like a beverage in small amounts throughout the day accompanying the prescribed doses of Chuan Qi (powder) and Wan Ling Dan. If the patient has a poor appetite, then you can add Xian Zha, Ji Nei Jin, and Da Huang (small dose of 5 fen).

Case Study #4: Elevated AFP and Low T-Pro Following Surgery

Q: I have a 46 y/o male patient with Hepatitis B virus (HBV) that deteriorated into liver hepatocellurar carcinoma (HCC) and an AFP level of 13000. Following partial hepatectomy, AFP levels dropped to 2000, GOT/GPT 35/50, and T-Pro 5.3. What's the best way to handle this case going forward?

A: AFP dropping from 13000 down to 2000 following surgical resection in a liver cancer patient indicates that the surgery was successful. However, the low T-Pro level suggests that the liver's function of protein absorption, storage, and release has been impaired. At this time, even if AFP was elevated it wouldn't definitively indicate liver cancer – it could also be a result of the intensive regenerative responses following hepatectomy.

Following hepatectomy the liver will undergo regenerative hyperplasia (benign) and generally will grow back to the original size within about 6 months. The rapidity of regenerative hyperplasia is reflected in the elevated AFP; however, AFP 2000 is still too high, so you should try bringing it down further.

I receommend the following two approaches: 1) If the patient has "not been" intubated, then you can prescribe Bu Zhong Yi Qi Tang (including large doses of Huang Qin) adding Yuan Hu, Mu Xiang, Ren Shen (powder), Chuan Qi (powder), Dan Shen, Dang Shen, and large doses of Fu Ling, Zhu Ling, Ze Xie, Bai Zhu, and Mu Dan Pi. You don't need to add Ma Huang, Xing Ren, Ting Li Zi, and Fang Ji, because patients undergoing this type of surgical resection almost never incur cardiopulmonary dysfunction (e.g., pleural effusion). 2) If the patient "has been intubated," then you can prescribe Chai Ling Tang adding Dang Shen, Dan Shen, Fu Ling, Bai Zhu, and Si Shen Tang (Huai Shan, Lian Zi, Qian Shi, Yi Ren, and Fu Ling), which will function to increase T-Pro. Adding large doses of Huang Qin, Mu Dan Pi, and "the Four Ling's" is aimed at both bringing down AFP and increasing T-Pro. If AFP drops down to 50~100, then the large doses of these medicinals can be discontinued; but if AFP initially drops to 500~800 and subsequently jumps back up again, then you need to add Ren Shen (powder), Gan Jiang, Fu Zi, and Yu Gui.

Case Study #5: Diffuse Hepatocellular Carcinoma (HCC)

Q: I have a patient whom has been diagnosed with diffuse HCC. Most recent lab results showed normal GOT/GPT, T/D Bil, and AFP levels; the patient sleeps well, but has a poor appetite; and stool 1x/day. I prescribed Chai Ling Tang adding Bai Zhu, Fu Ling, and Ze Xie (8 qian each), Huang Qin (8 qian), Huang Lian and Huang Bo (5 qian each), San Leng and E Zhu (4 qian each), Xu Duan and Qian Cao (4 qian each), Chuan Qi (powder) (3 qian), and Wan Ling Dan (6 pills/3x/day). Do you think this is a good formula?

A: Once an oncologist confirms the diagnosis of diffuse HCC, usually a very conservative "wait and see" approach will be adopted as opposed to aggressive treatment. And sometimes this "living with the condition" conservative approach really does extend the patient's survival period, while also sparing the patient of senseless, often agonizing, treatment– you could say it is the lesser of two evils.

Recently, I have treated a patient with a similar condition. The patient was admitted to the hospital on March 15 and two weeks later I was called on to make a hospital visit. After overhearing the doctor tell his family that "...currently there is no treatment available...he probably only has 3 to 6 months remaining...," the patient was so worried and full of anxiety that he experienced diaphragm contractions, shortness of breath, and distending pain all over his body. On March 27, I accepted the family's request to treat this patient and the next morning I had a formula decocted, sealed in packets, and sent over to the hospital. The patient only took one packet before suffering an outbreak of drug-induced (from Western medicine!) fulminant heptatitis with shortness of breath and panting. The attending physician originally diagnosed the condition as pleural effusion and had an X-ray taken in preparation for aspiration, but to his surprise there was no sign of effusion so he suspected the cause was from excessive administration of drugs. The previous drug regimen was discontinued, and instead, he was administered the opiod analgesic morphine, Thalidomide, diuretics (no edema, only distention), intravenous amino acid infusions, and interferon. Unexpectedly, the ensuing lab tests revealed a spike in GOT to 1000 and BIL also increased. I had no choice but to call the family and tell them to stop taking the Western medicine drugs, except for interferon (Lamivudine), which should be gradually discontinued as the GOT/GPT levels come down, and by all means start taking TCM medicinals as soon as possible. I prescribed Xiang Sha Liu Jun Zi Tang adding Si Shen Tang, Huang Qin, Mu Dan Pi, Chuan Qi (powder), "the Four Ling's," San Leng, and E Zhu.

It was obvious the attending physician lacked experience. Despite the patient having low T-Pro levels, once this doctor saw the elevated ammonia levels he immediately administered Lactulose and contraindicated the use of TCM medicinals. Other lab test results were as follows: GOT 800, ALB 3.4, WBC 25500, PLT 5000, T-BIL 17~18, BUN 52, and Cr 3. Other presenting symptoms were lower leg edema, petechiae, and ascites. You could tell right away that this patient could very well have "sepsis" or even drug-induced hepatorenal syndrome, hemolysis, or drug-induced fulminant hepatitis. The patient also received long-term administration of intravenous ALB and diuretics (oral and intravenous), which perpetuated a state of irreversible edema. Obviously, when you see a PLT count of only 5000 it is clear that sepsis may induce disseminated intravascular coagulation (DIC) and lead to death.

On April 7 the patient's wife came to my clinic seeking consultation and treatment for her husband. Though I knew this would be a tough case, I felt obligated to try my best. I prescribed Chai Ling Tang adding Huang Qin, Ze Xie, Fu Ling, and Mu Dan Pi (8 qian each); Ren Shen (powder) (3 qian); Lu Rong (1 qian); Gan Jiang and Fu Zi (3 qian each); and Da Huang (5 fen). I also explained the importance of having her husband continue the life-sustaining Western medicine treatment (e.g., infusions of whole blood and platelets), while "discontinuing" all the other drugs.

The patient's condition did improve some, but they didn't take my advice about discontinuing the other drugs. However, since I had clearly stated my position, I didn't feel it was appropriate to keep persisting. This is an experience that we can all learn from. For advanced stage cancer patients taking a conservative approach of "living with the condition" may be better than aggressive treatment. As for your prescription above, for the most part I approve, but if T-Pro and A/G levels are low it is best to add Si Shen Tang, Bai Guo, Dang Shen, and Ren Shen (powder). If the tumor undergoes rapid growth, then add large doses of Wan Ling Dan.

Case Study #6: Elevated AFP Levels

Q: I have a liver cancer patient who received a partial hepatectomy and now has an elevated AFP of 2000. The patient sought consultation from a South Korean TKM doctor of the Sasang Constitutional Medicine school and was told he had a Tai Yin constitution. The doctor advised him to eat more table salt to restore energy and strengthen his immune system. What are your thoughts on this approach?

A: If 1 month has already elapsed since partial hepatectomy and the AFP has only dropped from 2000 to 1000 then this indicates poor efficacy and inability to correctly identify the pattern and administer the appropriate treatment. My approach would be to prescribe Chai Ling Tang variant, which would improve the patient's condition in less than 3 weeks time. Remember! Following partial hepatectomy the liver will regenerate and thus you should expect AFP levels of anywhere from 30~200. Don't misinterpret this as an indication of liver tumor recurrence! And you don't need to add any special medicinals either! Just keep administering Chai Ling Tang variant (or other relevant formula such as Xue Ku Fang, Zhi Bo Di Huang Tang, or Xiang Sha Liu Jun Zi Tang variants, as along as it corresponds with the presenting symptoms and pattern identification). If AFP suddenly jumps to 500, or even higher to 1000 or 2000, then this clearly indicates liver tumor relapse. At this time, you must add large doses of anticancer medicinals and great heat yang-supplementing medicinals.

Case Study #7: Postoperative Hepatocellular Carcinoma (HCC) Multiple Metastases

Q: A 29 y/o female HCC patient underwent partial hepatectomy and later on peritoneal metastases was discovered, which resulted in another surgical resection. The surgeons allowed her father to observe the operation, and that's how the father observed firsthand that they had only resected a small piece of tissue "the size of a rice grain." He was astonished by this and would subsequently observe all of his daughters surgical procedures. A year later, another sugery was performed on her peritoneum and she also received targeted therapy with Tarceva at a lesion near her diaphragm. Another year passed and a massive tumor was found in the patient's pelvis for which she received radiotherapy. It wasn't until 4 years and 5 months after the patient was first diagnosed with cancer that she sought my consultation.

I prescribed Chai Ling Tang adding Bai Zhu, Fu Ling, Ze Xie, Gan Jiang, Fu Zi, Huang Qin, and Mu Dan Pi (8 qian each); Ma Huang (1 qian); Tao Ren (4 qian); Lai Fu Zi, Chen Pi, Ci Wan, and Kuan Dong Hua (5 qian each); Chuan Qi (powder); Wan Ling Dan; and Yu Sheng Wan. In July the patient had another surgery to resect most of the large tumors in the pelvis, but the tumor in the abdomen had grown larger. I suspected that the tumors on the peritoneum and diaphragm were related. Recently, the patient has presented with ascites and abdominal distension, but liver function tests are normal; stool normal (3~5 times/day; currently taking the stool softener and hyperammonemia drug Lactulose); appetite down a bit; and overall daily activities and function relatively normal. Please offer your advice and guidance on this case.

A: Patients having HCC with peritoneal metastases will inevitably present with ascites and abdominal distention. Also, since the surgical resection involved dissection of the abdominal muscles and peritoneum, absorption of nutrients will be compromised so you must focus on ensuring sufficient nutritional intake. Once T-Pro and Na levels drop, tympanites (known as qi gu, blood gu, and water gu in TCM classical pathologic terminology) will rapidly develop. Based on the patient's current condition, I agree with prescribing Chai Ling Tang variant, but it doesn't seem necessary to add Zi Yuan and Kuan Dong Hua. The key here is to monitor the T-Pro level and make sure to keep it in the normal range. Also, at the onset don't prescribe large doses of Gan Jiang and Fu Zi, because doing so may accelerate lymphatic fluid secretion and thus further obstruct the lymphatic system's capacity to reabsorb the fluid (ascites) in the peritoneal space. As for Ren Shen (powder), from the onset you should prescribe 3 g/3x/day; and only if T-Pro levels persistently remain low, should you consider adding larger doses.

Based on my experience, for abdominal tumors it's best to add Yuan

Hu, Mu Xiang, San Leng, E Zhu, Jiang Huang, Yu Jin, Bin Lang, and Sha Ren. Of course, other formula variants such as Tong Jing Fang adding Liang Jiang and Shan Dou Gen also have the actions of quickening the blood, transforming stasis, and breaking blood in the treatment of tumors. Regardless of which formula you choose, it is essential to add Da Huang in order to maintain low circulatory pressure and prevent the formation of blood stasis and hemorrhage in the GI tract. Remember! For medicinals that accelerate the metabolism and promote blood perfusion such as Ren Shen (powder), Gan Jiang, Fu Zi, Yu Gui, Huang Qi, and Dang Gui you should start out by prescribing small doses and increase incrementally. If you don't do so, this makes the patient susceptible to hemolysis, GI tract varices, and blood stasis of the endothelial cells and mucous membranes along the GI tract; or worse, it could lead to induration with profuse bleeding, shock, and even death. You must be vigilant!

Why is it that virtually all of my cancer treatment formulas contain Fu Ling, Ze Xie, Mu Dan Pi, Di Gu Pi, Da Huang, Huang Qin, and Chuan Qi (powder)? It's because these medicinals have anticancer properties and mutually interact (i.e., have a synergistic effect) with the capacity to repair normal cells, vasculature, lymphatics, and fluids; inhibit abnormal tissue, fluids, neoplastic progession and infiltration; and effectively restore physiological function throughout the course of disease.

Case Study #8: South Korea's Popular "Vegetarian Liver Cancer-Fighting Diet"

Q: Some food therapy books in South Korea have made bold claims into the efficacy of a "vegeterian liver cancer-fighting diet" declaring that if you eat vegetables (often raw) and grains like ashitaba (immortal grass), cale, dandelion, thistle, tomato, lotus root, Brewer's yeast, wheat germ, enzymes, red beans, and pearl barley your liver cancer will shrink. These books also list dozens of cases supposedly verifying its effectiveness. This line of reasoning doesn't mesh with modern medicine rationale. Is this just a fad or is it for real? What's your opinion?

A: I don't agree at all that liver cancer patients should rely solely on food to treat their condition, and eating vegetarian (particular a strict vegan diet) is an even worse idea. No matter what type of cancer it is the body needs adequate nutrients to put up a defense. This is evident in studies that have been done about cancer patients losing their appetites, develop a metabolic defect that causes body tissue to break down, and become severely malnourished following radiotherapy and chemotherapy. These patients simply waste away and die, but not from the cancer itself!

Eating a strict vegan diet over extended periods of time makes a person susceptible to low s-Pro and Hb levels. This is a particularly precarious situation for liver cancer patients who are already susceptible to hemolysis that may lead to hepatorenal syndrome (high BUN/Cr). Maintaining a long-term strict vegan diet makes the patient susceptible to irreversible ascites and pleural effusion, and with the presence of cerebral edema and high ICP (hepatic encephalopathy), this could lead to death. This is why it is unequivocably inadvisable for liver cancer patients to eat a strict vegetarian diet. The best diet for these patients includes grains and legumes like brown rice, pearl barley, and soybeans as staples; lots of nuts (all kinds); Si Shen Tang (Huai Shan, Qian Shi, Lian Zi, Yi Ren, and Fu Ling); fresh vegetables; and fish, meat, and eggs. For patients who are very weak, eating small amounts of Ren Shen (powder) is also a good idea.

The TCM approach to treating liver cancer is as follows: As long as there isn't an accumulation of fluid or stasis obstruction in the peripheral tissue around the tumor, typically the cancer will not rapidly progress and metastasize. If the patient still has a decent appetite without signs of wasting (cachexia) and abstains from making the often hasty and rash decision proponed their Western medical doctor for immediately receiving chemotherapy and radiotherapy, then simply prescribe water-disinhibiting by bland percolation, heat-clearing and toxin-resolving, and blood-quickening and stasis-transforming TCM medicinals. My personal preference for the treatment of liver cancer is Chai Ling Tang variant. Over the years, it has been the most effective formula I have prescribed for treating this pathocondition.

Section 8: Breast Cancer

Breast cancer is the most common type of cancer in women. However, the advancement of health education and advocacy has highlighted the importance of performing self-examinations and going for periodic screening examinations. This has resulted in early detection and initiation of treatment with more favorable outcomes. Typically, when a lump is found and a tumor suspected, most patients follow Western medicine protocol having the lesion resected and then receiving adjuvant radiotherapy and chemotherapy. This is when most patients seek TCM treatment, which provides effective relief of Western medicine therapeutic adverse effects, inhibits proliferation of cancer cells, prevents metastatic spread, and offers adjuvant and palliative treatment for late stage disease that improves quality of life.

Case Study #1: Frequent Massage for Postoperative Arm Lymphedema

Q: I have a breast cancer patient with arm lympedema (non-pitting). How would you treat this patient?

A: Postoperative lymphedema can be classified as qi vacuity with water amassment pattern. In addition to prescribing TCM medicinals for the treatment of this condition, it is imperative for the patient to perform massage techniques on the limb as well. Of course, having good posture and maintaining a healthy lifestyle is also important.

First, you should remind the patient that when lying down for sleep to position the arm either horizontally (perpendicular from body) or bend the elbow at a 90° angle with the palm facing upwards resting on a pillow or bedside table. Second, you should advise the patient to regularly perform massage, initially having a tui na (massage) therapist or physiotherapist conduct the procedure, and then once the patient understands the process, either have the patient do self-message or seek assistance from a close friend or family member.

Lymphedema massage should start at the back and shoulder near the region of Gao Huang (UB43) acupoint (where a myofascial "knot" will almost inevitably be found) manipulating until the hard "knotted" lump has softened, and then proceed massaging gently with the fingertips from the elbow up towards the back, from the wrist up to the elbow, and from the fingers up to the wrist with each repetition ultimtely directing the flow back up towards the centrally located healthy lymphatic vessels. Do this everyday, starting from the back and shoulder all the way down to the tips of each finger and back up again. Continue performing this daily massage until the swelling has resided and the limbs can function freely and unimpeded as normal.

As for TCM medicinals, you can prescribe Wu Ling San (Nephritis Formula) adding large doses of Huang Qi (starting out at 2 liang and gradually increasing to 4 liang), Yin Xin Ye (8 qian from the onset), Ren Shen (powder), and Chuan Qi (powder); or you could prescribe Gui Qi Jian Zhong Tang adding "the Four Ling's," Gan Jiang, and Fu Zi. After administering this formula for a period of time, you can determine the effectiveness of treatment by assessing whether hardness and tightness of the affected arm has been reduced and wrinkles in the skin appear. If so, continue administering this formula and the condition will continue to improve.

Case Study #2: Intermittent Upper Limb Lymphedema

Q: Following a lumpectomy (breast-conserving surgery) the patient developed lymphedema in the upper limb (same side as surgery). After performing massage the condition resolved, but a few days later the swelling returned? How should I approach this condition?

A: For treating lymphedema following lumpectomy you can consider prescribing either Wu Ling San (Nephritis Formula) adding large amounts of Huang Qi; or Bu Zhong Yi Qi Tang (with large doses of Huang Qi) adding Fu Ling, Ze Xie, Gan Jiang, Fu Zi, and Huang Qin. If after administering this formula for 1~2 weeks the edema persists and becomes even tauter, advise the patient to elevate the arm perpendicular to the body when lying down to rest or sleep. This simple measure is very helpful in improving the condition; in most patients the swelling will gradually go down. Don't worry!

Case Study #3: Acupuncture and Moxabustion Principles Following Surgery, Radiotherapy, and Chemotherapy

Q: Nowadays, it is common for many cancer patients and their families to seek TCM consultation and treatment to regulate the constitution following Western medical treatment (i.e., surgery, radiotherapy, chemotherapy). However, oncologists at most major hospitals are not supportive of this approach, and some categorically contraindicate the use of TCM medicinals. In recent years there have been growing numbers of successful cases applying an integrative TCM and Western medicine approach for the treatment of cancer. These successes are making headway, turning the tides from objections and biases into acceptance. Recently, the dean of a major South Korean university contacted me about collaborating on a paper entitled "Efficacy of acupuncture therapy on cancer patients." The purpose of this paper focuses on determining whether or not the administration of acupuncture treatment was effective at preventing and improving symptoms of breast cancer patients following Western medicine treatment (i.e., recection, radiotherapy, chemotherapy). I'd like to focus on the efficacy of preventing adverse effects of radiotherapy and chemotherapy, but I don't have enough experience in this area. I was hoping you could share your experiences and insights with me.

A: The efficacy of acupuncture treatment following chemotherapy and radiotherapy for malignant tumors is not very good. When administering acupuncture treatment you must be aware of several principles. The most important is warm needling (applying moxa cubes onto the handles of the needles), especially if the patient has received chemotherapy infusions for extended periods of time, which commonly causes phlebitis and damage to the vein at the site of the IV. Warm needling will also relieve postoperative pain and reduce the amount of time it takes for the swelling to go down following removal of the IV, improve hematopoietic function following chemotherapy and radiotherapy, and boost the immune system.

Useful acupoints to select are He Gu (LI4), Nei Guan (P6), Chi Ze (LU5), San Yin Jiao (SP6), Yin Lin Quan (SP9), Shou San Li (LI10), Zu San Li (ST36), Fei Shu (UB13), Pi Shu (UB20), Shen Shu (UB23), Tai Chong (LV3), Shen Men (HT7), Feng Chi (GB20), and Hou Xi (SI3). If there is lymphedema on the affected side, it is best to apply warm needling (moxa); and after you remove the needle make sure to press firmly on point of insertion.

During the acupunture treatment regimen, patients should not concomitantly receive Western medicine drug infusions; instead, they should be administered TCM medicinals. This will ensure the best results.

Case Study #4: Postoperative Ileal and Lung Metastases

Q: A 40 y/o female patient was diagnosed with left-sided breast cancer. Three years after undergoing mastectomy, follow-up examination revealed metastatic spread to the right ilium, and 1 year later metastatic spread to the lung was discovered. Over the past 3 years the patient has been receiving infusions of Taxol and Docetaxel in attempts to keep her condition under control. Originally, the treatment showed effectiveness, but these results have waned. Now, she has a cough with white foamy sputum, and was administered expectorant medication that improved her symptoms a bit. Caught up in her other health concerns and daily life, the patient recently realized that it had been 3 months since her last menstruation. Based on the patient's history, what's the best way to treat her?

A: For breast cancer patients with metastatic spread to the iliac and lung who receive long-term and repeated radiotherapy and chemotherapy cancer cells will tend to develop drug resistance. Once the lymph nodes, lymph ducts, and microvascular circulation undergoes fibrosis, induration, and stasis, there is no available Western medicine drug that offers efficacy. This is especially true for Taxol and Docetaxel, which can only reach the periphery of the tumor and is incapable of penetrating the cancerous tissue, so of course it is patently inneffective. Chemotherapy also causes endometrial inflammation that leads to atrophy and adhesions, and in more severe cases even the ovaries become inflamed and atrophy. Sometimes the toxicity of chemotherapy and radiotherapy will damage the liver, kidney, PNS, and CNS, which interferes with the gonadal axis secretory function inhibiting its natural feedback mechanism. I suspect these two factors could play a role in the patient's amenorrhea. The patient is only 40 y/o so I anticipate that following a TCM treatment regimen for a period of time her menstral cycle will regain normal function.

The metastatic spread to the lung presenting with white foamy sputum can be identified as water-cold shooting into the lung pattern and suggests the patient most likely has pleural or pericardial effusion. First, you should check to see if the patient has edema on the wrists and shins, if so, this is a sign that there is fluid build-up in the thoracic cavity and your initial prescription should be to disinhibit water in the thoracic cavity. Once the water has been disinhibited the tumor will become inactive.

As for TCM medicinals, I would prescribe Chai Ling Tang (large doses of Fu Ling and Ze Xie) adding Ma Huang, Xing Ren, Ting Li Zi (large dose), Fang Ji, Ren Shen (powder), Chuan Qi (powder), and Da Huang (small dose). Remember! At the onset you must "not" add Gan Jiang, Fu Zi, and Yu Gui; only after most of the water (fluid) has been cleared should you gradually add these great heat supplementing medicinals.

For bone metastais, Cu Lu Jiao still offers the best effectiveness in improving the patient's condition. If pleural effusion presents along with low levels of Hb, WBC, PLT, and T-Pro, then of course, you should immediately add large doses of Ren Shen (powder) (best to gradually add up to 5~7 qian), Cu Lu Jiao, Gan Jiang, Fu Zi, and Yu Gui. If there is metastatic spread to the bone of the lower extremities, then add Chuan Qi (powder), Niu Xi, and Di Long.

If it is only mild pleural effusion, then you can prescribe yang-supplementing, qi-supplementing, and blood-quickening and stasis transforming medicinals along with small doses of water-disinhibiting by bland percolation medicinals. These medicinals will soften the tissue surrounding the tumor; and if the patient decides to go ahead with chemotherapy and/or radiotherapy at that time, then the efficacy will be substantially enhanced. If pleural effusion does "not" present, then you could consider prescribing variants of either You Gui Yin, Shen Qi Wan, Zhen Wu Tang, or Shi Quan Da Bu Tang adding Ren Shen (powder),

Chuan Qi (powder), Huang Qi, Huang Qin, Huang Bo, and Lu Jiao. If Hb is low and CR high, then add Xi Lu Rong (powder). You could also consider adding Fu Ling, Ze Xie, Ting Li Zi, Cang Zhu, and Zhu Ling based on the presenting signs, symptoms, and pattern.

Case Study #5: Hormonal Therapy

Q: The patient is a 62 y/o female who began hormone replacement therapy (HRT) 11 years ago to treat what her doctors suspected were menopausal syndrome related symptoms (e.g. hot flashes, profuse sweating). Several years later a malignant tumor was discoverd in her left breast. Following surgical resection her doctor advised her to take Fareston (SERM) and an aromatase inhibitor. After taking the medication, the hot flashes increased in frequency to over 20 times per day, profuse sweating occurred at intervals throughout the day, and prior to attacks she would feel a prickly sensation in the skin all over her body. In hopes of relieving these symptoms, I recently prescribed Bu Zhong Yi Qi Tang adding Qing Hao, Di Gu Pi, and Zhi Mu, but it wasn't helpful at all. Do you think I have failed to accurately identify the patient's pattern? Would Jian Ling Tang variant be a better formula for her condition?

A: The patient's menopausal syndrome type symptoms of hot flashes and profuse sweating worsened after taking Fareston (a SERM class drug like Tamoxifen). The underlying pattern here is clearly yin vacuity, but I have provided a more detailed pattern identification analysis below. This condition can be identified as one of the following three patterns and treated accordingly:
1) Emotionally-derived: Chai Hu Long Gu Mu Li Tang adding Qing Hao, Zhi   Mu, and Di Gu Pi.
2) Kidney and liver yin vacuity and hyperactive yang pattern: Variants of either   Zhi Bo Di Huang Tang or Dang Gui Liu Huang Tang; or Ba Xian Chang Shou   Wan adding Zhi Mu, Huang Bo, Qing Hao, Di Gu Pi, Long Gu, Mu Li, Dai   Zhe Shi, Gan Cao, and Long Yan Gan.
3) Yang straying outward pattern: Jian Ling Tang (Gan Cao) adding Long Yan   Gan, Qing Hao, Zhi Mu, Di Gu Pi, and Huang Bo (in cases of severe heat   consider adding "the Three Yellows").
Based on your description, I would identify this patient as yang straying outward pattern, thus I would go with the Jian Ling Tang (Gan Cao) variant.

Case Study #6: Lung, Liver, and Lymphatic Metastases

Q: The patient is a 62 y/o female who was diagnosed with left-sided breast cancer and had surgical resection 3 years ago. This year she began having shortness of breath and heaviness in the chest so she went to have it checked out. Examination confirmed the cancer had spread to the lung, liver, and lymphatics. At this stage, what's the best treatment approach?

A: If the patient has already started chemotherapy, then I would prescribe Chai Ling Tang adding large doses of Fu Ling, Ze Xie, Ting Li Zi, Ma Huang, Xing Ren, Fang Ji, Da Huang, Ren Shen (powder), and Chuan Qi (powder); and if hematopoietic dysfunction presents, then add Gan Jiang, Fu Zi, Yu Gui, and Xi Lu Rong. If the pateint has not received chemotherapy, then you can still prescribe the above prescription subtracting Gan Jiang, Fu Zi, and Yu Gui and adding Tong Jing Fang instead. If there is metastases to the lymphatics presenting with swollen lymph nodes and tidal fever, then add Qing Hao, Zhi Mu, and Di Gu Pi. Shortness of breath suggests pleural effusion for which Chai Ling Tang variant (do "not" add Gan Jiang, Fu Zi, and Yu Gui) can be prescribed to relieve symptoms and allow the patient to live in harmony with this condition.

Case Study #7: Vegetarian Diet – Devastating for Chemotherapy and Radiotherapy Patients

Q: A 58 y/o female patient received treatment for breast cancer 7 years ago and it wasn't until a recent examination that multiple metastatic bone lesions were discovered. At the time of discovery, lab test results showed CA15-3 36 and WBC 4000. She decided to receive treatment with infusions of anticancer agents and oral aromatase inhibitors (already on her third different one). Currently, lab results show WBC 2100 and CA15-3 28.4, and a CT scan revealed metastatic spread to the skull. Other signs, symptoms, and history are as follows: reflux gastritis; Ca, P, and K levels are normal; and the patient has now begun a vegetarian diet. I prescribed Xiang Sha Liu Jun Zi Tang adding Gan Jiang, Fu Zi, Mu Dan Pi, Chi Shao, Cu Lu Rong, and Chuan Qi (powder). Do you think this will be effective?

A: Cancer patients must maintain healthy and balanced nutritional intake in order to overcome the side effects of chemotherapy and radiotherapy in order to prevent T-Pro and Hb levels from falling too low, which could lead to hemolysis and death. It really isn't good for cancer patients to maintain a strict vegeterian diet or suddenly change eating habits becoming a vegetarian as a result of cancer diagnosis. This is especially the case for vegetarians who receive chemotherapy. Chemotherapy inhibits a broad spectrum of metabolic and endocrine mechanisms causing severe inhibition of bone marrow function (hypoplasia and fibrosis), while the suppression of the kidney's capacity to secrete hormones such as granulocyte-colony stimulating factor (G-CSF) and EPO further leads to a poor blood picture. Once these physiological mechanisms have been disrupted, bringing the body back into homeostasis is very difficult. Thus, you should aggressively encourage your patient to at the very least eat plenty of eggs and milk along with a variety of nuts and grains (including brown rice, pearl barley, and soybeans), which are all high in vitamin B complex. You should also prescribe "starchy" TCM medicinals to promote appetite (e.g. Si Sheng Tang (Lian Zi, Qian Shi, Huai Shan, and Fu Ling)); Dan Shen, Dang Shen, and Ren Shen (powder) to improve hematopoiesis; and large amounts of Gan Jiang, Fu Zi, Yu Gui, and Cu Lu Rong. Administration of these medicinals follows the key treatment principle of "supplementing to benefit attacking and supplementing as a substitute for attacking."

For breast cancer patients who have received chemotherapy, if the CA15-3 levels are high this suggests potential for relapse. At this time, you can prescribe Xiang Sha Liu Jun Zi Tang variant; and if Gan Jiang and Fu Zi are added, you must remember to include appropriate amounts of "the Three Yellows" (to counterbalance the heat) along with Mu Dan Pi and Di Gu Pi. Remember! Monitoring and attempting to maintain CA15-3 within the normal range is a guiding principle in my treatment approach. If CA15-3 levels increase again, then this suggests that bone metastases has occurred and you can add medicinals such as Cu Lu Jiao, Yin Xing Ye, Chuan Qi (powder), Sheng Du Zhong, Di Long, Gou Ji, and Xu Duan. Bone belongs to the kidney and Cu Lu Jiao can inhibit the tumor vasculature from generating hormones inhibiting tumor angiogenesis and tumerogenesis, thus ensuring the tumor remains stalled in the G1 to G0 phase, unable to rapidly proliferate. In fact, the actions of other TCM medicinals such as "the Three Yellows," Mu Dan Pi, and Di Gu Pi function in the same way.

Case Study #8: Be Careful of Contracting HPV

Q: A 41 y/o female breast cancer patient contracted human papillomavirus (HPV) following radiotherapy and chemotherapy. I followed your advice by prescribing Xiao Chai Hu Tang adding large doses of Huang Qin (8 qian), Mu Dan Pi, Zhi Zi, Long Dan Cao, and Pu Gong Ying. After taking the formula for 1 month the HPV completely resolved. Thanks for your guidance!

A: Ah! Administering Xiao Chai Hu Tang adding Mu Dan Pi, Zhi Zi, Long Dan Cao, and Pu Gong Ying to successfully treat HPV in a breast cancer patient following radiotherapy and chemotherapy. Congratulations! This is a good case study. You should organize the material and submit it to a professional medical journal in South Korea or even an international publication.

Case Study #9: Acupuncture Treats HPV

Q: I followed your advice prescribing Xiao Chai Hu Tang adding Long Dan Cao along with acupuncture to treat a breast cancer patient presenting with flushing, hot flashes, and HPV infection following radiotherapy and chemotherapy. The treatment was very effective as the HPV tested negative.

The most noteworthy aspect of this case for me was the selection of acupoints for the treatment regimen— Feng Chi (GB20), Shen Men (HT7), Shao Fu (HT8), and San Yin Jiao (SP6)— needling 1x/week. After just 4 treatments (weeks) the condition had improved by over 70%. I intend to present these results at a TCM conference in the US.

A: Congratulations on your successful treatment of HPV, and I wish your presentation the best of success!

Case Study #10: Intermittent Plueral Effusion

Q: A 58 y/o female patient was first diagnosed with left-sided breast cancer, surgical resection was peformed, and 2 years later a 6 cm tumor was discovered in the right lung. After receiving radiotherapy and chemotherapy, the tumor shrank to 2 cm and the patient's condition relatively stabilized, but she was still hindered by the pleural effusion of the right lung. Examination did not reveal metastatic spread to the pleura and the patient didn't have the classic symptoms of intermittent fever, shortness of breath, or difficulty breathing when lying down. However, this pleural effusion problem remained intermittent with symptoms presenting at times and then resolving.

A: There are many potential causes of right lung pleural effusion, including spontaneous occurrence, infection, inflammation, trauma, cardiopulmonary disorder, uremia, sequelae of cirrhosis with ascites, immune system abnormalities, and cancer. If the patient has undergone treatment, the condition may become chronic with a small quantity of pleural effusion that typically does not produce obvious symptoms. I have come across something like this before with a patient having an air-filled cyst located between the lower lobe of the right lung and the diagphram, which was so large it had compressed the right lung down to the size of a fist. Despite the extent of this distortion, the patient didn't have any symptoms, and it was only upon routine physical examination that this abnormality was discovered. In any case, the best formula for treating right lung pleural effusion is still Chai Ling Tang variant adding large doses of Fu Ling, Ze Xie, Ting Li Zi, Fang Ji, Qing Hao, Zhi Mu, Di Gu Pi, Ren Shen (powder), and Chuan Qi (powder). For this condition, patients must take this formula for 3~6 months before administration can be gradually discontinued.

Case Study #11: Leukopenia Following Radiotherapy

Q: A 43 y/o breast cancer patient presented with leukopenia following radiotherapy. How should I treat this?

A: One of the potential adverse effects of radiotherapy is hematopoietic suppression. Fortunately, radiotherapy to the chest area in breast cancer cases is typically not as severe as irradiation to the bone marrow of the long bones! The cardiopulmonary system plays an integral role in hematopoiesis with the lungs secreting "precursors" to EPO, whereas the majority of "functional" EPO is secreted by the kidneys (with small portions secreted by the lungs, liver, fat, and marrow.) Lung and myocardium damage may occur when breast cancer patients undergo radiotherapy and thus cause anemia and leukopenia. These adverse effects can be effectively treated through an integrative TCM and Western medicine approach.

Case Study #12: Is Pregnancy Safe for Breast Cancer Patients Following Treatment?

Q: A 34 y/o breast cancer patient underwent mastectomy on her left breast followed up by radiotherapy, chemotherapy, and hormonal therapy. Now, she wants to get pregnant, but her oncologist strongly opposes this idea. What is your opinion?

A: Indeed, it is not advisable for breast cancer patients whom have been administered Tamoxifen following radiotherapy and/or chemotherapy to get pregnant right away. The reason is because the fetal cells differentiate rapidly very similar to cancer cells. Once a woman becomes pregnant, the high nutrient diet required provides ample sources of fuel for cancer cells to exploit, which can differentiate faster than fetal cells. This opens up the possibility for relapse and multiple metastases during gestation. This puts everyone involved in a difficult position. The best thing to do is temporarily hold off on pregnancy.

That doesn't mean she should never become pregnant. It's best for patients to wait until their breast cancer condition has stabilized. Once stabilized, discontinue the use of Tamoxifen and take either Ru Mo Si Wu Tang adding "the Three Yellows;" Di Gu Pi Yin variant; or Zhi Bo Di Huang Tang adding "the Three Yellows," Qing Hao, Zhi Mu, and Di Gu Pi. After a period of time, have lab tests taken to determine if the patient is hormone receptor-negative, and if so, continue administering TCM medicinals for 6 more months. At that time, the patient will be ready to prepare for pregnancy!

Case Study #13: Adverse Effects – Long-term Administration of Tamoxifen

Q: Why is it that over 70% of breast cancer patients who take Tamoxifen (SERM) for 1~2 years develop fatty liver, but their GOT/GPT levels are normal? What's the best way to approach this?

A: Long-term administration of Tamoxifen (SERM) may cause a number of side effects, including hepatitis, fatty liver, cirrhosis, neuropathy, edema, blood clots, and sometimes even endometrial cancer. These can all be identified as stasis heat with water amassment, and treatment is as follows: 1) Ru Mo Si Wu Tang adding "the Three Yellows," Mu Dan Pi, Fu Ling, and Ze Xie, which funtions to inhibit hormone receptor-positive response and reverts it to negative, while also lowering the CA12-5 and CA15-3 levels. Administration of this formula will eventually enable the patient to discontinue Tamoxifen; or 2) Includes various approaches each with distinct advantages and disadvantages that can be selected based on the individual patient's constitution and condition: a) Continue taking Tamoxifen while gradually reducing the dose; b) Administer TCM medicinals and discontinue Tamoxifen; or c) Wait until CA12-5 and CA15-3 levels return to normal before discontinuing Tamoxifen.

Case Study #14: TCM Medicinal Prescriptions Must Flexibly Respond to Patient's Condition

Q: I have a 62 y/o female patient with breast cancer that has already metastasized to the lung and left femur. She has received various regimens of radiotherapy and chemotherapy, and is currently taking Tamoxifen. Now, her WBC remains at low levels of 2000~2800, so I prescribed Xiang Sha Jun Zi Tang adding Gan Jiang, Fu Zi, Yu Gui, Ren Shen (powder), Chuan Qi (powder), and Dai Zhe Shi. I added Dai Zhe Shi because of her reflux esophagitis. After taking this formula her WBC level increased from 3000 to 6000 and the patient now wants to stop taking the TCM medicinals. What's your opinion on this case?

A: Congratulations on your patient's WBC increasing. If your patient wants to stop taking the medicinals now that would be fine. In the future, if she wants to continue with TCM treatment you must pay close attention to increases in the tumor markers CA12-5, CA19-9, CA15-3, and CEA.

If levels do rise above normal, then you should either subtract or reduce the dose of Gan Jiang, Fu Zi, and Yu Gui. Administration of "the Three Great Yang-Supplementers" may cause CA12-5, CA15-3, CEA, LDH, and CPK levels to rise; increase blood concentrations of calcium, potassium, and magnesium; and prompt peripheral blood stem cells to differentiate thus inducing tumor relapse.

The best thing to do if the aforementioned scenario of relapse does occur is to change the prescription to include blood-quickening, stasis-transforming, blood-cooling, heat-clearing and toxin-resolving medicinals such as Ru Mo Si Wu Tang adding "the Three Yellows," Bai Zhu, Fu Ling, Ze Xie, Mu Dan Pi, Yu Sheng Wan, and Wan Ling Dan. If tidal heat presents, then consider adding medicinals such as Qing Hao, Zhi Mu, and Di Gu Pi; or Chai Hu, Qin Jiao, Tian Men Dong, and Mai Men Dong.

The manifestations of pathoconditions are continuously changing and new Western medicine drugs are being developed every passing day. TCM prescriptions must also continuously evolve and adapt to the conditions, just as it is written in the *Book of Changes*:"If you can one day renovate yourself, do so from day to day, and let there be daily renovation." Another verse that resonates in a similar spirit is "Be diligent and alert from morning till night," which is also a core philosophical principle of traditional Korean medicine (TKM). But remember! You must always be discerning. Do not adjust the TCM formula contents too quickly or drastically and always carefully consider the results of biomedical lab tests (e.g., CBC, tumor markers) and other diagnostic tools. After all, these are the fundamental principles of an integrated TCM and Western medicine treatment approach, and combined with pattern identification provide the basis for which to fine-tune your prescriptions.

Case Study #15: Increased CA15-3 and Thrombocytopenia

Q: I have a 60 y/o female breast cancer patient with metastatic spread to the lung and femur. After taking Tamoxifen, lab tests showed CA15-3 1869 (normal range is lower than 25) and WBC 2400. I prescribed Ru Mo Si Wu Tang adding Huang Qin (1 liang), Huang Lian, Huang Bo, and Dai Zhe Shi (5 qian), Mu Dan Pi and Chi Shao (8 qian), and Wan Ling Dan (5 pills/3x/pay). However, up to now there have not been noticeable results. Is this because it is a chronic intractable disease? Please offer your invaluable advice and guidance.

A: For breast cancer patients with lung and skeletal (femur) metastases who have taken Tamoxifen but still are hormone receptor-positive, it isn't necessarily appropriate to prescribe Ru Mo Si Wu Tang variant. Bone belongs to the kidneys so Ru Xiang and Mo Yao aren't the best choices. You should change your formula to either Zhi Bo Di Huang Tang or Tong Jing Fang adding "the Three Yellows," Qing Hao, Zhi Mu, Di Gu Pi, Cu Lu Jiao, and large doses of Wan Ling Dan. Regardless of the formula you choose, make sure to include combinations of blood-quickening and stasis-transforming medicinals such as Sheng Du Zhong, Sang Ji Sheng, Liu Ji Nu, Du Niu Xi (or Huai Niu Xi). If water amassment presents, then add Fu Ling, Bai Zhu, Ze Xie, Ting Li Zi, and Fang Ji.

Case Study #16: Lung Metastases – Focus on Increasing WBCs

Q: I have a 61 y/o female breast cancer patient with lung (right lung tumor 5.5 cm) and vertebral metastases (discovered during TomoTherapy). Lab results: WBC 2500 and monocyte 13% (9%~11%). The patient has no presenting symptoms. What treatment approach would you consider for this patient?

A: Typically, for breast cancer patients with lung metastases and lab tests showing WBC 2500 and monocyte 13% following chemotherapy, you can simply focus on increasing the levels of ANC (absolute neutrophil count) and LYM (lymphocytes) to normal range. Monocyte levels will naturally follow suit, so you don't need to worry about them. Your focus should be on increasing the WBC count!

For malignancy of the lung, I generally prescribe Chai Ling Tang as the main formula adding Ren Shen (powder) and Chuan Qi (powder). If chemotherapy is not administered, WBC levels should quickly rebound. If the patient takes Chai Ling Tang variant concomitantly with chemotherapy and the WBC drops once again, then it is tyically very difficult for TCM medicinals to restore normal WBC levels. At this time, it is necessary to add small doses of Gan Jiang, Fu Zi, and Yu Gui to the main formula.

Case Study #17: Bone Metastases – Add Lu Jiao

Q: A breast cancer patient with bone metastases presented with elevated $Ca2^+$ after being administered Fareston (SERM). After adding Cu Lu Jiao to the formula, the hypercalcemia and related symptoms have resolved. Do you think the CT/PET imaging will reveal that the bone tumor has disappeared?

A: Adding Cu Lu Jiao can prevent breast cancer from spreading to the bone, but if Hb, PLT, WBC, and T-Pro levels are low you must first nourish kidney yin and abate steaming bone heat by also adding Ma Huang, Di Long, Niu Xi, and Sheng Du Zhong (or Jin Mao Gou Ji). If the patient has poor appetite and T-Pro and A/G levels are low, then you should change the formula to either Xiang Sha Liu Jun Zi Tang or Bu Zhong Yi Qi Tang adding Huang Qin and Mu Dan Pi. If BUN/Cr levels are high, then first add Gan Jiang, Fu Zi, and Yu Gui; if the condition does not improve, then add Ren Shen (powder), Chuan Qi (powder), and Lu Rong (powder); and if there is still no improvement, then treat this condition as renal failure adding other anticancer medicinals.

Case Study #18: Colorectal Metastases – Nausea and Vomiting Following Chemotherapy and Radiotherapy

Q: Colorectal metastasis was discovered in a 55 y/o female breast cancer patient following radiotherapy and chemotherapy. After receiving 5 infusions of chemotherapy she experienced vomiting and retching. The patient is a very sensitive person to begin with. She has a poor appetite, cannot tolerate foods with peculiar smells or flavors, and virtually everyting she eats makes her feel nauseous; even plain white rice makes makes her want to retch. She has sought treatment from numerous TCM and Western medicine doctors, but nothing has been effective. Her bowel movements vary, sometimes 1 stool/1~2 day(s) and others 3~4 stools/day. How would you approach this case?

A: This patient sounds like she fits the classic description of "cancer neurosis." Some people will have extreme reactions in response to the stimulus of radiotherapy and chemotherapy. In this situation, to stop vomiting and retching I like to prescribe Ban Xia and Fu Ling (powdered medicinals, 2g each/3~4x/day); and once the vomiting and retching subsides, then I would prescribe either Ban Xia Hou Po or Gan Mai Da Zao Tang combining Ban Xia Hou Po Tang. Ban Xia and Fu Ling are virtually flavorless, but if the patient still thinks Fu Ling has an unappealing flavor, then just prescribe Ban Xia by itself, it is "absolutely" flavorless. Once the patient's symptoms improve, then you can gradually add in antiemetic medicinals (formulas) that are sweet in flavor. Once the patient is able to tolerate the sweet-flavored antiemetic medicinals, then proceed to gradually add the slightly more robust flavors of Xiang Sha Liu Jun Zi Tang variant. This formula is the ideal formula because of its function as an antiemetic, improving appetite, promoting the absorption of nutrients and medicinals, and also supplementing the kidney and dispersing swelling.

Prescribing Xiang Sha Liu Jun Zi Tang variant at this time will prove effective in remedying the adverse effects of radiotherapy and chemotherapy, helping the patient overcome the discomforts and enabling her to complete the scheduled radiotherapy and chemotherapy regimens. During the Xiang Sha Liu Jun Zi Tang phase of treatment, if hematopoietic dysfunction presents and this formula proves ineffective at remedying the condition, then you can add Ren Shen (powder), Dan Shen, and Dang Shen; and if this is still ineffective, then you can go ahead and add small amounts of Gan Jiang, Fu Zi, and Yu Gui.

Section 9: Other Types of Cancer

Case Study #1: Tonsillar Cancer – Salivary Gland Hypofunction, Xerostomia, and Aguesia Following Chemotherapy and Radiotherapy

Q: Ten years ago this patient was diagnosed with tonsillar cancer. Following surgical dissection, radiotherapy, and chemotherapy, the patient experienced salivary gland hypofunction, dry mouth (xerostomia), loss of taste (aguesia), and right-sided neck pain and stiffness. My idea is to prescribe Xue Ku Fang variant. Do you think this is a good choice?

A: Virtually all patients receiving chemotherapy and radiotherapy for cancers of the head, neck, and mouth will experience the adverse effects of losing the sense of taste (aguesia), dry mouth, and salivary gland hypofunction (or complete loss of secretion). These conditions require the inclusion of great yang-supplementing medicinals. Yes, you can presribe Xue Ku Fang, but you should also add Gan Jiang, Fu Zi, Yu Gui, Huang Qin, Tian Ma, and Ge Gen. For patients currently receiving radiotherapy and chemotherapy, you can prescribe Sha Shen Mai Men Dong Tang adding Jie Geng and Ke Zi; and if salivary secretions have dried up, then add Gan Jiang, Fu Zi, Yu Gui, Huang Qin, Ren Shen (powder), and Chuan Qi (powder). Both of these formulas are effective in improving the patient's condition. You can reassure the patient that positive results will be noticeable after taking these medicinals for about 3~5 weeks. However, it will take at least 6 months of ongoing administration to completely remedy this condition.

Case Study #2: Gastrointestinal Cancer – Pancreatic and Lymph Node Metastases

Q: A 58 y/o male patient was diagnosed with gastric cancer and colorectal cancer and immediately underwent partial gastrectomy and colectomy. Not too long after surgery pancreatic and lymph node metastases were discovered and the patient received 3 targeted therapy treatments. Recently, follow-up examination revealed metastatic spread to the abdominal cavity and the patient is currently being administered polysaccharide K (PSK). He is still able to go on hikes in the hills and doesn't have ascites or lymphedema. How would you treat this condition? Please offer your guidance and instruction on this case. Thank you!

A: In general, the most important concern for advanced cancer patients is to maintain a good appetite. With a good appetite and positive attitude nutrients will be efficiently absorbed and the patient will be able to continue maintaining a relatively good quality of life. With this in mind, if the patient can still take food, then you can consider prescribing Ban Xia Tian Ma Bai Zhu San, Bu Zhong Yi Qi Tang, Xiang Sha Liu Jun Zi Tang, or Chai Ling Tang variants. You can add medicinals such as Shan Dou Gen and Liang Jiang; Gan Cao, Hong Zao, and Long Yan Rou; and Xian Zha and Ji Nie Jin. Remember! Regardless of which formula you choose, the addition of Chuan Qi (powder), Yu Sheng Wan, and Wan Ling Dan is essential for this treatment regimen.

Ban Xia Tian Ma Bai Zhu San can remedy stomach cold and poor appetite induced by anticancer agents. If necessary, you can add Gan Cao, Hong Zao, and Long Yan Gan. Formulas such as Shen Ling Bai Zhu San, Si Shen Tang, and Shui Lu Er Xian Dan are all moderate in nature (neither hot nor cold) and are appropriate for maintaining health, increasing appetite and absorption of nutrients, and boosting the body's natural capacity to fight cancer. If levels of the tumor markers CEA, CA72-4, and CA19-9 are increased, then you should subtract Gan Jiang and Fu Zi and instead add large doses of "the Three Yellows."

Case Study #3: Cervical Cancer – Colorectal Metastases

Q: Today a female patient visited my clinic who was first diagnosed with cervical cancer and after surgical resection follow-up examinations revealed colorectal metastases. She received chemotherapy without effective results and then became infected with pulmonary tuberculosis. Right now the symptoms are as follows: inhibited defecation (constipation), poor appetite, dry mouth, numbness in the upper and lower limbs, insomnia, and lab tests show tumor markers SCC antigen 48.1 and CYFRA 21 at 9.7. I prescribed Sheng Yu Tang adding Chuan Qi (powder), Da Huang, and Yu Sheng Wan (2 pills/day). Originally, I was thinking about prescribing Ru Mo Si Wu Tang variant, but decided not to because of problems with digestion. I think the most difficult aspect of colorectal cancer is trying to get the tumor to shrink. Please offer your guidance and instruction on this case. Thank you!

A: SCC and CYFRA 21 are lung cancer tumor markers and don't correlate with colorectal metastases. CEA and NSE are also referenced for lung metastases so it would appear that these results could suggest more than infection with pulmonary tuberculosis. As for TCM medicinals, I would prescribe Chai Ling Tang adding Qing Hao, Zhi Mu, Di Gu Pi, Gan

Jiang, Fu Zi, Yu Gui, Xian Zha, Ren Shen (powder), and Chuan Qi (powder). Remember, start out with small doses of Gan Jiang, Fu Zi, and Yu Gui (2~3 qian each), waiting until tidal fever and night sweats subside and then increase to 5 qian or even higher; and you can also consider adding Wan Ling Dan for its potent anticancer actions.

Case Study #4: Prostate Cancer

Q: Is PSA a useful indicator for diagnosing and monitoring patients for prostate cancer?

A: Right now PSA offers the highest specificity of any tumor marker. The problem with accuracy is that patients with prostatitis will also test high PSA levels (false-positive test result) and sometimes PSA levels are normal in people who really do have prostate cancer (false-negative test result). But overall, I would say PSA is accurate at least 70%~80% of the time.

TCM identifies prostate cancer as liver channel damp-heat pouring downward pattern, requiring the administration of either Long Dan Xie Gan Tang, Zhi Bo Di Huang Tang, Zhi Zi Bo Pi Tang, or Huang Lian Jie Du Tang variants. All of these formula variants are effective. Just make sure that the formula includes Long Dan Cao (5~8 qian), Huang Bo (5~8 qian), and Chuan Qi (powder); and if the patient has endured this condition for a long period of time, then add Long Yan He and Chuan Lian Zi. Remember! Patients with chronic constipation often have blood amassment in the urinary bladder that causes bilateral pain in the pubic bones, so you will need to add either Tao Ren Cheng Qi Tang or Di Dang Tang, making sure to incrementally increase the dose of Da Huang to maintain 3~5 stools per day.

Case Study #5: Swollen Neck Lymph Nodes

Q: A 37 y/o female patient explained that she has had swollen lymph nodes in her neck since she was 20 y/o. After taking TCM medicinals for 6 months the swellings disappeared. Is it possible for this condition to be completely cured in such a short period of time?

A: If the lymph node swelling disappeared, then it is most likely not of malignant origin. Typically, benign cervical lymph node swelling (simple goiter) can be identified as Shao Yang heat pattern or caused by infection, including infections of the cervical lymph nodes, ears, nose, mouth, teeth, and lungs. If you accurately prescribe TCM medicinals based on assessment of the signs and symptoms and pattern identification, then you most certainly can expect to see rapid treatment results.

Case Study #6: Non-Hodgkin's Lymphoma (NHL)

Q: A 70 y/o female patient was diagnosed with non-Hodgkin's lymphoma (NHL) and she presented with swelling on the left side of her nose. She is currently receiving chemotherapy and her WBC count is slightly low, but she has a good appetite. Is it necessary for NHL patients to receive chemotherapy?

A: If the diagnosis of non-Hodgkin's lymphoma is indeed accurate, then you can follow the Shao Yang heat pattern treatment approach. You can prescribe either Xiao Chai Hu Tang, Di Gu Pi Yin, or Xi Niu Di Huang Tang variants adding Qing Hao, Zhi Mu, Di Gu Pi, Huang Qin (and/or Huang Lian and Huang Bo), Chuan Qi (powder), Yu Sheng Wan, and Wan Ling Dan. If soft, diffuse swelling of lymph nodes present, then add Si Ling Tang or Wu Ling San adding Huang Qin (large doses), Mu Dan Pi, and Di Gu Pi.

If chemotherapy induces leukopenia, then you should add Ren Shen (powder) and Chuan Qi (powder), which should produce a rapid increase in the WBC count. If the WBC count does not increase, then add Gan Jiang, Fu Zi, and Yu Gui. Remember! Once chemotherapy has been discontinued, then you must "subtract" Gan Jiang, Fu Zi, and Yu Gui; otherwise, the lymph node enlargement may return.

Case Study #7: Multiple Spinal Cord Tumors

Q: I have a 38 y/o male patient with a 2 cm x 1 cm coccygeal vertebrae tumor that was discovered 5 years ago. Recently, he had experienced back pain and difficulty rotating his torso. An MRI was performed revealing the presence of 5 variably sized tumors in other parts of his spine. This is a classic case of multiple spinal cord tumors. What's the best way to treat this condition?

A: If the patient does not undergo surgery, then simply prescribe either Ru Mo Si Wu Tang or Di Gu Pi Yin variants. If the patient undergoes surgery, then after the operation administer either (Yu Sheng) Paralysis #2 Formula (Shi Quan Da Bu Tang Variant) or (Yu Sheng) Paralysis #3 Formula (You Gui Yin Variant). Depending on the patients presenting symptoms and progress, you can also consider adding Di Long, Ma Huang, Lu Jiao, and Wan Ling Dan.

Case Study #8: Cervical Artery Aneurysm

Q: An MRI revealed the presence of a cervical carotid artery aneurysm that appeared to be on the verge of rupturing. Do you think the patient should undergo bypass surgery? Or should he just take Aspirin and glycerin? Please offer your guidance and instruction on this case.

A: Among cervical segments of the external carotid, internal carotid, and vertebral arteries, the vertebral artery is the most important. Once the vertebral artery becomes occluded or ruptures virtually every case leads to severe disability with high mortality rates. Right now the only Western medicine drug option a patient with a cervical artery aneurysm has is to take antihypertensive medication to control blood pressure. As far as the options you provided in your letter, I think that a surgical procedure offers the best potential outcome, whether its with coil embolization, titanium clips, or CyberKnife, but they all have their own risks.

The use of anticoagulants like Aspirin is "absolutely contraindicated"; not only are they ineffective, worse, they can induce hemolysis and rupture of aneurysms in other parts of the body. Bypass surgery is also not advisable because the cervical artery would need to withstand enormous pressure and adequate extracorporeal circulation would be a challenge during the operation. Also, the materials used for the bypass surgery would not last for much more than 10~20 years, either becoming damaged or dislodged and likely causing sudden death.

As for TCM treatment, I would prescribe long-term administration of Ru Mo Si Wu Tang, Sheng Yu Tang, or Bu Yang Huan Wu Tang variants, which focuses on preventing rupture by maintaining low blood pressure and vascular wall elasticity and tenacity.

Case Study #9: Syringoma – TCM Treatment

Q: A 48 y/o female patient explained that since about the age of 30 y/o syringomas began appearing on both of her lower eyelids; and she underwent laser surgery to remove them, but the growths reappeared. Now, she has numerous growths appearing on her forehead and cheeks and wants to try treating this condition with TCM medicinals. Would Ma Xing Yi Gan Tang variant be effective at preventing the spread of these growths? Why do these growths continue proliferating in her sweat glands? Some reports from TCM doctors in China advocate using large doses of Xia Ku Hua. Do you think this is an effective approach?

A: Most patients with syringoma don't have the patience for TCM treatment. If the patient is compliant in taking Ma Xing Yi Gan Tang variant for long durations, this formula can definitely improve this condition. You can talk with your patient and suss out the situation. Regarding reports from China advocating the efficacy of Xia Ku Hua, I don't oppose giving it a try, but you must remember that Xia Ku Hua will lower T3 and T4, so it should not be prescribed for patients with low thyroid hormone levels (hypothyroidism).

Instead of Xia Ku Hua, I would consider including combinations of the following medicinals for more effective and quicker results – Zao Ci, Ci Ji Li, Ye She Mei, Que Bu Ta, Lu Lu Tong, and Yao Ren Gou. You can also consider selecting combinations of Mu Dan Pi, Bai Xian Pi, Zhi Ke, Chen Pi, Cang Bai Pi, and the leaves of citrus fruit plants such as oranges, tangerines, Buddha's hand, pomelo, and grapefruit.

Section 10: Therapeutic Side Effects and Novel Therapy

Case Study #1: Radiotherapy-induced Salivary Gland and Gustatory Nerve Damage

Q: I provided acupuncture treatment (acupoints: Tian Chuang (SI16), Tian You (SJ16), Yi Feng (SJ17), He Gu (LI4), and Xia Guan (ST7)) to a patient presenting with xerostomia following radiotherapy. After four treatments (1 per week), the patient had noticeably increased salivary flow, but the patient's sense of taste (hypoguesia) was still impaired (everything tastes bitter). The patient has a very poor appetite, and oddly the only dish he likes to eat is fried saucy noodles, anything else is hard to swallow. Why would this be?

A: For patients incurring xerostomia and hypoguesia following radiotherapy, as long as they can still discern some flavor (e.g. bitter), then this indicates gustatory nerve damage is mild and gradual recovery eminent. Continue with the acupuncture treatment, but I recommend adding moxa for quicker results. I would also recommend prescribing an orally adminstered dual supplementation of qi and blood TCM formula adding yang-supplementing medicinals such as Shi Quan Da Bu Tang adding Tian Men Dong, Mai Men Dong, and Huang Qi (2~4 liang each); Gan Jiang, Fu Zi, and Yu Gui (5~8 qian each); and Ren Shen (powder) and Chuan Qi (powder). This approach should facilitate quick recovery of gustatory sense for spicy and sweet flavors and promote increased salivary flow rate. At the onset, the patient may experience profuse salivory secretions, and then the patient will gradually regain capacity to draw in and swallow the saliva like normal.

Difficulty swallowing is likely caused by damage to the cranial nerves in the brainstem that control swallowing. The patient probably likes to eat fried saucy noodles because this dish is moist so all the patient has to do is lift up his head and let the noodle covered in sauce flow down his esophagus. Remember! You still need to prescribe TCM medicinals to ensure complete recovery of nerve function, and this will require continuous administration over a long period of time. If the patient takes TCM medicinals for a period of time, shows improvement, and then decides to discontinue treatment, at some point the incompletely healed nerves will likely begin regressing into a progressive atrophy.

I have a classmate whom had difficulty swallowing food nearly 20 years after receiving radiotherapy to the neck, and he refused to have an NG tube inserted. In the end, he suffered from severe depression and died of starvation (basically, committing suicide). Inserting an NG tube or undergoing a percutaneous endoscopic gastronomy (PEG) procedure would have enabled the patient to continue taking TCM medicinals through the feeding tube, which would have allowed at least partial recovery and extended his life. I advise you to continue striving to help this patient provide the best care possible.

Case Study #2: Chemotherapy-induced Peripheral Neuropathy of the Upper and Lower Limbs

Q: Among the cancer patients I have treated, many of them have experienced peripheral neuropathies of the upper and lower limbs and urticaria (sometimes so severe that their entire body is swollen) following chemotherapy. How should I treat this condition?

A: Peripheral neuropathy following chemotherapy can be identified as qi vacuity pattern. Simply add large doses of blood-quickening and blood transforming medicinals into your main formula, such as Huang Qi (up to 2 liang), and you will quickly see positive results. For drug-induced urticaria (wind papules), you can bleed (above, on, and below) Da Zhui (DU14) and the well points of the three yang channels (hands and feet); needle Feng Chi (GB20), Shou San Li (LI10), Zu San Li (ST36), Tai Chong (LV3), and He Gu (LI4); and add Lu Lu Tong, Ma Huang, and Gui Zhi, along with large doses of Huang Qin and Sheng Shi Gao to your main formula. This approach will effectively remedy the patient's condition in a short period of time.

Case Study #3: Immunotherapy (Biologic Therapy)

Q: Immunotraherapy (biologic thepy) involves drawing blood from a patient, cultivating the immune system components, and then transfusing them back into the patient. Is this an effective treatment solution? Thanks for sharing your knowledge and advice!

A: Immunotherapy involves drawing a patient's blood, adding oxygen and exposing it to ultraviolet light or other irradiation, and then transfusing it back into the patient's body. For some patients this method can be very effective, but it does come with the risk of causing an allergic reaction, and in severe cases, cerebrovascular, CNS, cardiovascular, and peripheral nerve disorders. Types of immunotherapy include: monoclonal antibodies (e.g., Avastin, Erbitux, Herceptin), non-specific immunotherapies (e.g., interferons, interleukins), and cancer vaccines. Some Western medicine physicians will also concomitantly administer immunosuppressants (e.g., corticosteroids, MTX, cyclosporine) as anticancer agents.

2. HEAD AND CEREBROVASCULAR DISEASES

This chapter includes cases on Parkinson's disease (PD), Alzheimer's disease (AD), CSF hypovolemia, cerebral atrophy (encephalatrophy), senile tremor, essential tremor, cerebral infarction, and periodic paralysis among others. Many potential causes of spasms, twitches, and tremor will be presented along with effective methods of treatment.

Case Study #1: Sex Headaches (Coital Cephalgia)

Q: A 48 y/o female patient came to my clinic with the chief complaint of getting headaches during sexual intercourse. She explained that recently during intercourse she felt stiffness and pain in the right side of her neck and a sharp pain in her right Tai Yang (EX-HN5), which occasionally extended up to Shuai Gu (GB8). The first time this happened the pain so bad she even checked into the emergency room (ER), but was too embarrassed to fully explain the circumstances. It has happened 3 times up to now. She wants to know the cause, if it could be life-threatening, and what she can do, if anything, to prevent these headaches.

A: Sex headaches most often occur in men, especially in those who are overworked and stressed out. It is relatively rare for this to occur in women. The cause similarly could be from overwork, stress, or emotionally-derived; however, the possibility of cerebral aneurysm can't be ruled out, so you should advise her to have an MRI performed. I have treated several patients with this condition and even presented one of the cases when I was invited to share my clinical experiences treating vertigo, dizziness, and headache at the International Symposium of Traditional Korean Medicine held in South Korea. I discussed the administration of either Jian Ling Tang, Wen Dan Tang, Ru Mo Si Wu Tang, or Da Chai Hu Tang adding Tian Ma and Wu Zhu Wu to treat these conditions. If an MRI does reveal a cerebral aneurysm in your patient, then surgery should be immediately performed, either undergoing open craniotomy to clip the aneurysm or endovascular repair using a titanium coil or coil and stenting to "plug up" and prevent the aneurysm from rupturing. Otherwise, a life-threatening rupture could occur at any moment. You must be vigilant!

As I understand, cerebral aneurysms usually occur along a loop of arteries that run between the underside of the brain and the base of the skull. Any type of excessive tension or stimulation, not just during sexual intercourse, can cause pulstaing pain. A cerebral aneurysm is an extremely dangerous condition that must not be taken lightly and when it comes to health there is nothing to be shy about. What you should do now is urge your patient to get a functional MRI (fMRI) and angiography performed as soon as possible, and also prescribe mild TCM medicinals to ensure her condition remains stabilized. Your formula should include Cang Zhu, Fu Ling, and Ze Xie add large doses of "the Three Yellows." It is not advisable to prescribe blood-quickening and stasis-transforming medicinals such as Chuan Qi (powder).

If you want to gain further insight into this condition you can check out a book called *When the Air Hits Your Brain: Tales of Neurosurgery* by Frank Vertosick, Jr., MD. There is a section that presents a case involving mortality from an "accidentally ruptured aneurysm." This is a critical condition. When you receive this letter you should immediately contact your patient and strongly advise her to get examined as soon as possible; and if tests do confirm cerebral aneurysm, then seek immediate treatment.

Case Study #2: Parkinson's Disease (PD)

Q: This is the first Parkinson's disease (PD) patient I have treated. I prescribed Bu Yang Huan Wu Tang adding Gan Jiang, Fu Zi, Yu Gui, Huang Qin, Ren Shen (powder), and Lu Rong (powder). I also needled Feng Chi (GB20), He Gu (LI4), Zu San Li (ST36), Tai Chong (LV3), and Tou Lin Qi (GB15). I added Tou Lin Qi (GB15) because I recently read that research indicates this acupoint improves blood circulation to the brain. The patient currently takes 2 dopamine pills per day. Please share with me your experiences in treating this condition – treatment approach, formula variations, prognosis, etc. Thank you again!

A: I am thrilled that you have embarked into the fascinating realm of neurology! The prevalence of Parkinson's disease (PD) will continue increasing in the future, so you should keep pace with the latest discoveries and developments in this field. For this condition acupuncture assumes a complementary role combined with the primary treatment of TCM medicinals. Indeed, Tou Lin Qi (GB15) may also be effective, but in my experience Feng Chi (GB20) is the essential acupoint for treating this condition. As for TCM medicinals, you can incrementally increase the doses of Gan Jiang and Fu Zi. But remember! Don't overdo it with these great heat yang-supplementing medicinals! Even if CNS symptoms (e.g., tremor, rigidity) are severe, with administration of Madopar at 6~8 times or more per day, the maximum dose I would prescribe is 7 qian. Also, for Ren Shen (powder) you should incrementally increase the dose up to 4~5 qian. By administering this integrated approach, the side effects (e.g., dyskinesia) of the Western medicine drugs can be remedied, enabling the patient to walk with greater stability and maintain more fluid functional movement.

Case Study #3: Limb Tremor – Early Sign of Parkinson's Disease?

Q: I have a 53 y/o female patient presenting with tremor in the left hand, and its more pronounced in cold weather and when she is fatigued. The patient had similar symptoms previously when she had frozen shoulder on her left arm, but that condition has already resolved. This winter after the first big cold front the tremor in the fingers of her left hand intensified. Based on my limited experience treating other Parkinson's disease (PD) patients in which this type of tremor presented at the onset, I suspect that this patient is also presenting with an early sign of PD. Thus, I prescribed Ban Xia Tian Ma Bai Zhu San adding Quan Xie, Wu Gong, Bai Jiang Can, Yu Sheng Wan, and Niu Huang Qing Xin Wan. After taking this formula her symptoms improved dramatically. Please share your views and advice on this case.

A: Yes, this case does sound like it's Parkinson's disease (PD), and the formula you prescribed should definitively be effective. However, Niu Huang Qing Xin Wan is very expensive, and unless the patient is financially capable, she won't be able to take this for very long. PD is not a condition that can be cured in a short period of time. It is a chronic condition that requires long-term administration of medicinals in order to prevent further degeneration, improve symptoms, and ensure a good quality of life. The long-term administration of Bu Yang Huan Wu Tang adding Gan Jiang, Fu

Zi, Huang Qin, and Ren Shen (powder) offers excellent efficacy for the treatment of PD. This is the simplest and best approach I have found for the treatment of PD.

Case Study #4: Early-Onset Parkinson's Disease

Q: A 35 y/o female patient came to my clinic presenting with finger tremor and chest distention. The patient said that prior to getting married about 10 years ago any time she felt excessive nervousness or anger the fingers of her right hand would shake. About 1 year after marriage her symptoms gradually worsened. Recently, she experiences resting tremor even in the absence of emotional swings or pressure, and she also feels distention in the chest and sighs frequently. I diagnosed this condition as Parkinson's disease (PD) and prescribed Ban Xia Tian Ma Bai Zhu San adding Huang Qi (2 liang), Ban Xia, Fu Ling, Ren Shen (powder), and Chuan Qi (powder) (large dose of 3 qian). Do you think this is a good approach?

A: Hand tremor in a 35 y/o patient does suggest early-onset Parkinson's disease. You can prescribe Bu Yang Huan Wu Tang adding Gan Jiang, Fu Zi, Yu Gui, Ren Shen (powder), and Chuan Qi (powder). You don't need to prescribe "the Three Insects." For frequent sighing and distention in the chest, you can add large doses of Ren Shen (powder) (start out with 3 qian gradually increasing to 5 qian) and Huang Qi (start out with 2 liang incrementally increasing by 1/2 liang doses up to 4 liang) to remedy these symptoms. For Parkinson's patients suffering from depression, you can consider adding medicinals such as Yu Sheng Wan, Hong Zao, Long Yan Gan, or You Gui Yin (pulverized raw powder) to your treatment regimen.

Case Study #5: Hemilateral Edema – It's Not Alzheimer's Disease!

Q: A 70 y/o male patient began having symptoms of slow and slurred speech and motor function impairment. He was diagnosed with Alzheimer's disease (AD) by a Western medical doctor and hasn't shown any discernible improvement after taking medication for many years now. Recently, he visited me seeking treatment for right-sided edema of the arms and legs. I prescribed Wu Ling San (Nephritis Formula) adding large doses of Huang Qi, Yin Xing Ye, Dan Shen, Chuan Qi (powder), Tian Ma, Ren Shen (powder), Cang Zhu, Fu Ling, and Ze Xie. Do you think this is a good approach?

A: Current research by medical professionals indicate that Alzheimer's disease (AD) (previously known as senile dementia) results from abnormalities in neurons in the brain and specifically how these neurons connect. The rate at which AD progresses varies among individuals. Symptoms may develop (degenerate) slowly over a period of years, but will be very pronounced in later stages with relatively rapid degeneration. Typically, from the first onset of symptoms (e.g., motor function impairment, behavior and personality changes, mild memory loss (forgets where keys are placed)) to the moderate stage (e.g., decision-making, language skill impairment) may occur slowly over a period of years. But from the moderate stage to the late stage (e.g., severe memory loss (fails to recognize friends and family) and severely impaired cognitive and motor function) this pathocondition usually develops rapidly over a 6-month period. In my opinion, it is highly unlikely that 10 years have elapsed and the patient remains in the same cognitive and motor function state. To me, this suggests that the diagnosis of AD is inacccurate. These types of symptoms (e.g., forgetfulness, memory loss, loss of directional sense, disorientation, expressive aphasia) are more aptly diagnosed as chronic cerebrovascular disease, chronic CNS disorders, or cerebral atrophy. Hemilateral edema has nothing to do with Alzheimer's disease; most likely it is due to nutritional imbalance, remaining in a sitting position for too long, or other systemic disease (e.g., renal disease). I agree with the approach of "first treating the edema," but suggest you change the formula to Bu Yang Huan Wu Tang combining Si Ni Tang adding large doses of Ren Shen (best to use raw ginseng pulverized into powder, gradually increasing the dose up to 5~8 qian), Chuan Qi (powder), and Huang Qin.

Case Study #6: Parkinson's Disease, CSF Hypovolemia, or Cerebral Atrophy?

Q: A 57 y/o male patient with neck rigidity so tight it causes extension (head tilted back) didn't feel up to making a visit to my clinic in person so a family member sought my consultation instead. The patient's history is as follows: Three years ago he began having tremors in his fingers, and over the past month neck rigidity has become so severe that his neck involuntarily remains in an extended position. Even when he uses his hands to draw his neck forward, not long after, the neck will gradually slide back into extension. It is difficult for him to get around and that's why he doesn't want to leave the house. During the past few days his neck has been gradually angling to the left side. I am concerned that he may be showing early signs of Parkinson's disease (PD).

A: Involuntary extension of the neck and spasms suggest CSF hypovolemia or cerebral atrophy. As for treating this condition with TCM medicinals, you can prescribe You Gui Yin combining Bu Yang Huan Wu Tang adding Ren Shen (powder) and Chuan Qi (powder). In the past, I have also had successful results prescribing Ban Xia Tian Ma Bai Zhu San adding Huang Qi (serving as the sovereign medicinal), Ren Shen (powder), Chuan Qi (powder), "the Three Insects," and Lu Rong (powder). You can consider both of these approaches based on your patients presenting patterns, signs, and symptoms.

Case Study #7: Cerebral Atrophy, Parkinson's Disease, or Atypical Parkonsonism?

Q: Four years ago the patient first experienced symptoms of lower limb flaccidity, slow and disjointed speech (expressive aphasia), and hand tremor on exertion, prompting him to get examined at a hospital. MRI findings resulted in the diagnosis of cerebral atrophy, and after receiving years of ineffective Western medical treatment, he lost faith in their approach. The patient has a good appetite and nutritional intake and his stool is normal. Do you think this diagnosis could be accurate? How should I treat this condition? What's the prognosis? If the symptoms are remedied, can the brain function also be restored to normal?

A: Based on your description of his symptoms, it doesn't sound like he has cerebral atrophy. It seems more likely to be "atypical Parkinsonism" and specifically vascular Parkinsonism (aka multi-infarct Parkinsonism) involving progressive aratherosclerosis and embolization. You can prescribe Bu Yang Huan Wu Tang adding Gan Jiang, Fu Zi, Huang Qin, Ren Shen (powder), Chuan Qi (powder), and Yu Gui. The condition should gradually stabilize over time. If you want to gain a more in-depth understanding of this condition, I highly recommend reading the book *Application of Integrated TCM and Western Medicine in the Treatment of Neurological Diseases* (實用中西醫結合神經病學)..

Case Study #8: Essential Tremor among the Elderly

Q: A 75 y/o female patient began having tremors in her upper and lower limbs about ten years ago. At first, these tremors only occurred when she was in stressful situations and under exertion, and the left side was much more pronounced. When she is at rest there is no tremor and she doesn't have any motor, speech, or cognitive impairment. Could this be Parkinson's disease (PD)?

A: There are many potential causes of arm and leg tremor with the most common being physiological factors, cerebrovascular and CNS disorders, cerebral atrophy, cerebellar disorders, chorea (dyskinesias), and Parkinson's disease. One of the main symptoms of Parkinson's disease is hand tremor, which is usually a resting tremor that classically presents as a "pill-rolling" action of the hands, and typically tremor in the legs is rare up until the late stages when some patients develop a shuffling gait. The tremors presenting in chorea (dyskinesias) occur when the body is engaged in movement or action. However, TCM treatment for all of these conditions is very similar – based on the same pattern identification and treatment principles. You can prescribe Bu Yang Huan Wu Tang adding Gan Jiang, Fu Zi, Yu Gui, Ren Shen (powder), Chuan Qi (powder), and Huang Qin as the main formula. If the patient presents with spleen and stomach vacuity, then you can consider prescribing either Bu Zhong Yi Qi Tang, Shen Ling Bai Zhu San, Xiang Sha Liu Jun Zi Tang, or Ban Xia Tian Ma Bai Zhu San adding in the remaining medicinals from the main formula (Bu Yang Huan Wu Tang variant).

Case Study #9: Lower Jaw and Upper Limb Tremor – "Not" Essential Tremor of the Elderly

Q: An 83 y/o female patient began having tremors in her lower jaw and right upper limb. Generally, the tremor only occurs when she feels nervous or under stress and not in the process of speaking; it doesn't occur when she is at rest or talking. Drinking a small amount of alcohol also tends to help remedy the condition. I diagnosed her condition as essential tremor of the elderly and prescribed Bu Yang Huan Wu Tang adding "the Three Insects," Qi Cao, Ren Shen (powder), Long Yan Gan, and Yu Sheng Wan. The patient has taken this formula for over 2 months without any discernible effects. Please advise me on this case. Thank you!

A: Your description of this patient's condition suggests that this 83 y/o elderly woman likely has developed chorea. Treatment will require long-term administration of TCM medicinals; results will take some time to appear and considering her age this will be a challenge! Your goal should be aimed at remedying the symptoms and slowing the rate of degeneration. If you can achieve this feat, you will be acknowledged as a "master" physician in the medical field. You should provide her with psychological support and emphasize the importance of staying active, eating healthy, and getting good sleep. Remind her that in old age minor ailments are inevitable and the best approach is a positive attitude. Let's go!

Case Study #10: Lower Jaw Spasms and Twitching

Q: A 73 y/o female patient began having involuntary spasms in her lower jaw 10 years ago. Recently, the condition has intensified over the past two weeks to the point where, aside from subsiding during sleep, her lower jaw continuously has spasms and twitching. However, it doesn't affect her speech, and her blood pressure and stool are normal. Plesae share your views on this case. Thank you!

A: An elderly female patient presenting with lower jaw spasm and twitching clearly indicates some type of "extrapyramidal" involvement. The TCM classical pathologic terminology for this condition is "spasm" and "tugging and slackening (clonic spasm)," which is now commonly described as Parkinsonism. You can precribe either Bu Yang Huan Wu Tang or Gui Qi Jian Zhong Tang adding Gan Jiang, Fu Zi, Yu Gui, Quan Xie, Wu Gong, Bai Jiang Can, Huang Qin, Ren Shen (powder), Chuan Qi (powder), and Yu Sheng Wan (Remeber! It is imperative to add Yu Sheng Wan for this type of condition!). You can also administer acupuncture (warm needling) selecting Feng Chi (GB20), He Gu (LI4), and Zu San Li (ST36). Treating this condition will take a long time and a lot of patience, but eventually this approach should produce effective results.

Case Study #11: Posterior Cerebral Artery "Beating Like a Drum"

Q: The patient's BP is normal, and he doesn't have headaches nor neck pain and stiffness. It's just that his posterior cerebral artery (PCA) pulsates forcefully and frequently and sometimes it almost feels as if it's "beating like a drum." Why would this be? How should I treat ths condition?

A: A PCA pulsating too quickly and too strongly indicates the condition arises from yang hyperactivity of the urinary bladder channel. In severe cases, patients will be able to hear their heartbeats "beating like a drum." There are many potential causes for this with the most common being sleep deprivation, excessive sexual activity, or both of these together, which makes this condition even more likely to arise. Treating this condition requires the prescription of quieting the spirit with heavy settling medicinals such as Jian Ling Tang adding Gan Cao and Long Yan Gan. If the pulse pounds so forcefully that it "beats like a drum," then add "the Three Yellows"; and if headache presents, then add Tian Ma. If indeed your patient suffers from sleep deprivation and excessive sexual activity, you could also consider adding Zhi Mu and large doses of Huang Bo, or instead prescribe Zhi Bo Di Huang Tang adding Sheng Mu Li and Sheng Long Gu. The most important advice you can give your patient is to get enough sleep (it's optimal to get in 8~10 hours of sleep every night!).

Case Study #12: Cerebellar Atrophy and Cerebral Infarction Inducing Dizziness

Q: A heavy-set male patient with high blood pressure, who says he still enjoys "his share of alcohol," recently went for a medical examination due to frequent dizziness. MRI results revealed cerebral infarction and cerebellar atrophy. Stool and urine is normal. Please offer your advice and guidance on treating this patient.

A: Both cerebrovascular and brain stem infarction can cause dizziness, and cerebellar atrophy will present as balance and gait disorders often manifesting in apprehension of and difficulty walking downhill or down stairs even though the slope is only slight. For the treatment of dizziness caused by cerebral infarction I can suggest three approaches: 1) Bu Yang Huan Wu Tang adding Gan Jiang, Fu Zi, Yu Gui, Tian Ma, Huang Qin, Chuan Qi (powder), and Ren Shen (powder); 2) Ban Xia Tian Ma Bai Zhu San adding large doses of Tian Ma and Huang Qi along with Chuan Qi (powder), Chi Shao, and Yin Xing Ye; and 3) If visceral agitation presents, then prescribe Ban Xia Tian Ma Bai Zhu San adding Gan Cao, Long Yan Rou, and Hong Zao. All of these formula options should produce effective results.

Case Study #13: Cerebral Infarction Complicated by Hydrocephalus

Q: A 62 y/o male patient suffered from cerebral infarction and received treatment. Then, 6 months later hydrocephalus arose with secondary cerebrovascular infarct and mild hemorrhage. I prescribed Bu Yang Huan Wu Tang variant. After taking this formula for 3 months, the symptoms of heaviness of the entire body and mental fogginess dramatically improved, helping him make close to a full recovery. Yesterday his daughter called notifying me that her father has been lethargic and clumsy over the past month, prompting another MRI that showed signs of hydrocephalus, but without increased ICP and no fever. Do you think this could be cerebral atrophy? How should I treat this?

A: For cerebral infarct complicated by hydrocephalus, you can consider prescribing either Wu Ling San (Nephritis Formula) adding Da Huang, Ren Shen (powder), and Chuan Qi (powder); or Ban Xia Tian Ma Bai Zhu San variant adding Ren Shen (powder) and Chuan Qi (powder). If there is constipation, then add large doses of Da Huang (gradually increasing the amount up to about 8 qian); and if the patient is still unable to pass stool, then add Pu Xiao (starting out at 5 fen incrementally increasing until the patient is able to pass stool everyday). Typically, in hydrocephalus patients cortical thinning and atrophy occurs in both hemispheres; and if adhesions form, then increased ICP will present.

Case Study #14: TIA – A Type of Cerebral Infarction

Q: A 65 y/o male patient suffered from stroke and sudden collapse, and after this incident he continues experiencing temporary loss of consciousness during sleep at least once a month. What is the etiology of these blackouts (syncope)? Is it caused by cerebral infarction?

A: Repeated bouts of passing out or collapse (syncope) following a stroke results from a type of cerebrovascular infarction, the correct medical term for this is transient ischemic attack (TIA), also called a "mini-stroke." To treat this condition, you can prescribe Bu Yang Huan Wu Tang variant, and considering South Korea's cold climate it would be best to add Gan Jiang, Fu Zi, Yu Gui, Huang Qin, Ren Shen (powder), and Chuan Qi (powder). If the patient experiences periodic paralysis, then you should have the patient get a blood test to determine further modifications to your formula.

Case Study #15: Nocturnal Cramps – Periodic Paralysis "Not" Cerebral Infarction

Q: In recent years at nighttime during sleep a 66 y/o female patient has been experiencing frequent cramps throughout her entire body (especially in her arms and legs). She had an MRI performed and was diagnosed with a lacunar infarct. Following several months of Western medicine drug treatment the cramps continued to occur (though with lesser intensity). And now she has the sensation of ants crawling under her skin (formication). Do you think this could be a side effect of Western medicine drug treatment? How would you approach treatment of this patient's condition?

A: It sounds to me like this patient has periodic paralysis and not cerebral infarction, and the "ants crawling" sensation is phantom itch. I base this presumption on the fact that if it was cerebral infarction causing her symptoms she would have these attacks the entire day and they should be even more severe during the day when she is active; these symptoms wouldn't just manifest at nighttime! Also, cerebral infarction generally would involve motor function impairment of the extremities, and the absence of these symptoms indicates that your patient's condition has nothing to do with cerebral infarction. You should advise your patient to have lab tests done on her Na and K levels. In cases of hypokalemic-induced attacks, the patient can take oral potassium chloride supplements and avoid carbohydrate-rich meals and strenuous exercise; and in cases of hyperkalemic-induced attacks the patient can eat carbohydrate-rich, low-potassium foods, and avoid strenuous exercise and fasting. Another helpful bit of dietary advice is telling her to buy salt-free soy sauce. As for TCM medicinals, I would prescribe either You Gui Wan or Shen Qi Wan variants.

Case Study #16: Climacteric Hypertension Inducing Headache

Q: A 51 y/o female patient sought my consultation for the treatment of climacteric hypertension with headache. Just as I have done in the past for similar pathoconditions, I prescribed Jian Ling Tang adding Zi He Che. Unexpectedly, the patient's blood pressure rose even higher. Why would this happen?

A: Prescribing Jian Ling Tang variant for climacteric hypertension inducing headache is an accurate pattern identification. If your patient's blood pressure increased, then I would try adding Qing Hao, Zhi Mu, Di Gu Pi, Long Yan Gan, and Gan Cao to your original formula. If headache presents, then add Tian Ma, Chuan Qi (powder), Wu Zhu Yu, and Yu Sheng Wan. Or you could change the main formula to either Di Gu Pi Yin, Zhi Bo Di Huang Tang, Bu Yang Huan Wu Tang, or Wen Dan Tang adding Long Gu, Mu Li, Tian Ma, Qing Hao, Zhi Mu, and Di Gu Pi.

3. CARDIOVASCULAR DISEASES

There is more to the etiology of cardiovascular disease than just angina pectoris and myocardial infarction. For instance, anemia can also cause arrhythmia and sweating from the chest (heart) region. The key is to be aware of these complexities and nuances in order to accurately diagnose and effectively treat pathoconditions of the cardiovascular system.

Case Study #1: Palpitations and Tachycardia – Wolff Parkinson White Syndrome

Q: A 26 y/o male patient experienced symptoms of palpitations and tachycardia and thus went for an examination. He was diagnosed with Wolff Parkinson White (WPW) syndrome. Two years ago, the patient had a surgical procedure done on his heart. Since then, he has been taking Western medicine drugs continuously over the past two years, yet he still frequently has palpitations and tachycardia. These attacks are very painful and distressing. What would you do for this patient?

A: WPW syndrome is a a type of atrioventricular reentrant tachycardia in which there is an extra electrical pathway of the heart. Regardless of the type of surgical procedure or catheter ablation Western medicine performs, TCM treatment is pretty much the same. I would prescribe either Xiao Chai Hu Tang combining Long Gu Mu Li Tang; Jian Ling Tang adding Gan Cao, Long Yan Gan, Huang Qin, Mu Dan Pi, and Zhi Zi; Gan Mai Da Zao Tang combining Ban Xia Hou Po Tang; or Wen Dan Tang adding Long Gu and Mu Li. The patient's symptoms will be relieved and gradually resolved.

Case Study #2: What Is Wolff Parkinson White Syndrome?

Q: A friend of mine has had a feeling of oppression in the chest since childhood, but never underwent any special investigations or treatment. Recently, his company provided free medical examinations for employees and this is when he was diagnosed with Wolff Parkinson White (WPW) syndrome, a condition that commonly causes chest pain and tightness, palpitations, and tachycardia among other symptoms. His Western medical doctors recommended having a catheter ablation procedure performed, otherwise ventricular fibrillation (VF) may arise and rapidly lead to sudden cardiac arrest and death. However, the only symptoms the patient has are occasional palpitations and these really don't affect normal livelihood and quality of life at all. Is this condition really as severe as the Western medical doctors say it is? Considering the potential complications of surgery, what advice should I give him? Forego surgery and solely administer TCM medicinal treatment? Or go ahead with the surgery first and then administer TCM medicinal treatment to regulate his constitution?

A: If you are certain about the WPW syndrome diagnosis, I am not opposed to performing the catheter ablation procedure. This is a relatively minor procedure that is in principal very safe. As for TCM medicinals, you can prescribe either Zhi Gan Cao Tang or Gan Mai Da Zao Tang combining Ban Xia Hou Po Tang; or Zhi Bo Di Huang Tang or Wen Dan Tang adding Fu Ling and Hou Po (large doses each), Long Gu, and Mu Li. All of these variants should provide effective results.

Case Study #3: Coma Following Cardiac Arrest

Q: A patient is now comatose after incurring a cardiac arrest, but stimulus to the fingers did elicit a contraction response. What's the best approach for treating this pathocondition? How long does it usually take for the patient to regain consciousness? Thank you for your ongoing guidance and advice.

A: This cardiac arrest comatose patient you refer to most likely results from the ensuing cerebral hypoxia brought on by impaired circulation. You can prescribe Bu Yang Huan Wu Tang adding Gan Jiang, Fu Zi, Yu Gui,

Huang Qin, Ren Shen (powder), and Chuan Qi (powder). After administering this formula for a period of time the patient will show gradual improvement and eventually regain consciousness. After regaining consciousness the patient will feel sluggishness and weakness with limp limbs, weak neck, inability to lift eyes upwards, and drooling similar to that of a stroke patient. Assess the patient's condition after administering the above formula for 1 month, and if there hasn't been much progress, then change the formula to You Gui Yin adding Huang Qi, Ren Shen (powder), and Chuan Qi (powder). If there is neck and lumbar weakness, start out by adding Xi Lu Rong (powder) (5 fen) (incrementally increasing the dose by 5 fen each time up to as much as 3 qian per day). The patient's family must have patience. This treatment regimen will take time, but gradually the patient will achieve substantial recovery of functional capacity and increased quality of life.

Case Study #4: What is Marfan syndrome?

Q: I have a 13 y/o female patient whom is 178 cm tall with disproportionately long arms and legs. Recently, she has experienced shortness of breath during activity and thus her mother brought her in for a visit. Ten years ago her father suddenly died as he was eating dinner and on his death certificate the cause was determined to be a ruptured aneurysm. Ever since then she has been worried about following in his fateful footsteps. Five years ago (8 y/o), she experienced irregular heartbeats, prompting a thorough examination and subsequent diagnosis of heart valve disorder. Considering her disproportionately long arms and legs and concomitant heart condition her doctors suspected Marfan syndrome, but since there were no other specific symptoms to support this diagnosis she was advised to return for follow-up investigation every 6 months. Please share with me your knowledge of Marfan syndrome? What kind of treatment and/or advice can TCM provide?

A: Marfan syndrome is a genetic disorder of the connective tissue caused by defective genes and commonly leads to abnormalities in the limbs, eyes, and internal organs (i.e., heart). Most patients will present with a distinguishing feature of long arms that extend down near their knees. In classical TCM texts, this condition is described as "abnormal contention," or to use a more contemporary and colloquial description "out of sync;" and many famous leaders, both civic and military, were described as possessing this feature (such as the legendary character Liu Bei in *Romance of the Three Kingdoms* with "arms and legs that hung beyond his knees). As for your patient, if she doesn't present with any symptoms, then treatment is unnecessary. If symptoms do arise, then simply identify the pattern and treat the symptoms accordingly. For instance, if cataracts present, then treat the cataracts or if cardiovascular disorders present, then treat the cardiovascular disorders and so on. Usually, these complications will not cause mortality, but patients with this condition can expect a slightly shorter life span than average (late 60s). There is no evidence whatsoever that her father's aneurysm had anything to do with Marfan's, so she doesn't need to worry about that at all! If taking TCM medicinals would make the patient feel at ease, then you can prescribe long-term administration of Bu Yang Huan Wu Tang variant. If edema presents, add Bai Zhu, Fu Ling, Ze Xie, Ren Shen (powder), and Chuan Qi (powder).

Case Study #5: Angina Pectoris (Stable Angina), Psychosomatic Disorder, or Esophageal Ulcer?

Q: A 43 y/o male patient has experienced pain and discomfort in his chest for the past 3 years. He was diagnosed with angina pectoris by Western medical doctors and administered treatment with nitroglycerin and anticoagulants. Three months ago at nighttime while in bed he incurred an attack of sudden, severe pain in his chest with the pain radiating to his left-side pericardium channel. At other times following this initial attack he would experience similar sudden episodes of pain when at rest, which forced him to check into the emergency room (ER) on numerous occasions. Previously these episodes would only occur at night or dawn with the chest pain lasting for increasingly longer durations. A recent episode lasted 6 hours and went unremedied despite taking medication and receiving an injection. Do you think this patient's condition could be improved by having a surgical procedure performed?

A: From your description, it sounds like this patient may not actually be suffering from angina pectoris; instead, his symptoms may derive from psychoneurosis or psychosomatic disorder. I recommend you prescribe a spirit-calming formula and try to help him open up and resolve underlying psychological issues. By doing so, the patient's condition should improve. There are so many of these types of cases nowadays.

Other considerations for this patient's condition could be gastroesophageal reflux disease (GERD) induced esophageal ulcer; intake of oral medication without adequate water or while eating, resulting in the pill or capsule sticking to the mucous membrane and causing erosion; or these episodes may stem from the habit of eating a "bedtime snack" of spicy (chili pepper) and sour scalding hot soup right before bed, inducing acid reflux and resulting in these "attacks" at nighttime. For these types of conditions, you can prescribe Bu Yang Huan Wu Tang adding Ban Xia, Fu Ling, Lai Fu Zi, Hai Piao Xiao, "the Three Yellows," Yuan Hu, and Mu Xiang. However, it is important to sip and gargle the decocted liquid and make sure it is taken either cold or at room temperature. You could also needle acupoints Tai Chong (LV3), Zhong Feng (LV4), Zu San Li (ST36), Nei Guan (PC6), and Shen Men (HT7) as well.

Case Study #6: Arrhythmia Resulting from Anemia

Q: Last year a 38 y/o male patient suffered from acute lower limb edema, difficulty breathing (dyspnea), and oliguria (urine output below 500cc). He went to the hospital for examination where he was prescribed diuretics and antihypertensives and advised to maintain a low-salt diet. His symptoms resolved and subsequently aspirin was also prescribed. Currently, the patient has no symptoms and a cardiac contractility of 15% (normal range 55% ~75%). He wants to take TCM medicinals to regulate his constitution. Do you have any advice or suggestions?

A: The patient's signs and symptoms suggest chronic heart failure with anemia, and the patient may also have mild lung blood depression (stasis) and obstruction (e.g., pericardial effusion, pleural effusion). For this condition, you can prescribe Bu Yang Huan Wu Tang adding Gan Jiang, Fu Zi, "the Four Ling's," Ting Li Zi, Fang Ji, Huang Qin, Ma Huang, Xing Ren, Ren Shen (powder), and Chuan Qi (powder); or Wu Ling San (Nephritis Formula) (including large doses of Fu Ling and Ze Xie) combining Bu Yang Huan Wu Tang adding Ting Li Zi, Fang Ji, Ma Huang, Xing Ren, Ren Shen (powder), and Chuan Qi (powder). Remember! Regardless of which formula you choose, it is essential to add Ma Huang and Xing Ren for this pathocondition. This will require long-term administration up until CT scan images reveal no pericardial or pleural effusion and the patient is able to exercise normally (consisting of walking at a slow pace for a mininum of 3~5 hours) without experiencing any discomfort or noticeable symptoms. That's when you know the patient's condition has been successfully treated, and at that time, you can gradually discontinue administration of TCM medicinals.

Case Study #7: Sweating from the Chest – One of the Sweating in the

Five Hearts

Q: A 73 y/o male patient presented with mitral valve insufficiency (left atrial hypertrophy), arrhythmia, and occasional shortness of breath, and has been receiving treatment with Western medicine drugs for many years now. Recently, he has experienced profuse sweating from the chest and is concerned the condition could get worse, so he came to me for consultation. He hopes to wean away from Western medicine drugs taking TCM medicinals instead. What is your opinion? Would Fu Ling Bu Xin Tang variant be effective?

A: Sweating from the chest is one of the sweating in the five hearts, but it doesn't have any specific correlation with mitral valve insufficiency (left atrial hypertrophy), arrhythmia, and occasional shortness of breath. If this condition derived from heart disease, the sweating would occur over the entire body and not just in the chest region. If the condition resulted from pleural effusion, sweating would flow profuse as rain and the patient would have difficulty breathing while lying in a recumbent position. The key is that for any of these conditions you can prescribe either Di Gu Pi Yin adding Zhi Mu, Qing Hao, and Sheng Mu Li; or Xiao Chai Hu Tang adding Qing Hao, Zhi Mu, and Di Gu Pi. In the most severe cases, you can administer Jian Ling Tang (w/ Gan Cao) adding Zhi Mu, Huang Bo, Qing Hao, Di Gu Pi, and Long Yan Gan. These formulas should be able to improve symptoms of profuse sweating.

Case Study #8: Coronary Artery Disease (CAD) (aka Ischemic Heart Disease (IHD))

Q: Coronary artery disease (CAD) can be life-threatening if blood flow to the heart is severely blocked, thus I am always particularly vigilant when treating these patients. I have treated a number of patients with this condition, from milder cases (i.e., arrhythmia, ischemia of coronary arterioles and capillaries) to severe cases (i.e., 80% coronary artery blockage), but unfortunately have never had very effective results. Please share your experience and offer advice about treating this condition.

In the past, for patients with severe cardiac ischemia I usually prescribe Bu Yang Huan Wu Tang adding Gan Jiang, Fu Zi, Yu Gui, Chuan Qi (powder), and Ren Shen (powder) for a duration of 2 weeks to 3 months. For arrhythmia and ischemia of the coronary arterioles and capillaries, I prescribe the same main formula (including a large dose of Huang Qi (2.5 liang)) adding Gan Jiang, Fu Zi, and Yu Gui (1 liang each), Huang Qin, Ren

Shen (powder), and Chuan Qi (powder) for a duration of 1 1/2 months. Do you have any suggestions about any changes that should be made to these treatment regimens?

A: Bu Yang Huan Wu Tang is the most effective formula for coronary artery disease (CAD). If you have already prescribed large doses of this formlula and have not had effective results, then you can try having the patient soak this formula (decocting pieces) in rice wine for 30 minutes up to 2 hours prior to decocting. This will increase the potency of these medicinals' active constituents, direct the medicinals into the upper burner, and enhance the overall blood-quickening and channel and network vessel-freeing capacity of this formula.

Remember! You don't need to add such a large dose (1 liang each!) of Gan Jiang, Fu Zi, and Yu Gui for most cases. Sometimes if the dose is too large, paradoxically, it will act to inhibit heart function, resulting in PR interval lengthening, slow heart rate, irregular heartbeats, and sometimes even causing vasospasms. The best method is to start out at 5 qian each and maintain this dosage for 2~3 months, while continuing to assess the patient's condition. If there isn't much improvement, then increase to 6 qian. Similarly, in another 2~3 months, if there still is not a lot of improvement, then increase to 7 qian. Gradually increasing the dose is particularly relevant for Fu Zi due to its toxic nature: long-term administration in large doses may induce adverse effects of slow heart rate, irregular heartbeats, dizziness, blurry vision and confusion, weakness of limbs, and cold sweats. By starting out prescribing small doses, allowing the body to adapt, and then gradually increasing the dose, you can alleviate the potential for these adverse effects. You can also consider adding Fu Ling, Ze Xie, Ting Li Zi, and Fang Ji to help neutralize the toxicity of Fu Zi. If the patient presents with pericardial effusion and/or cardiopulmonary disease, then you must add Ma Huang into your formula.

Case Study #9: Lower Limb Edema – Heart Disease or DVT?

Q: A 60 y/o female patient has left-sided lower limb edema. Following examination by her Western medical doctors, no specifc etiology was identified, so they prescribed diuretics. She took the medication, but the condition remained the same. That's when she came to me for consultation. This symptom has been present for over 1 year, and palpation on her shin revealed pitting edema that looked similar to lymphedema. Do you think this could be elephantitis or deep vein thrombosis (DVT)?

A: Lower limb edema could be a result of heart disease with most cases arising from pericardial effusion, cardiopulmonary congestion (static blood), and pleural effusion. For the treatment of water accumulation and static blood, you can prescribe either Chai Ling Tang or Wu Ling San (Nephritis Formula) adding large doses of Fu Ling, Ze Xie, Ting Li Zi, Fang Ji, Ma Huang, Chuan Qi (powder), and Ren Shen (powder). For longstanding (chronic) disease you should also add Gan Jiang, Fu Zi, Yu Gui, and Huang Qin. Another approach would be to prescribe Bu Yang Huan Wu Tang adding Cang Zhu, Fu Ling, Ze Xie, Ting Li Zi, Fang Ji, and Ma Huang; and if heat presents, then add Huang Qin, Mu Dan Pi, Zhi Zi, Qing Hao, Zhi Mu, and Di Gu Pi. Remember! Chronic conditions eventually evolve into cold pattern, and thus you must add Gan Jiang, Fu Zi, Yu Gui, and Huang Qin (as a counterbalance) into the main formula.

This patient's condition doesn't sound like elephantitis nor DVT to me. In patients with lower limb "venous" thrombosis (aka deep vein thrombosis (DVT)), dark pigmentation will appear and during the earlier stages the skin is softer and looser; and in patients with lower limb "arterial" thrombosis, the skin is hot, red, hard and swollen. "Venous" thrombosis (aka DVT) can be identified as qi and blood vacuity with yang vacuity and water amassment pattern: the longer the patient stands or walks the greater the swelling, the swelling does not resolve easily, and the skin surrounding the thromosed vessels tends to be itchy and tingly. "Arterial" thrombosis can be identified as stasis heat pattern, over time the condition will evolve into true cold false heat pattern, and eventually in longstanding conditions it evolves into yang vacuity pattern. In both "venous" (aka DVT) and "arterial" thrombosis, a patient who may have enjoyed walking before, now finds herself feeling fatigued and in pain only after a short stroll. If the condition worsens, patients with lower leg thrombosis may incur leg muscle atrophy and weakness.

Case Study #10: Hyperglycemia Following Coronary Artery Stent Placement

Q: A 45 y/o male patient explained that 3 years ago he suffered from an acute myocardial infarction (MI) and received treatment that included placement of a coronary artery stent. Following surgery the patient developed hyperglycemia (AC 200~300), prompting his doctors to prescribe Diaben (Glyburide), but this treatment was not effective. Subsequently, he later suffered from gout, facial palsy, glaucoma cataracta viridis (green cataract), and has distending pain in both eyes. How would you treat this patient?

A: I have already explained this to you previously on numerous occasions. Putting it simply, as explained previously, there are many precipitating factors for the presentation of hyperglycemia that you must consider; it can be caused by more than islet cell inflammation, atropy, and tumors. For example, excessive release of glycogen and muscle glycogen or excessive absorption by the intestinal mucosa; dysfunction of hypothalumic endocrine regulation; vascular endothelial growth factor (VEGF), erythrocyte deformability, and lack of vascular permeability; or even vasculitis, myocarditis, and cardiac hypertrophy are all possibilities. Sometimes there is interference in the feedback system of the glycagon control centers in the brain, which essentially fools the brain into thinking that there is a deficiency so it works overtime to make up for the perceived loss by secreting large amounts of glycogen and muscle glycogen. Tears, burns, contusions, and inflammation of the striated muscle, skeletal muscle, cranial nerves, and marrow; and tumors and edema that induce hemolytic reactions, including leukemia, can all cause hyperglycemia. Therefore, you can see it's necessary to clearly determine the etiology and pathomechanisms involved in order to conduct accurate pattern identification as the basis for determining effective treatment.

If this patient's condition really did result from coronary artery stent placement, then it can be identified as heart stasis heat and static blood with water amassment pattern; if it's pericardial effusion inducing panting and palpitations or myocardial stasis swelling and hypertrophy, then it can be identified as qi vacuity, stasis blood, and water amassment pattern; or if the patient has been administered either TCM or Western medicine anti-inflammatory, antipyretic, anticoagulant, or diuretic medication for long durations without effectiveness, then this can be identified as cold damp with stasis heat pattern. All of these various patterns require the administration of different TCM medicinal treatment approaches.

Generally, for stasis heat pattern you should prescribe blood-quickening and stasis-transforming medicinals such as Di Gu Pi Yin or Ru Mo Si Wu Tang adding "the Three Yelows"; Niu Jiao Di Huang Tang or Liang Ge San; or Zhi Zi Bo Pi Tang or Zhi Zi Chi Tang.

For water amassment pattern, it is essential to include Fu Ling, Zhu Ling, Ze Xie, Ting Li Zi, and Fang Ji in your main formula. For pericardial effusion, prescribe either Chai Ling Tang or Wu Ling San combining Bu Yang Huan Wu Tang; or Ling Gui Zhu Gan Tang, Mu Fang Ji Tang, or Fang Ji Huang Qi Tang.

For cold damp with stasis heat you should prescribe Wu Ling San (Nephritis Formula) combining Bu Yang Huan Wu Tang adding Ting Li Zi, Fang Ji, Ma Huang, Ren Shen (powder), Chuan Qi (powder), Sang Bai Pi, and Sheng Shi Gao; or add Mu Dan Pi, Huang Qin, Huang Lian, Huang

Bo, and Zhi Zi. If blood glucose levels still doesn't come down, then add Bai Jiang Can (or Wan Jiang Sha); Nu Zhen Zi; or Long Yan Gen. These TCM formula variants are specifically for cardiac related hyperglycemic conditions. Obviously, hyperglycemia resulting from other organs, pathomechanisms, and patterns may require different treatment approaches.

4. VASCULAR DISEASES IN OTHER PARTS OF THE BODY

Many sudden onset maladies are caused by vascular disease. If a person's visual field suddenly darkens and partial loss of vision occurs, this suggests the onset of either "ocular stroke" or retinal detachment. If a person walks even a short distance and experiences pain in their leg(s) that requires rest in order to continue, this most likely indicates intermittent claudication....

Case Study #1: Retinal Vascular Occlusion (Ocular Stroke)

Q: One month ago a 43 y/o female patient visited my clinic complaining of partial vision loss in one of her eyes. She explained that roughly 6 months ago she was walking to her car and suddenly "half the sky turned dark" in one of her eye's field of vision. She rushed to the hospital where Western medical doctors diagnosed her with retinal vascular occlusion ("ocular stroke") and subsequently received treatment for 5 months without substantial improvement in her vision. That's when she decided to seek TCM consultation. I prescribed Bu Yang Huan Wu Tang adding large doses of Yin Xing Ye (8 qian), Gan Jiang, Fu Zi, Yu Gui, Huang Qin, Ren Shen (powder), Chuan Qi (powder), Fu Ling, and Ze Xie. Unfortunately, this formula has not produced very effective results; she still has partial vision loss. Do you have any suggestions? Is it possible to effectively treat this condition?

A: Retinal vascular occlusion is also known as "ocular stroke." Just by the name you know the etiology and pathomechanisms are similar to cerebrovascular attack (CVA) (aka "stroke"), and so is the treatment approach. In the treatment of stroke, the process is always slow, and even slower for ocular stroke; it will take at least 3~5 months before you will see any noticeable improvement. That has been my experience treating this condition...patience...patience...and there will be gradual improvement. Prescribing Bu Yang Huan Wu Tang variant is the right approach, just have patience!

Case Study #2: Intermittent Claudication

Q: What is the etiology of intermittent claudication? Is it another kind of vascular occlusion? How should I treat this condition?

A: "Intermittent" means occurring occasionally or at intervals and "claudication" means to limp or walk with difficulty. This is a peripheral vascular disease (PVD) in which blood vessels are either narrowed or blocked. For those afflicted with this condition, walking for a period of time will induce pain, achiness, fatigue, cramping, and/or a burning sensation in the leg(s) to the point the person must stop and rest for a while before they can continue on again.

The etiology of intermittent claudication is varied with some of the more common causes listed here: peripheral vasculature (arterial and venous) of the leg may become narrow and spasm; pain reflex resulting from administration of oral psychotropic drugs (gate control theory); and CNS (brain, brainstem, spinal cord) damage that leads to neural pain transmission to the leg with these "pain signals" remaining in the pain memory centers and thus manifesting as phantom pain (central memory theory). The swelling and pain arising from narrowing and spasm of an artery will typically be accompanied by heat and the skin will feel tauter upon palpation, whereas the swelling and pain arising from narrowing and spasm of a vein will feel suppler without pronounced heat (slightly cool). In the presence of fatigue, aching, and/or pain after walking for moderate periods of time, you must first rule out the possibility of brain tumor and neuropathy before the diagnosis of intermittent claudication can be made.

Nearly all patients with intermittent claudication present with water amassment. Thus, when treating this condition you must differentiate between stasis heat with water amassment pattern and qi vacuity with cold stasis and water amassment pattern. For stasis heat pattern, prescribe Ru Mo Si Wu Tang adding Huang Qin, Huang Lian, Bai Zhu, Fu Ling, Ze Xie, and Chuan Qi (powder); bleed the well points of the affected limb; and administer acupuncture (needling) on corresponding distal acupoints. For qi vacuity with cold stasis and water amassment pattern, prescribe either Bu Yang Huan Wu Tang or Ru Mo Si Wu Tang adding Gan Jiang, Fu Zi, Huang Qin, Bai Zhu, Fu Ling Ze Xie, and Chuan Qi (powder); and administer acupuncture (warm needling) on corresponding distal acupoints.

Regarding the possiblity of intermittent claudication being caused by "pain signals" remaining in the pain memory centers and thus manifesting as phantom pain, you must sill differentiate between drug-induced and CNS damage. For drug-induced phantom pain, once the body develops tolerance the phantom pain will gradually resolve; and if these symptoms do not resolve, then advise the patient to change medication. For CNS damage inducing phantom pain, this condition will gradually resolve as the lesion heals. This type of phantom pain is unique in that every 3~4 weeks there will be recurring episodes of intensified pain for 1~2 days, and every 2.5~3 months there will be a period of about 2 weeks with symptoms of intensified, severe pain. After enduring a few of these intensified periods, the symptoms will rapidly improve up until there is no longer a "pain signal" of this memory stored in the brain. At this time, the symptoms of intermittent claudication will be remedied.

Case Study #3: Varicose Veins (VV) and Deep Vein Thrombosis (DVT)

Q1: A 47 y/o female patient presented with swelling and bruising on both shins with symptoms more prevalent and pronounced when her legs are draped in a sitting position. I diagnosed this condition as varicose veins (VV) with concomitant deep vein thrombosis (DVT) and prescribed Wu Ling San (Nephritis Formula) adding large doses of Huang Qi, Fu Ling and Ze Xie along with Yin Xing Ye, Chuan Qi (powder), Dang Gui, Chuan Qiong, Sheng Di Huang, and Chi Shao. Do you think this is the right approach?

A1: This is an excellent approach for treating VV and DVT, but this case clearly indicates swelling following thrombosis as opposed to thrombosis following swelling, so you only need to make sure to add large doses of Huang Qi and just standard doses of Bai Zhu, Fu Ling, and Ze Xie. Also, to accelerate the dissipation of swelling you can administer acupuncture (warm needling) on corresponding distal extremity acupoints.

Q2: After taking the TCM formula, the swelling in both lower legs improved, but the right leg still had slight swelling and the patient also felt fatigued. Her husband had heard people say, "If you don't have surgery for varicose veins you are susceptible to blood clots that could get stuck in your lungs and cause death." Thus, fearing the possibilty of pulmonary embolism, he encouraged his wife to have a surgical procedure performed. Surprisingly, her condition worsened following surgery (spinal anesthesia was administered) to the point where simply sitting for 30 minutes would result in lower leg swelling and discomfort. So she came back to see me again hoping that TCM treatment would help improve her condition. Is Bu Yang Huan Wu Tang variant still the right formula to prescribe at this time?

A2: Increased swelling following surgery for varicose veins (VV) is mainly due to compromised venous and lymph return. Deep vein thrombosis (DVT), as the name indicates, involves deeper veins and has risks of serious complications. Your treatment objective is to stimulate lower limb circulation, promoting venous return and preventing lymph and fluids from pooling. Yes, you can still prescribe Bu Yang Huan Wu Tang adding Gan Jiang, Fu Zi, Cang Zhu, Fu Ling, Ze Xie, and Huang Bo; or consider prescribing Wu Ling San (Nephritis Formula) combining Bu Yang Huan Wu Tang adding large doses of Gan Jiang, Fu Zi, and Yu Gui. Administer this formula up until the patient is able to walk continuously for long periods without resting or sit continuously for up to 2~3 hours without swelling or stiffness. That's when you know the condition has been cured. Naturally, during the treatment regimen you should also urge the patient to walk for at least 1 hour every day to promote circulation, preventing blood, fluid, and lymph from pooling the legs.

This condition has nothing to do with spinal anesthesia. It is caused by severely compromised venous return resulting from surgery. After any surgical procedure lasting an extended period of time venous return will likely be inhibited and swelling of the lower limbs may occur. For your patient, you must immediately stimulate lower limb circulation and promote venous return, preventing lymph and fluids from pooling. If left untreated, severe cases of DVT can lead the formation of a blood clot (thrombus) that could become dislodged and result in pulmonary embolism and fatality. You must be vigilant!

Case Study #4: Deep Vein Thrombosis (DVT)

Q: A 50 y/o female patient developed symptoms of lower leg swelling and went for examination upon which she was diagnosed with deep vein thrombosis (DVT). Soon after she received vascular surgery and was administered Coumadin (warfarin). Follow-up examination revealed no obstruction in the iliac vein, but the smaller venules located below Wei Zhong (UB40) are still blocked. I happened to be reading a thesis from abroad about brain tumors sometimes causing this type of condition. Is this a viable scenario? What formula should I use to treat this condition?

A: DVT can be identified as heat stasis and cold stasis pattern. For heat stasis pattern, you can prescribe Ru Mo Si Wu Tang adding Huang Lian, Mu Dan Pi, Niu Xi, and Chuan Qi (powder); acupuncture Tai Chong (LV3), Zhong Feng (LV4), and Di Wu Hui (GB42; and bleed the well points on the affected limb(s). For cold stasis pattern, you can either prescribe the same main formula used for heat stasis pattern adding Gan Jiang, Fu Zi, and Yu Gui; or change the main formula to Bu Yang Huan Wu Tang adding Gan Jiang, Fu Zi, Yu Gui, Huang Bo, Ni Xi, Chuang Qi, Cang Zhu, Fu Ling, and Ze Xie; and administer acupuncture (warm needling) at the distal extremity acupoints mentioned above. Typically, cold stasis feels cool and supple on palpation and responds well to TCM treatment (medicinals and acupuncture) with swelling gradually dispersing and the limb feeling light and uninhibited.

Most cases of DVT result from disorders of the heart and cerebral vasculature. Typically, a thrombus (clot) forms in the brain or neck vasculature, breaks away to form an embolus, and then flows downstream causing venous blockage (thrombosis) that results in DVT. Blockage can occur in the arms and legs, but most often it occurs in the legs: this is due to the basic principle "water flows downstream." Once the blood clot is carried down to the lower extremities, if the patient leads a sedentary lifestyle and doesn't get enough exercise (e.g., doesn't even regularly walk a significant distance), then there is an increased possibility of blockage and subsequent swelling. Two factors that make countries such as Korea and Japan particularly susceptible to DVT are cold winters and the habit of sitting cross-legged. *The Yellow Emperor's Inner Cannon* specifically mentions "a lack of walking (circulation)" as a factor involved in "crippling wilt," so you can see clearly here that aside from eating healthy, walking (exercise) and maintaining good circulation (e.g., not sitting cross-legged) are essential for the prevention of DVT.

Case Study #5: Hyperlipidemia

Q: A 56 y/o female patient explained that she has many relatives whom have become afflicted with chronic disease (e.g., liver, heart, diabetes) at around her age, and some have been fatal. With this family history, she has lived health consciously and goes for periodic medical checkups. Despite having only slightly elevated total cholesterol (T. Chol), triglyceride (TG), and blood sugar levels, she is still worried and wants to take TCM medicinals to regulate her constitution.

On the patient's initial consultation her lab tests showed T. Chol/TG 264/232 and GLU AC 184. I have been administering Sheng Yu Tang adding Xian Zha, Ji Nei Jin, Chuan Qi (powder), Huang Qin, and Tu Si Zi for a two-month period now. During her subsequent visits lab test results were (second visit) 256/155 and 175; (third visit) 238/203 and 129; and (fourth visit) 275/274 and 143. Do you think this is a good approach for treating hyperlipidemia? Please share your experiences in treating this condition?

A: This prescription is very good. However, you must be aware of a typical pattern that evolves when attempting to lower T. Chol, TG, GLU, BUA, BUN, and Cr levels. Initial treatment will usually result in successfully lowering these levels down to a threshold before rebounding (not as high a before), leveling off for a period, and then progressively declining again. This is the body's natural protection mechanism working here, ensuring that vital functions are maintained within viable homeostatic parameters and protecting the body against abrupt and dramatic changes that could be life-threatening. This is why it's safer and more logical to administer natural, multi-action, and reversible treatment that adheres to the body's protection mechanism. Once these physiological markers reach a threshold and level off, the only way to go beyond is change the formula or increase the dose.

Generally, for severe ascendant hyperactivity of liver yang, liver channel stasis obstruction, or deficiency of lipid metabolizing enzymes in the liver that leads to increased T. Chol and TG levels, you can prescribe either Long Dan Xie Gan Tang; Huang Lian Jie Du Tang; or Da Chai Hu Tang adding blood-quickening and stasis transforming medicinals such as Chi Shao, Xian Zha, Dan Shen, Gu Sui Bu, Sang Ji Sheng, and Niu Xi.

For patients with "idiopathic" hypercholesterolemia and hypertriglyceridemia, this condition can be identified as yang straying outward pattern. By "idiopathic" I mean that at some point in life the patient's lipid metabolism centers in the brain have been disrupted by toxin; the remnants (i.e., body or fragments) of culled virus or bacteria disrupts the hosts metabolism; or the body produces too many antibodies which interferes with the normal functioning of the endocrine system making it errantly think that it needs to produce large amounts of cholesterol and triglycerides in order to synthesize and produce cells, antibodies, antigens, and complements resulting in overabundance. For patients with this type of yang straying outward pattern, you can prescribe either Jian Ling Tang or

Jian Ling Tang adding Huang Lian Jie Du Tang; Chai Hu Jia Long Gu Mu Li Tang; Zhi Bo Di Huang Tang; or Huang Lian Jie Du Tang adding Sheng Mu Li, Sheng Long Gu, Xian Zha, Dan Shen, and Chi Shao. All of these formulas will achieve effective results.

If the condition is caused by increased instestinal lipid absorption, then it can be diagnosed as either blood amassment and abiding stool or dry repletion and stomach repletion. Mild cases can be idenfitied as stomach heat food accumulation and oil accumulation pattern; and severe cases can be identified as Cheng Qi Tang pattern. You can consider prescribing either Cheng Qi Tang, Ge Gen Qin Lian Tang, Huang Lian Jie Du Tang, Qing Wei San, or Bai Hu Tang adding Lai Fu Zi, Ji Nei Jin, Mai Ya, Gu Ya.

In rare instances, a patient will develop hyperlipidemia as a result of an insufficient amount of digestive enzymes produced in the pancreas, stomach, and bile (liver). This condition can be indentified as binding depression of the spleen qi pattern. Formulas containing Shen Qu with its actions of resolving depression, dispersing food, and opening the stomach (promoting digestion) can be prescribed to treat this condition.

In summary, regardless of the underlying cause, TCM can effectively treat hyperlipidemia (hypercholesterolemia and hypertriglyceridemia). Just remember! Don't discontinue TCM formula administration immediately after T. Chol and TG levels decrease. You must continue administering the formula for 1~2 more months to make sure levels don't rebound. Once your certain acceptable levels are being maintained, then you can gradually reduce the dose until the formula is completely discontinued.

Case Study #6: Gangrene – Poor Circulation of the Lower Limbs

Q: A 48 y/o patient presented with darkened (black) skin on his left lower leg. The skin doesn't feel hot upon palpation and he has numerous large venous aneurysms bulging in this leg as well. The patient explained that he has been afflicted with this condition for 20 years and has been evaluated and treated by many specialists at major hospitals, but nothing has proven effective. Upon closer observation his left lower leg is thinner than his right and the tissue feels noticeably tighter. I suspect the patient has gangrene, but I am not sure if it should be classified as cold type or heat type. Please offer your guidance and advice on this case. Thank you!

A: Based on the symptoms you have described, it sounds like cold type, but you must carefully differentiate between the skin discoloration of venous aneurysms (darkened skin with bruised appearance surrounding the site of the vessel) and gangrene (below a specific borderline the entire lower extremity appears dark purple or black, almost like pig blood cake or charcoal). If the leg is cool upon palpation and the tissue tight, then this can be identified as congealing cold pattern. For this pattern, you can prescribe Dang Gui Si Ni Jia Wu Zhu Yu Sheng Jiang Tang adding Fu Zi, Huang Qin, Ren Shen (powder) and Chuan Qi (powder); and if edema presents following administration, then also add Fu Ling and Ze Xie.

If the skin color is purplish brown or black colored and putrid-smelling, purulent, and bloody discharge oozes from the tissue (serosanguineous discharge) that smells like a dead carcass, this can be identified as heat toxin with blood stasis pattern, requiring administration of Xian Fang Huo Ming Yin or Ji Sheng Jie Du Tang adding Pu Gong Ying and Huang Qin. If the skin color is pale and lusterless, then this can be identified as congealing cold and you can prescribe Gui Qi Jian Zhong Tang. In addition, you should advise your patient to get lab tests done for BUN, Cr, WBC, PT, and APPT; and also maintain a healthy lifestyle that includes adequate sleep, diet, and moderate exercise if possible.

5. HEAD AND NECK DISORDERS

Office workers and "smartphone users" are the demographic that most commonly experience stiffness, soreness, and aches in the head, shoulder, neck, and upper back region. However, there are many other potential causes of head and neck pain that you must be careful not to overlook!

Case Study #1: Foot Tai Yin Phlegm Reversal Headache

Q: Today a female patient visited my clinic complaining of malaise saying that she "just didn't feel right all over." She explained her symptoms as follows: fatigue, distention and fullness in the lower abdomen (stool and urine normal), neck pain, lower back soreness, and increased perspiration (when fatigued). She has been seeking consultation and treatment from both Western medicine and TCM doctors, but nothing has been effective. Some TCM doctors said her condition was caused by postpartum wind and Western medicine doctors diagnosed her with chronic pelvic inflammationatory disease (PID). I did note that during her visits to my clinic, these symptoms never seemed to be bothering her too much. What is your opinion about this case?

A: During the process of making a diagnosis it is imperative to consider a full spectrum of potential pathologies based on both TCM pattern identification and Western medicine diagnostic tools and lab test results. For instance, it sounds to me like this patient who was diagnosed with chronic PID actually has "Foot Tai Yin phlegm reversal headache." Aspects of this condition can be classified in Western medicine pathological terms as a psychosomatic disorder. I recommend prescribing Ban Xia Tian Ma Bai Zhu San adding Gan Cao, Long Yan Gan, Sheng Du Zhong, Yuan Hu Suo, and Mu Xiang. If copious amounts of vaginal discharge (leukorrhea) presents, then add Sheng Mu Li, Bai Guo, and Yu Sheng Wan. If increased perspiration persists, then add Ma Huang Gen (or Qing Hao) and Zhi Mu. This approach should result in effective results.

Case Study #2: Psychosomatic Disorder, Fibromyalgia, or Foot Tai Yin Phlegm Reversal Headache?

Q: Three years ago a 42 y/o male patient began having sudden attacks of neck stiffness and pain that radiated to the chest on both sides, the right eye socket, both shoulders, and the posterior aspect of the elbow (near Ching Leng Yuan (SJ11) acupoint). This pain was described as severe with episodes occurring 2~3 times per week and the pain was worse at night. Occasionally, the patient felt hot flashes and dizziness, muzziness, headache, and blurred vision. Results of an MRI indicated no abnormalities in his cervical spine. In attempts to remedy these symptoms, the patient has received frequent injections of muscle relaxants and analgesics and has been taking oral sedatives for a long period of time. Western medical doctors diagnosed him with psychosomatic disorder and fibromyalgia.

Do you think this patient could be suffering from cerebral atrophy or upper cervical spine problems? I carefully examined the MRI image myself and couldn't see any noticeable compression on the spinal cord or nerve roots. Please share your views on this case.

A: It sounds to me like this is another case of Foot Tai Yin phlegm reversal headache. Again, you can prescribe Ban Xia Tian Ma Bai Zhu San adding Gan Cao; Hong Zao; Long Yan Gan; large doses of Tian Ma (at least 1 liang); Gan Jiang, Fu Zi, and Wu Zhu Yu (5 qian each); Du Zhong (4 qian); and Yu Sheng Wan. You can also administer acupuncture selecting Feng Chi (GB20), Feng Fu (DU16), Wan Gu (GB12), Guan Yuan Shu (UB26), He Gu (LI4), Hou Xi (SI3), Zan Zhu (UB2), Si Zhu Kong (SJ23), and Ting Gong (SI19)

Case Study #3: Intractable Headache, Uterine Fibroids, and Endometrial Hyperplasia

Q: A 49 y/o female patient (a Western medical physician) has suffered from intractable headaches since she was a child. She explained that each time an episode occurs the excrutiating distending pain in both eyes inhibits eye muscle rotation and they remain fixed for 2~3 days before pain-free, normal movement is again possible. A couple of years ago she incurred an abrubt elevation in blood pressure (190/110), but after being administered the vasoconstrictor angiotensin II receptor blockers (ARB) her systolic pressure dropped down to 140. A few months ago she experienced 2 weeks of continuous menstrual dribbling and went for an examination. The exam revealed numerous uterine fibroids. The largest fibroid was 6~7 cm in diameter and excessive menstrual bleeding had caused a decrease in Hb to 9 and insufficient Fe levels. With so many different types of presenting symptoms, I am not sure where to focus my treatment on. What would you do?

A: My impression is that the patient's gynecological symptoms are primarily induced by sleep deprivation combined with endometrial hyperplasia and blood stasis. Whereas the intractable headache, eye pain, and dizziness that have occurred since childhood most likely stem from cerebrovascular or brainstem circulatory irregularities inhibiting blood flow.

I would prescribe Ru Mo Si Wu Tang combining Wen Dan Tang adding Tian Ma (large dose), Ze Xie, Ce Bo Ye, Ou Jie, Chuan Qi (powder), Huang Qin (at least 8 qian), Huang Lian, and Huang Bo. If the patient still has continuous menstrual dribbling, then mix Zhu Sha (powder) into the Chuan Qi (powder), and also administer acupuncture selecting Tai Chong (LV3), Zhong Feng (LV4), and San Yin Jiao (SP6). This approach should effectively stanch bleeding as well as promote good sleep and reduce the severity of her headaches. It is best for the patient to take this formula until the uterine fibroids comletely disappear and the endometrial hyperplasia resolves, which generally takes about 6~10 months. Remember! During the first 1~2 months of taking the formula the uterine fibroids will appear "haloed" on CT scan images, enlarging at the onset and then gradually shrinking in size until they disappear. In the absence of the fibroids and hyperplasia, the patient will be primed for pregnancy so advise her to use contraception, unless of course, she wants to have a child.

Case Study #4: Swollen Lymph Node in Neck

Q: A 38 y/o male patient recently came down with a cold and not long after discovered a slightly swollen nodule on the left side of his neck (near Tian Rong (SI17) and Tian Chuang (SI16) acupoints) with tenderness upon palplation. He doesn't have a fever. How would you treat this condition?

A: For a swollen nodule on the left side of the neck, I would prescribe Xiao Chai Hu Tang adding Huang Qin (large dose), Qing Hao, Zhi Mu, and Di Gu Pi. You can also acupuncture the Shao Yang channel and bleed the three yang channel well points of the four limbs. This approach should quickly resolve this condition.

Case Study #5: Elderly Patient Unable to Rotate Neck

Q: A 68 y/o male patient explained that starting 3 or 4 years ago he began having difficulty rotating his neck. He had a number of MRIs and CT scans performed but nothing wrong could be found; and he was treated by both TCM and Western medicine doctors without success. Could this condition have derived from a transient ischemic attack (TIA) or cerebrovascular accident (CVA)?

A: It's possible that this patient contracted tuberculosis (TB) at some point in his life, which resulted in a chronic cough that put wear-and-tear on his trachea and neck and shoulder muscle tissues. After the TB infection resolved into a calcified granuloma, the tissues of the neck and shoulders and trachea underwent fibrosis, leaving his neck too stiff and rigid to rotate. This is just one possibility that you can follow-up on. If you do determine that this is the cause, then you can prescribe either Ba Xian Chang Shou Wan, Mai Men Dong Tang, or Bai He Gu Jin Tang adding Qing Hao, Yuan Shen, Zhi Mu, Di Gu Pi, and Chuan Qi (powder). You can also advise the patient to eat fresh South Korean homegrown Bei Sha Shen (Coastal Glehnia Root) and Hei Da Gen [aka Ge Gen; a popular, inexpensive, and widely available "hangover" elixir in Korea] and lots of water chestnuts and Chinese turnips. His condition should show improvement with this approach.

Case Study #6: Nuchal Rigidity

Q: A 39 y/o female patient explained that since about 1 year ago every time she lay flat on her back (supine position) her legs spontaneously raise upwards, reaching a maximum height of 50 cm at its most extreme. When this happens the patient has tried laying both hands on her abdomen and pressing down on Tian Shu (ST25), but it has not been helpful. Lying down in other positions or during any other activity she doesn't experience any problems, only in a supine position. She has already had an MRI performed on her neck and lumbar regions, which revealed no compression or other abnormalities. The only other significant complaint the patient mentioned was a stiff neck. Do you have any ideas or suggestions about this case?

A: These symptoms suggest increased intracranial pressure (ICP) that puts excessive pressure on the foramen magnum and thus induces nuchal rigidity (stiff neck) (or "stretched stiffness of the nape and back" in classical TCM pathological terminology). This condition can be identified as repletion or non-repletion pattern. For repletion pattern, you can prescribe Da Chai Hu Tang; Huang Lian Jie Du Tang combining Wu Ling San; or Jian Ling Tang combining Huang Lian Jie Du Tang adding Cang Zhu, Fu Ling, and Ze Xie. For non-replete pattern, you can consider prescribing Ban Xia Tian Ma Bai Zhu San variant; and for patients with hydrocephalus, you can prescribe Wu Ling San (Nephritis Formula) adding Mang Xiao and Da Huang.

6. AUTOIMMUNE DISEASES

There are many types of autoimmune diseases. This chapter will only focus on several of the most common and difficult to treat conditions including rheumatoid arthritis (RA), systemic lupus erythmatosus (SLE), and purpura. There are a lot of products on the market touting their capacity for "boosting the immune system," when in fact, autoimmune diseases arise from an overactive immune system in which the body's command and control centers become confused and errantly attack itself. The body clearly doesn't need to be "boosted" – what it needs is "balance."

Section 1: Rheumatoid Arthritis (RA)

Case Study #1: Five Approaches to Treating RA

Q: A 35 y/o female patient said that 5 years ago she began feeling aches and soreness in joints all over her body, and these symptoms were worse at night. Finally, it got to the point where she really couldn't stand it anymore and went to see a rheumatologist at a major hospital. She was diagnosed with rheumatoid arthritis (RA) and immediately began taking medication to treat this condition. After four years of continuous administration, she doesn't feel that the treatment has been very effective overall, so she decided to try TCM treatment.

Right now the patient's condition is as follows: Aching, red, and swollen joints with symptoms increasing in severity at night, while remaining relatively symptom-free during the daytime; occasionally at nighttime she has indigestion and incontinence; pulse – stringlike and fine; and stool normal. I prescribed Feng Shi Fang increasing the dose of Ma Huang to 3 qian. After 2 weeks of administration, the effects have not been noticeable. Please share your experiences and advice about treating this condition. Thank you!

A: In classical TCM pathological terminology rheumatoid arthritis (RA) correlates with "wind-damp traveling influx (moving impediment)" or "joint-running wind." For the majority of cases, this pathocondition is not that difficult to effectively treat; it just takes some time! Critical factors that will impact the outcome of treatment are the following: 1) the patient must be willing to accept the long-term TCM treatment regimen and encounter slight discomfort along the way; and 2) whether or not the patient has already been administered Western medicine RA drug treatment for a long duration. It's been my experience that patients whom do not receive Western medicine RA drugs, and instead solely receive TCM treatment, were more likely to show marked improvements in their symptoms and get this condition under control at the soonest in about 3 months. If the patient has been administered various types of potent anti-inflammatory and analgesic Western medicine medication, then it will take at least 6 months before seeing effective results. For those who are very sensitive to pain and unwilling to accept a bit of discomfort, the treatment regimen will take longer for results to appear.

Five approaches I most often use in the treatment of RA:

1) Administer bleeding at the site of swollen and painful joints and also Da Zhui (DU14) (above, at, and below the acupoint); and acupuncture (needle) the acupoints He Gu (LI4), Feng Chi (GB20), Zu San Li (ST36), Yang Ling Quan (GB34), and Jue Gu (GB39).

2) For acute flare ups presenting with severely swollen and painful joints that the patient finds unbearable, prescribe Huang Lian Jie Du

Tang combining Wu Ling San adding Ma Huang.

3) If the patient's RA condition has already entered the chronic stage, then prescribe (Yu Sheng) Hyperactive Immune Formula.

4) If the patient has been receiving TCM treatment for a long duration with effective results (no longer has red and swollen joints), the patient still must continue taking the formula for 2~3 more months until the aching and pain resolves to the point the patient only feels slight tigtness during work or other activity. At this point, you can change the formula to variants of Zhi Bo Di Huang Tang or Zuo Gui Yin and administer it for about 2 weeks, assessing to make sure there is no joint swelling; and if not, then gradually add incremental doses of Gan Jiang, Fu Zi, and Yu Gui.

5) If you are treating the patient during the initial flare up prior to receiving treatment with Western medicine RA drugs or if the patient has never received treatment with Western medicine RA drugs that tend to mask the symptoms, then this condition is called the "essential state," which is easier to treat. In the absence of Western medicine RA drug intervention, advise the patient to perform lab tests on rheumatoid factor (RF), ESR, and C-reactive protein (CRP). If ESR and CRP levels are elevated, then the condition can be identified as yang hyperactivity pattern, requiring administration of heat-clearing and toxin-resolving medicinals adding exterior effusion medicinals such as Hyperactive Immune Formula adding Ge Gen and Ma Huang or Ge Gen Tang adding "the Three Yellows," Qing Hao, Zhi Mu, and Di Gu Pi. If ESR and CRP levels are normal, but rheumatoid factor (RF) is (+), then prescribe Ma Gui Wen Dan Tang or Gui Zhi Jia Ling Zhu Fu Tang adding Huang Qin and Shi Gao. This should resolve the patients symptoms and effectively control the condition.

Case Study #2: Scan Image Reveals Joint Inflammation

Q: A 44 y/o female patient came to my clinic for an initial consultation 6 months ago complaining of morning stiffness, tenderness, and swelling in the joints of every finger. I prescribed Huang Lian Jie Du Tang combining Wu Ling San variant and her symptoms completely resolved. However, the patient was worried that she might have inherited "intractable" rheumatoid arthritis (RA) since a relative of hers had been afflicted with RA over 15 years without any improvement. With this in mind, the next time she had an episode of joint stiffness, tenderness and swelling she made an appointment with a rheumatologist, had a blood test, and performed an MRI. Results revealed hypointensity in the wrist joint and glenohumeral joint (sites where she had experienced tenderness and pain). Her doctors suspected RA and administered drug treatment, but after 3 months of treatment the patient didn't feel there was any noticeable improvement so she returned for another TCM consultation. I started her out with Zhi Bo Di Huang Tang variant and 2 weeks later her joint pain resolved. She had a blood test performed with results showing RF, CRP, and ESR normal, but she hasn't had another MRI performed. I am still uncertain if she actually has RA or not.

I think this patient may have avascular necrosis caused by insufficient blood supply to the joints, and not RA. Please offer your respected advice and opinion on this case. How would you treat this patient?

A: Strictly speaking rheumatoid arthritis (RA) is not a hereditary condition, though there is a genetic presdisposition making certain people's immune system more susceptible to external contraction (e.g., viral and bacteria infections). In TCM, RA can be identified as heat with mild exterior pattern and it's relatively easy to remedy. If severe swelling and heat present, then add large doses of "the Three Yellows," Qing Hao, Zhi Mu, and Di Gu Pi, administering this formula until the symptoms resolve and both rheumatoid factor (RF) and ESR levels are normal. At this time, the patient can discontinue Western medicine RA drugs as well. Remember! For patients who have never been administered Western medicine RA drugs, effective results from TCM treatment will appear even faster!

The hypointensity appearing on the CT scan and MRI images is most likely a result of arthritic degeneration and not ischemic necrosis. You can look at it like "the sediment and mud that deposits between architectural structures following a severe flood." Don't worry about this "sediment," just continue prescribing the heat-clearing and toxin-resolving and blood-quickening and stasis-resolving medicinals (and possibly in some cases also add yin-supplementing medicinals). This approach will successfully prevent inflammation from recurring, while the body will naturally do the rest by gradually reabsorbing the metabolic waste ("sediment") from previous inflammatory episodes, putting the body back on the track of recovery.

Case Study #3: Differential Diagnosis – Periodic Paralysis (PP), Subacute Combined Degeneration (SCD), Ankylosing Spondylitis (AS), and Rheumatoid Arthritis (RA)

Q: A 24 y/o female patient came to my clinic complaining of left-sided hemilateral pain. In her childhood she experienced severe abdominal pain on numerous occasions and in high school she experienced left ankle pain following a fever. Later in life left-sided joint pain gradually developed in her upper limb, lower limb and jaw. At that time, lab test results showed rheumatoid factor (RF) 735, HLA-B27 (+), and low K+. Despite being administered various Western medicine drugs, her condition has continued to deteriorate. Over the past several years she has felt generalized weakness and lack of strength, especially in her legs. The patient has seen numerous TCM and Western medicine doctors, but no one has been able to diagnose her condition. Do you think this could be rheumatoid arthritis (RA), periodic paralysis (PP), or subacute combined degeneration (SCD)? I want to prescribe Gui Qi Jian Zhong Tang combining Chai Hu Jia Long Gu Mu Li Tang, Yu Sheng Wan, and Huo Luo Dan. Please offer your perspectives and advice on this confusing case. Thank you!

A: Ah! The presentation and treatment approach of these conditions are all significantly different. These conditions are clearly distinguishable based on evaluation of lab tests, diagnostic tools, and clinical presentation.

Rheumatoid arthritis (RA) can be identified as yang hyperactivity pattern, exterior-interior triple burner repletion heat with exterior pattern, and steaming bone heat pattern. For the treatment of this condition you can prescribe Hyperactive Immune Formula (including large doses of "the Three Yellows," Qing Hao, Zhi Mu, and Di Gu

Pi) adding Mu Dan Pi, Shan Zhu Yu, and Ma Huang.. This formula should be administered continuously up until the ESR, CRP, and RF levels test (-); at that time, you can advise the patient to gradually reduce and eventually completely discontinue Western medicine drugs.

A definitive diagnosis of periodic parlysis (PP) can be made only if blood test results show normal levels of K, T3, and T4 with either elevated or decreased levels of TSH. If the patient tests HLA-B27 (+), then this strongly suggests ankylosing spondylitis (AS). For AS patients whose condition has progressed to the stage of vertebrae fusions (aka "bamboo spine") and hunchback, then you can prescribe Shi Quan Da Bu Tang or You Gui Yin adding Ma Huang, Du Zhong, Niu Qi, Di Long, Gan Jiang, and Yu Gui. Long-term administration of this formula will prevent further deterioration and gradually improve the patient's condition.

During the administration of TCM medicinals all of the key blood test levels will be elevated (don't worry about this!): just continue administering the formula. The patient's agonizing symptoms of stiffness, aching, and pain in the torso, shoulders, upper back, and lumbar regions will quickly be relieved and strength and flexibility improved. At this time, it's fine if the patient wants to continue taking Western medicine drugs (e.g., NSAIDs, TNF, corticosteroids, interferon, Methotrexate (MTX)). Of course, the optimal scenario is for the patient to gradually reduce the drug dosage up until complete discontinuation is achieved, though this process will take a long period of time.

If increased ESR, RF, and HLA-B27 levels persist after administering yang supplementing medicinals for a period of time, then this can be identified as true heat pattern and you need to add large doses of Huang Qin (or Huang Lian) and Huang Bo to the main formula above or change the formula to (Yu Sheng) Hyperactive Immune Formula adding Ma Huang, Gui Zhi, Niu Xi, and Sheng Du Zhong.

If the patient has not been administered MTX, and increased ESR, RF, and HLA-B27 levels persist, then this can be identified as exterior-interior triple burner repletion heat with exterior wind heat pattern. For this pattern you should prescribe either (Yu Sheng) Hyperactive Immune Formula, Huang Lian Jie Du Tang, or Ge Gen Qin Lian Tang adding Ma Huang (or Ge Gen), Qing Hao, Zhi Mu,

Di Gu Pi, Sheng Du Zhong, Niu Xi, Huo Luo Dan, and in some cases Wan Ling Dan. Administer this formula up until the blood test results are normal.

If K and T4 levels are low, then you must supplement yang, qi, and blood; conversely, if K and T4 levels are high, then you must prescribe heavy settling and heat abating medicinals; and if K and T4 levels are normal, then you must carefully consider the possibility of damp heat, qi vacuity, or dryness pattern, adjusting your formula accordingly. For instance, if damp heat pattern presents then prescribe either Er Miao San, San Miao San, Si Miao San, or Jia Wei Er Miao San; and if dry pattern presents, then prescribe either Qing Zao Jiu Fei Tang, Bai He Gu Jin Tang, or Ba Xian Chang Shou Wan.

Subacute combined degeneration (SCD) is a rare disorder of the spine, brain, and nerves, which is caused by vitamin B12 deficiency. Symptoms involve weakness, abnormal sensations, cognitive dysfunction, and vision difficulties. For details about this disorder you can reference the *Application of Integrated TCM and Western Medicine in the Treatment of Neurological Diseases* (pgs. 620~625). My personal approach is to prescribe either Gui Qi Jian Zhong Tang, Shi Quan Da Bu Tang, or You Gui Yin adding Huang Qi, Ma Huang, and Di Long. Or for certain cases you can prescribe Xue Ku Fang combining Si Ni Tang adding Huang Bo (or Huang Qin) and Huang Qi. Also, advise the patient to eat plenty of liver and garlic and supplement with B-complex vitamins (the TCM medicinal Dang Gui contains an abundance of B-complex vitamins (including B12), vitamin A, and vitamin E among other nutrients!).

Case Study #4: Ankylosing Spondylitis (AS)

Q: A 34 y/o female patient began experiencing lower back pain in her teens, but subsequent medical tests and examinations were unable to pinpoint a cause. After her second child was born, the pain became even more severe. Two years ago she went for another evaluation and was diagnosed with ankylosing spondylitis (AS). She doesn't take regular medication for this condition, but when symptoms become unbearable she does take corticosteroids. Two months ago she once again began experiencing left-sided lower limb and finger numbness, right-sided neck pain, and lower back pain. The last time she took corticosteroids she was initially reluctant because it made her gain weight, but the pain was too much to endure so she did anyways. However, this time it wasn't nearly as effective at relieving her pain, so she decided to seek TCM treatment. Do you have any suggestions or advice about treating AS?

A: That sounds like the typical history and presentation of an AS patient. In recent years, this condition has become much more prevalent in Taiwan. A key determinant for pattern identification and treatment of this condition is whether HLA-B27 is positive (+) or negative (-).

If HLA-B27 is (-), and the patient complains of soreness and backache after sleeping in cold weather or even air conditioning, then the condition could simply be identified as cold impediment of the urinary bladder channel. If is HLA-B27 (-), but the history and presentation of symptoms are the same as AS, then Western medical doctors will typically still administer corticosteroids, MTX (a disease-modifying antirheumatic drug (DMARD)), quinine, and potent analgesics. If HLA-B27 is (+), then the condition can be identified as cold impediment of the urinary bladder channel with exterior pattern. In these patients, stiffness of the spine extends all the way up to C1 and C2, and in severe cases fusion, dislocation, and fracture will occur resulting in upper limb weakness, limp paralysis, limp wilting back and legs, and hunchback. Pain in the sternum and ribs can become so unbearable that it may cause breathing difficulties. This condition can be identified as cold strike with exterior and qi vacuity pattern for which you can prescribe either Shi Quan Da Bu Tang, You Gui Yin, Du Huo Ji Sheng Tang, or San Bi Tang adding Ma Huang, Di Long, Lu Jiao, Gan Jiang, Fu Zi, Yu Gui, and Huo Luo Dan. Also, administer acupuncture (warm needling) selecting acupoints Feng Chi (GB20), Hua Tuo Jia Ji Xue (EX-B2), Shen Shu (UB23), Guan Yuan Shu (UB26), Huan Tiao (GB30), Ba Liao (UB31~34), Yang Ling Quan (GB34), and Jue Gu (GB39).

If HLA-B27 is (-), simply prescribe You Gui Yin variant, administer acupuncture (warm needling), and advise the patient to get enough sleep (at least 8~10 hours per day), dress warmly, and regularly exercise (e.g., swimming, walking). Also, tell the patient to eat sensibly (no dietary restrictions) and lead a normal sex life (just don't overindulge!). If the patient also presents with tearing on exposure to wind, then add large doses of Ma Huang and Bai Zhi. Continue long-term administration of TCM medicinals and acupuncture, and when the pain resides the patient may gradually discontinue the use of corticosteriods.

If the vertebral joints feel hot and swollen upon palpation, the patient has night sweats, HLA-B27 (+), and CRP, ESR, and RF are all elevated, then this condition can be identified as yang hyperactivity pattern indicating that the immune system is in the midst of a hyperactive episode, overreacting and "attacking" the vertebral joints. For this condition, you can prescribe formula variants such as Hyperactive Immune Formula, Huang Lian Jie Du Tang, Ge Gen Qin Lian Tang, Da Qing Long Tang, or Yang Dan Tang. Just make sure your formula includes Sheng Du Zhong, Niu Xi, Ma Huang (or Ge Gen), Qing Hao, Zhi Mu, Di Gu Pi, Mu Dan Pi, and Chi Shao. You can also bleed Da Zhui (DU14) (above, at, and below) and administer acupuncture on the acupoints Feng Chi (GB20), Wei Zhong (UB40), Hou Xi (SI3), and Guan Yuan Shu (UB26).

Case Study #5: Zygomatic (Cheek) Bone Swelling – Don't Prescribe Feng Shi Fang

Q: A 28 y/o male patient was diagnosed with rheumatoid arthritis (RA) at the age of 13. Over the past 2 years he has felt aches and pain in the muscles of his entire body. Western medical doctors diagnosed him with polymyalgia rheumatica and he has been on medication to control this condition since then. Three months ago, the right side of his face below the zygomatic (cheek) bone suddenly swelled up. His doctors recommended surgery, but the patient was concerned his face may become disfigured, so he came to me seeking TCM treatment instead. I prescribed Huang Lian Jie Du Tang adding Qing Hao, Zhi Mu, Di Gu Pi, Mu Li, and Tao Ren. Please offer your invaluable advice on this case. Thank you!

A: Rheumatoid arthritis (RA) can be identified as hyperactivity yang pattern. Unless the patient has been (or is currently being) administered corticosteroids or MTX (both have immunosuppressive effects), then don't prescribe (Yu Sheng) Feng Shi Fang. The reason is because it derives from Huang Lian Jie Du Tang and thus contains Zhi Zi. Long-term administration of Zhi Zi will tint the skin of some people a "greenish" color, especially the face and torso.

A student of mine, Dr. Cheng, Shu-mei first discovered this phenomenon during clinical treatment and research. She observed patients with overactive immune systems (e.g., Sjogren's) and rheumatoid arthritis (RA) had a heightened pigment absorption sensitivity. When these patients were adminstered TCM formulas containing Zhi Zi, their skin gradually acquired a noticeable "greenish" tint. However, quite the opposite, when TCM formulas containing Zhi Zi are administered for hepatitis patients (e.g., hyperbilirubinemia) their jaundice ("yellowish" skin coloration) is effectively abated.

This "greenish" skin discoloration can be reversed by simply discontinuing use of the Zhi Zi containing formula for a period of time or subtracting Zhi Zi from the formula altogether. For your patient, I would stay on the safe side; you don't want to give him any more challeges to overcome. Prescribe Huang Lian Jie Du Tang (substracting Zhi Zi) adding Qing Hao, Zhi Mu, and Di Gu Pi. This is essentially the composition of a signature formula that I have recently designed called (Yu Sheng) Hyperactive Immune Formula, offering excellent efficacy without the potential for unsightly side effects.

For those patients who have been administered corticosteroids without effectiveness, I have had great results prescribing Zhi Bo Di Huang Tang adding Ma Huang, Sheng Shi Gao, and Wan Ling Dan, which will keep RF, ESR, and CRP in check. Once ESR and CRP return to normal levels, even though RF may still be elevated, you can advise the patient to gradually reduce the dosage of analgesics, anti-inflammatories, MTX, and corticosteroids. If the patient incurs a mild relapse along the way, then simply add large doses of "the Three Yellows"; and bleed Da Zhui (DU14) (above, at, and below) and the well points of the corresponding channels presenting with pain or discomfort.

Section 2: Systemic Lupus Erythamatosus (SLE)

Case Study #1: Three Keys to Treating SLE

Q: This 22 y/o female is my first systemic lupus erythamatosus (SLE) patient. Two months ago a butterfly rash appeared on her face along with generalized joint pain, and lab tests showed RF 120. Currently, she is taking prednisolone 2 pills/day. What is the best approach for treating SLE (treatment regimen, duration of time needed for efficacy to appear in the TCM treatment of joint symptoms, skin symptoms, etc.)?

A: According to Western medicine's perspective, systemic lupus erythamatosus (SLE) is an autoimmune disease similar to rheumatoid arthritis (RA). Determining a diagnosis requires performing basic tests on ANA, C3 and C4, and RF levels. If SLE has been accurately diagnosed, the TCM treatment approach involves long-term administration of TCM medicinals, healthy lifestyle and nutritional intake, and making sure the body is warm (e.g., thermal underwear, heating). In my clinical experience, administration of approximately 185 packets (fastest 75 packets and slowest 615 packets) will effectively remedy this condition to the point that enables the patient to discontinue use of Western medicine drugs; and approximately 320 packets (fastest 82 packets and slowest 795 packets) will effectively cure this condition to the point that enables the patient to discontinue use of TCM medicinals. The patient will be able to lead a normal life without having to take drugs or medicinals.

It is commonly known that the long-term administration of Western medicine drugs (mainly corticosteroids) in the treatment of SLE can lead to ischemic necrosis of the joints, retinal detachment, Raynaud's syndrome, nerve atrophy, and renal failure. Based on my clinical experience, TCM can be administered to effectively treat SLE and its complications. It just takes some time and a lot of patience!

These are the three formulas I most commonly administer for the treatment of SLE patients:

1) Xiang Sha Liu Jun Zi Tang adding Gan Jiang, Fu Zi, Yu Gui, Huang Qin, Huang Qi, Tu Si Zi, Ren Shen (powder), and Chuan Qi (powder).

2) You Gui Yin adding large doses of Gan Jiang, Yu Gui, Ren Shen (powder), Chuan Qi (powder), and Huang Qi.

3) If autoimmune hemolytic anemia (AIHA) presents, then subtract Chuan Qi (powder) and add Zhu Qi and Xi Lu Rong (powder); or change the formula to Sheng Yu Tang adding Gan Jiang, Fu Zi, Huang Qin, Tu Si Zi, Ren Shen (powder), Xi Lu Rong (powder), and Zhu Qi (Zhu Jie Qi).

Remember! Make sure to add appetite promoting (stomach opening) medincals, Yu Sheng Wan, and also Huo Luo Dan to remedy pain. If uremia presents, then add large doses of Fu Ling, Ze Xie, and Ting Li Zi; if pleural, pericardial, or mediastinal effusion present, then change the formula to Wu Ling San (Nephritis Formula) (including large doses of Fu Ling and Ze Xie) adding large doses of Ting Li Zi and Fang Ji along with Ren Shen (powder) and Chuan Qi (powder); if anemia presents, then add Xi Lu Rong (powder). Administer this formula until the C3/C4 levels return to 100/15; that's when you can begin discontinuing administration of prednisolone.

Also, in cold temperatures the patient may feel discomfort in the fingers (Raynaud's phenomenon (secondary Raynaud's)). Raynaud's phenomenon requires the administration of Wu Zhu Yu Tang, but this formula is very bitter, pungent, and spicy, and some patients cannot tolerate the flavor. This is why I have Wu Zhu Yu Tang processed into pills, so the patient can simply add it into a decocted TCM formula, thus ameliorating the unpalatable flavor. South Koreans generally like to eat spicy foods and drink alcoholic beverages, so during cold weather months decocted Wu Zhu Yu Tang would probably provide a palatable solution!

Case Study #2: SLE – Mediastinal Effusion Indicates Chronic Renal and Brain Damage Stage

Q: A 38 y/o female patient of mine has been living with systemic lupus erythamatosus (SLE) for many years. After being diagnosed with this disease 10 years ago, she received inpatient care at a hospital for 3 months until her condition stabilized and then was administered 20 mg of predinsolone daily to keep the disease in check. Five years ago, she experienced a sudden onset of palpitations along with swollen extremities, right-sided jugular veinous distention, shortness of breath, and dry cough. Examination results revealed costal and pericardial effusion for which she was administered high dose intravenous corticosteroid therapy daily on an outpatient basis as well as oral diuretics. The patient's relatives couldn't stand seeing her in this condition and came to me wondering if TCM treatment could get her back to normal.

A: When SLE presents with pleural effusion it usually indicates the disease has already entered the renal (e.g., interstitial nephritis, nephrotic syndrome, membranous GN, renal failure) and brain (e.g., CNS, behavioral, memory) damage stage. At this time, you must keep an eye out for elevated BUN/Cr levels, cerebrovascular disease, and CNS disorders. My treatment approach is to prescribe either Xiang Sha Liu Jun Zi Tang or Ban Xia Tian Ma Bai Zhu San variants adding large doses of Fu Ling, Ze Xie, Ting Li Zi, and Fang Ji. If uremia presents, then add Ding Shu Xiu and Ren Dong Teng along with Tu Si Zi, Huang Qi, Gan Jiang, Fu Zi, Yu Gui, Ren Shen (powder), Chuan Qi (powder), Xi Lu Rong (powder), Da Huang (adding incremental doses of 5 fen until 2~3 stools/day are maintained), and Ma Huang (3 qian, but in cold climates like South Korea you may need to add more).

Case Study #3: SLE – Acupuncture and TCM Medicinals

Q: A 33 y/o female SLE patient has decreased C3/C4 levels. Since receiving a definitive diagnosis, she has been taking prednisolone and quinine to control her condition (3 pills(5mg)/day). However, despite this treatment her condition has been getting worse and now she wants to try TCM treatment. Her symptoms are as follows: cold, painful knees; and since she stopped taking her Western medicine drugs the generalized joint pain worsens during menses, but she doesn't have swelling. While administering acupuncture treatment, it was difficult inserting the needle into Xi Yan (EX-LE5) and Du Bi (ST35); it felt like something was blocking the way. Could this be synovial adhesion? I prescribed Hyperactive Immune Formula adding Rou Gui, Gan Jiang, and Tian Xiong (aka Fu Zi) (starting out with small doses and incrementally increasing). Do you think this is the right approach?

A: Once an SLE patient is administered prednisolone, the condition can be identified as either yang vacuity pattern or true cold false heat pattern; and at this time, the patient can discontinue administration of quinine, but not prednisolone. First, prescribe kidney yang-supplementing medicinals to dispel cold stasis and cold-damp, along with swelling-dispersing, heat-abating, and dampness-disinhibiting medicinals for a period of time. Then, advise the patient to try discontinuing prednisolone. If after a period of 1~2 weeks the patient doesn't present with any significant discomfort, then continue with this approach of administering only TCM medicinals.

Remember! As a general rule, I wouldn't needle directly into the joints of SLE patients, because it could result in rupture of a synovial cyst or cause infection. For this type of joint pain and swelling, I would prescribe large doses of "the Three Yellows" and " the Four Ling's"; and of course you could add Qing Hao, Zhi Mu, and Di Gu Pi; and Gan Jiang, Fu Zi, and Yu Gui.

However, based on your description of this patient, she has decreased C3/C4 and HB levels. If that is the case, then you shouldn't increase the dose of "the Three Yellows" and "the Four Ling's"; instead, simply add yang-supplementing medicinals into your cold stasis formula and add larger doses of Gan Jiang, Fu Zi, and Yu Gui, and a small dose of Ma Huang.

Case Study #4: SLE and Idiopathic Thrombocytopenic Purpura (ITP)

Q: A 22 y/o female SLE patient experienced malaise and went to the hospital for an examination. Results of lab tests revealed PLT count of only 30,000 and her doctors diagnosed her with idiopathic thrombocytopenic purpura (ITP).

Three months later she suffered from enteritis and diarrhea and her PLT count continued to spiral downward, thus she was admitted to the hospital for treatment. Despite being administered intravenous immunoglobulin (IVIG) and intravenous corticosteroids, her PLT continued falling down to 5,000 before her diarrhea symptoms began showing improvement. The patient has been in the hospital for 3 weeks now receiving PLT infusions 2x/day, but her body has been disposing the PLTs as fast as they can be administered, making the treatment ultimately ineffective. She has been plagued by a persistent cough, nausea, and fever, and it looks like she may be about to pass away. Please offer your guidance and advice on this patient's condition.

A: SLE patients are susceptible to hemolytic disorders. The presence of severely low PLT count (thrombocytopenia) resulting from immune system malfunctions causing the body to errantly destroy platelets is called idiopathic thrombocytopenic purpura (ITP). As for TCM medicinal treatment, you can can prescribe (Yu Sheng) Sheng Yu Tang. If the patient has been administered corticosteroids, then this condition requires the prescription of medicinals that treat either spleen yang vacuity with cold stasis pattern or kidney yang vacuity with cold stasis pattern. At this time, advise the patient to reduce the dose of corticosteroids (Do not completely discontinue administration!) and as the PLT count returns to normal levels, then gradually reduce the corticosteroid dose further until it is eventually discontinued. If after discontinuing corticosteroids the PLT count again gradually decreases, then simply prescribe (Yu Sheng) Sheng Yu Tang variant to bring the PLT back up and maintain normal levels.

During the onset of idiopathic thrombocytopenic purpura (ITP), when the immune system is attacking renegade antibodies that have attached to platelets throughout the entire body, or during the acute heat stage of external contraction, you can add Qing Hao, Zhi Mu, Di Gu Pi, Mu Dan Pi, and Chi Shao. However, as the condition evolves into later, chronic stages, you must stop administering these types of vacuity heat-clearing, summerheat-resolving, and blood-cooling medicinals. These medicinals should only be prescribed in the presence of Shao Yang heat, steaming bone, taxation heat, late afternoon tidal heat (fever), night sweats, or meningitis in patients with autoimmune disorders.

Case Study #5: Rheumatoid Arthritis (RA) and Systemic Lupus Erythamatosus (SLE)

Q: I have a 34 y/o female patient diagnosed with RA and SLE. Her chief complaint is generalized aches and redness, heat, and swelling at the deltoid muscles of both shoulders (Bi Nao (LI14)), and lab tests results were as follows: RF 28, C3/C4 54/9, and WBC normal. What are the distinguishing diagnostic features of these two conditions and should different approaches be used for treatment?

A: First of all, they are both autoimmune diseases, and you can assess blood tests to make a diagnostic distinction between RA and SLE. A distinguishing diagnostic feature of SLE patients is low C3/C4 levels; whereas rheumatoid factor (RF) levels may or may not be high, and if high, it won't be as high as in RA patients. Also, in SLE patients, ANA and anti-dsDNA will be positive; CRP and ESR levels may be normal, high or low; and LDH and CPK levels may be high. In RA patients, during the initial onset and flare-ups, ESR and CRP will be increased, and only when the disease has spread to the heart and vasculature will changes in PT and APTT occur. For details about these autoimmune diseases and more, you can reference *Harrison's Principles of Internal Medicine*.

If you determine that the diagnosis of SLE is indeed correct, and the patient has not taken corticosteroids or MTX, then prescribe Hyperactive Immune Formula (including large doses of at least 8 qian for each medicinal); and if joint swelling and pain present, then add Ma Huang (and/or Ge Gen). The redness, heat, and swelling near Bi Nao (LI14) sounds like it might be vasculitis, and if so, then add Chuan Qi (powder) and Dan Shen, which will gradually resolve the inflammation. Remember! Any type of massage or manipulation, and even local bleeding is contraindicated for this condition; and if you do bleed, then bleed the well points of the fingers. Also, the normal range for C3/C4 is at least from 80~140 and 10~40 respectively.

Section 3: Idiopathic Thrombocytopenic Purpura (ITP)

Case Study #1: It's Probably Purpura

Q: A 26 y/o female patient explained that "her face broke out into a pimply mess" (actually seborrheic dermatitis) so she decocted some San Bai Cao (*Saururus chinensis (Lour.) Baill.* (aka Asian lizard's tail)) at her own discretion. Not long after taking this decoction, she experienced hematuria and bleeding gums prompting her to get examined at a hospital. The doctors diagnosed idiopathic thrombocytopenic purpura (ITP) and simply prescribed corticosteroids to maintain a stable PLT count. Eight months passed without elevation of the PLT count. Her doctors thought the condition was severe enough to warrant splenectomy, but the patient didn't want to have this done and instead continued corticosteroid administration. Follow-up examination one year later showed a PLT count of about 5,000 and the patient occasionally experienced bleeding gums, hematuria, nosebleeds (epistaxis), and excessive bruising (purpura) on the medial side of the elbow joint. I prescribed Xiang Sha Liu Jun Zi Tang adding Gan Jiang, Fu Zi, Yu Gui, Huang Qin, Zhi Zi, and Han Lian Cao. Please share your views and advice about this case. Also, do you think San Bai Cao (Chinese Lizarbtail, Saururus chinensis (Lour.) Baill.) could cause idiopathic thrombocytopenia purpura (ITP)?

A: I don't think San Bai Cao had anything to do with your patient's condition. San Bai Cao is a heat-clearing and toxin resolving and bone and sinew consolidating medicinal. The only scenario I could imagine this medicinal having any possibility of inhibiting PLT production is if the patient took enormous doses (up to 500g~1,000g of raw dried herb) over a long period of time. Based on your description of the patient's symptoms, it clearly indicates she has purpura.

A characteristic feature of purpura is "spontaneous external bleeding," which involves mild spontaneous bleeding from the gums, nasal cavity, skin, etc. In Western medicine, this condition is classifed as resulting from either low platelet counts (thrombocytopenic purpura), which is more commonly seen in young women, or normal platelet counts (nonthrombocytopenic purpura), which is more commonly seen in the elderly with fragile blood vessels (senile purpura). As for TCM treatment, I would prescribe (Yu Sheng) Sheng Yu Tang adding Gan Jiang, Fu Zi, Yu Gui, Huang Qin, Ren Shen (powder), Huai Niu Xi, Xi Lu Rong (powder), and Zhu Jie Qi. For Xi Lu Rong (powder) and Zhu Jie Qi start out with 1 qian and gradually increase the dose, and since Zhu Jie Qi tends to cause diarrhea add Cang Zhu and Ze Xie to counteract this potential side effect. Remember! You should not prescribe Chuan Qi (powder) or Zhi Zi for this condition, but Han Lian Cao is fine.

If the patient is being administered Western medicine drugs such as MTX and corticosteroids, once the patient begins taking the TCM formula you can advise her to first discontinue MTX and when PLT levels increase up to the 10,000~20,000 level, then advise her to gradually discontinue corticosteroids.

Case Study #2: What Is Idiopathic Thrombocytopenic Purpura (ITP)?

Q: It seems that the prevalence of idiopathic thrombocytopenic purpura (ITP) is increasing, especially among children. Incidences of ITP cases are being reported all over the Internet, but the only available Western medical treatment is intravenous immune globulin (IVIG) or Rho (D) immune globulin (WinRho), corticosteroids, and vitamin supplements. A lot of parents have been contacting me for advice and consultation wondering if TCM could provide effective treatment.

Please share your experiences in treating idiopathic thrombocytopenic purpura (ITP). Why are increased incidences of this disease occurring? What types of patterns does this condition manifest? Aside from prescribing (Yu Sheng) Sheng Yu Tang for treatment, are there any yang vacuity type patterns I should be aware of? What is the best treatment approach?

A: Idiopathic thrombocytopenic purpura (ITP) is also called immune thrombocytopenic purpura (ITP) or simply purpura. As the name implies, this condition results from either a descrease in PLT count or the inability of PLT to return to normal levels resulting in thrombocytopenic symptoms. Purpura can be classified as either thrombocytopenic purpuras (low platelet counts) or nonthrombocytopenic purpuras (normal platelet counts). Nonthrombocytopenic purpuras most commonly occur in the elderly whom tend to have fragile vessels or others with severe combined immunodeficiency (SCID), known colloquially as "bubble boy disease." Thrombocytopenic patients commonly present with splenomegaly caused by increased destruction and sequestration of platelets that may result in severe hepatosplenomegaly, which is very difficult to treat and why some Western medicinal doctors recommend splenectomy. In TCM, hepatosplenomegaly can be identified as heat pattern or blood vacuity with heat pattern and treated with Gui Pi Tang or Jia Wei Gui Pi Tang variants.

The high living standards and medical advancements of modern civilization have made it possible to control or cure many previously intractable diseases with drugs. However, many of these "wonder drugs" also happen to be toxins that may harm the body if administered in high doses or over long periods of time. One such complication is damage to the platelets that causes drug-induced hemolysis. Chemotherapeutic agents that kill cancer cells (and healthy cells too) wreak the most havoc followed by analgesics (e.g., NSAIDS), anti-inflammatories, quinine, aspirin, acetaminophen, anticonvulsants, etc. Of course, prolonged and serious illness such as cancer, severe hemorrhage, malaria, hemolytic liver diseases (e.g., cirrhosis, hepatic carcinoma, fulminant hepatitis), and excessive weight loss (anorexia) or long-term strict vegan diet causing malnutrition and bone marrow suppression will also lead to thrombocytopenia. There is also a type of dengue fever in temperate climate regions such as South Korea that, especially if contracted a second time, commonly leads to severe thrombocytic purpura.

The following are TCM medicinal treatment approaches for certain types of conditions associated with thrombocytompenia:

1. Chronic exposure to malaria may lead to hepatosplenomegaly.

The classical TCM pathologic term for this disease is "mother-of-malaria." In the early stage, prescribe either Xiao Chai Hu Tang, Chai Hu Gui Zhi Tang, or Chang Shan Wan; and for "interupt malaria" prescribe large doses of vacuity heat-clearing, summerheat clearing, and malaria-treating type medicinals (e.g. Qing Hao).

2. Insufficient production of thrombopoietin by the kidneys, long-term administration of chemotherapeutic agents, losing excessive weight (e.g., anorexia, cachexia), or long-term strict vegan diet resulting in malnutrition and bone marrow suppression can all be identified as kidney yang vacuity pattern. For treating this condition, you can prescribe either You Gui Yin, Shen Qi Wan, Shi Quan Da Bu Tang, or Ren Shen Yang Rong Tang adding Ren Shen (powder), Xi Lu Rong (powder), Zhu Qi, Gan Jiang, Fu Zi, Yu Gui, and Huang Bo.

3. Insufficient production of thrombopoietin by the liver can be identified as liver blood vacuity. For treating this condition, you can prescribe (Yu Sheng) Sheng Yu Tang adding Gan Jiang, Fu Zi, Yu Gui, Ren Shen (powder), Chuan Qi (powder) (or Zhu Qi), Xi Lu Rong (powder), and Huang Qin (or Huang Bo).

4. Contraction of dengue fever for a second time can be identified as exterior blood heat pattern. For treating this pathocondition, you can prescribe either Di Gu Pi Yin, Xiao Chai Hu Tang, or Yin Qiao San adding Qing Hao, Zhi Mu, Di Gu Pi, Yin Hua, Lian Qiao, Ou Jie, and Ce Bo Ye; or possibly consider combinations of medicinals such as Mu Dan Pi, Zhi Zi, Shi Shang Bo (aka Cui Yun Cao, Herba Selaginellae Doederleinii), Ji Xue Teng, and Luo Shi Teng.

5. The most difficult of these pathoconditions to treat are the hemolytic type presenting in cirrhosis, hepatic carcinoma, and fulminant hepatitis. Treatment of acute hepatitis is less demanding and easier to control and stablize. Patients with cirrhosis must be administered TCM medicinals for a long duration before resolving and then continue taking medicinals for at least another 6 months to 1 year to ensure the condition remains stabilized and is eventually completely remedied. Hepatic carcinoma requires long-term administration of TCM medicinals and follow-up evaluation.

6. For patients with drug-induced hemolytic pathoconditions, you can prescribe (Yu Sheng) Sheng Yu Tang or You Gui Yin variants. For patients with leukemia, renal cancer, and myeloma: in the acute stage, you should prescribe either Tong Jing Fang adding Huang Bo,

Qing Hao, Zhi Mu, and Di Gu Pi; or Zhi Bo Di Huang Tang variant; and in the chronic stage, you should prescribe either Zhi Bo Di Huang Tang, Dang Gui Liu Huang Tang, or Zuo Gui Yin variants. For patients presenting with thrombocytopenia resulting from repeated administration of radiotherapy and chemotherapy, if immature cells are "not" found in the blood and abnormal cells are "not" found in bone marrow aspiration, then prescribe You Gui Yin variant.

Case Study #3: Gong Zhen Dan - It's Not Sheng Yu Tang!

Q: I have an idiopathic thrombocytopenic purpura (ITP) patient with the following history:

The patient originally presented with PLT 7000. After taking a TCM formula (Gong Zhen Dan) that I did not prescribe, it increased to 27000; then 2 weeks later PLT fell to 5000, and the patient took more Gong Zhen Dan; and after another 2 weeks PLT jumped back up to 65000 and 87000. But just as before, 2 weeks later PLT dropped back down to 5000. This patient has an inexorable superstitution about the "elixir" Gong Zhen Dan. I have told the patient over and over again that Gong Zhen Dan will only provide "ephemeral" efficacy, but he just doesn't believe me. As you advised, the last time the patient visited I prescribed (Yu Sheng) Sheng Yu Tang adding Gan Jiang, Fu Zi, Yu Gui, Ren Shen (powder), and Xi Lu Rong (powder). Do you have any further advice on this patient?

A: Unfortunately, for this type of obstinant patient sometimes the only "medicine" that seems to work is having the patient find out for themselves what can happen when you don't listen to the "doctor's advice." Why would the PLT go up and down like a roller coaster ride? Gong Zhen Dan contains Xi Lu Rong (powder), Dang Gui, Shan Zhu Yu, and She Xiang, which all promote an increase in hematopoietic function; however, if corticosteroids are discontinued, then PLT levels will gradually fall back down again. Also, the dose of each medicinal is small with the effects relatively slow to appear; and nowadays She Xiang is usually synthetically manufactured, which has reduced its efficacy in the treatment of hematological disorders. In the past, many TCM doctors have proposed prescribing Shi Quan Da Bu Tang , You Gui Yin, or Xiang Sha Liu Jun Zi Tang adding Gan Jiang, Fu Zi, Yu Gui, Huang Qin, Ren Shen (powder), Xi Lu Rong (powder), Tu Si Zi, Huang Qi, and San Qi (or Zhu Qi). I have tried some of these approaches, but none has provided the effectiveness of (Yu Sheng) Sheng Yu Tang. One of my patients has been completely cured using this formula, going nearly 20 years now without a relapse.

Despite the patient's obstinance, my advice is to try again, firmly stating your case and assuring him that Sheng Yu Tang variant provides the best treatment for quick and sustained results. For even faster results try adding wine-soaked Zhu Qi (powder) 1 qian/day. Remember! For Xi Lu Rong (powder) start at 1 qian, don't add large doses too quickly; instead, first wait for the PLT to increase up until it plateaus and once the PLT remains at that plateaued level for about 3~5 weeks without rising, then you can begin adding large doses of Gan Jiang, Fu Zi, and Yu Gui. If at that point PLT levels do not rise, then you can gradually add 5 fen incremental doses of Xi Lu Rong (powder) (these small incremental increases will alleviate the potential for loose stools and overstimulation causing insomnia).

Case Study #4: Sheng Yu Tang - It's the Best!

Q: I have a patient diagnosed with idiopathic thrombocytopenic purpura (ITP). Both the patient and family members are very concerned about this condition and want to know specifics about the integrated TCM and Western medicine treatment approach: What Western medicine drugs should I take? When is the best time to discontinue taking the drug(s)? What is the plan if the PLT count falls again and the condition worsens? What is the role of TCM treatment if splenectomy is performed? Also, what is this Zhu Jie Qi medicinal anyways? If I don't have access to Zhu Jie Qi can I use Han Lian Cao instead?

A: Normally, all you need to do for positive results is prescribe (Yu Sheng) Sheng Yu Tang adding Gan Jiang, Fu Zi, Yu Gui, Huang Qin, Ren Shen (powder), Zhu Qi, Xi Lu Rong (powder), and Tu Si

Zi. If the patient has been administered corticosteroids or testosterone and has had blood transfusions, then the above formula will increase PLT up to around 200,000 within 1~3 weeks; and after 2~3 more weeks of administering this formula, then you should advise the patient to begin gradually reducing the doses of Western medicine drugs. If these drugs are discontinued too quickly, the TCM medicinals don't have enough time to rejuvenate the hematopoietic function of the bone marrow and compensate for the natural release of thrombopoietin by the kidneys, thus resulting in an initial decline followed by a subsequent rebound. In the great majority of cases, once you bring the PLT count back up to normal levels, the PLT count will remain sustained with relapse only rarely occurring.

As for splenectomy patients, if the PLT count is still low, then continue prescribing (Yu Sheng) Sheng Yu Tang variant. If splenitis or splenomegaly present, resulting in excessive platelet destruction, this is when you should prescribe Gui Pi Tang variant adding combinations of medicinals such as Mu Dan Pi, Zhi Zi, Gan Jiang, Fu Zi, Yu Gui, Huang Qin, Ren Shen (powder), Zhu Qi, and Xi Lu Rong (powder); or consider changing the formula to You Gui Yin variant instead.

Zhu Qi (aka Zhu Jie Qi) is the root of Sou Shan Hu (Radix Zanthoxyli austrosinensis) and appears in the book *Selected Medicinal Plants of Yunnan*.

Case Study #5: ITP in Menopausal Patient with Vaginal Bleeding

Q: I have been treating a 55 y/o female idiopathic thrombocytopenic purpura (ITP) patient for several months now, prescribing (Yu Sheng) Sheng Yu Tang adding Gan Jiang, Fu Zi, Yu Gui, Huang Qin, and Xi Lu Rong (powder) (each 6g); Ren Shen (powder) (3g); Han Lian Cao (6g); and Tu Si Zi (10g). I have been following up and evaluating her PLT count every 2 weeks with the results listed below:
  1st month: 5000→67000→3000
  2nd month: 3000→85000→5000
  3rd month: 5000→110000→10000

Her last menses was 3 years ago, so it was presumed she had entered menopause, but unexpectedly her menstrual cycles started up again (after taking (Yu Sheng) Sheng Yu Tang the patient felt mild fullness in her lower abdomen). Please share your views and advice about this patient's condition.

A: The dramatic fluctuations (sharp spikes and declines) in platelet count (thrombocytopenia) is likely due to excessive vaginal bleeding (menorrhagia) caused by endometrial hypertrophy. All you need to do is add Fu Ling, Ze Xie, Ou Jie, and Ce Bo Ye or consider adding a small dose of Zhu Sha (powder) to the mix. Technically, you can prescribe up to 12g per day of Zhu Sha, because this mineral medicinal is very dense by weight. Your plan should be to first reduce and check menstrual bleeding since this will enable the PLT to sustain high levels. Your treatment appears to be very effective, many patients would have dropped down to a low of 3000 ~5000, but your patient has leveled off at a minimum of 10000. Good work! Actually, it is not that uncommon for a 55 y/o women who has been menopausal for 3 years to have menses again. Adding Zhu Sha (powder) and large doses of Huang Qin and Huang Bo should stop the menstrual cycle (and bleeding) and also ensure that the PLT count does not drop back down again.

Case Study #6: Why Is the Fluctuation in PLT Count So Extreme?

Q: I am treating a 35 y/o female idiopathic thrombocytopenic purpura (ITP) patient with infertility whom has undergone intrauterine insemination (IUI) on two occasions. Last year in October she experienced sudden onset of high fever prompting her doctor to prescribe drug treatment that proved ineffective. She still had a fever after 10 days of drug administration so she was admitted into the hospital where low platelet count was discovered. In the hospital, she was administered 10 mg per day of corticosteroids and eventually her PLT rose back up to 170000 after which she was released from the hospital. However, her concerns over side effects of long-term corticosteroid administration prompted her to stop taking this medication, substituting it with another type. After switching medications, her PLT suddenly dropped to 3000 and due to persistent, severe nosebleeds she was admitted into the hospital again where corticosteroids and immunoglobin were administered. Her condition stablized once again, but after being released from the hospital she developed mild hepatosplenomegaly and continued taking oral corticosteroids, giving her the classic "moonface" appearance. Please offer your advice and guidance on this case?

A: Idiopathic thrombocytopenic purpura (ITP) patients who rely on corticosteroids to increase PLT above 100000 must "not" immediately stop taking corticosteroids. These patients must wait at least 3~5 months with PLT levels reaching between 150000~400000 before gradually reducing the dose by small incremental amounts. Remember! Hematopoietic function runs the risk of being dramatically suppressed unless a gradual approach to reducing and eventually discontinuing corticosteroid administration is employed.

Case Study #7: Splenectomy – Eliminates Platelet Destruction and Sequestration

Q: Right now I am treating five different idiopathic thrombocytopenic purpura (ITP) patients; all are taking cortiscosteroids and some have received splenectomies. An increasing number of potential patients are contacting me inquiring about TCM treatment for this condition. Among these patients, some are antinuclear antibody (ANA) positive and/or anti-dsDNA antibody positive, and another has Von Willebrand's disease. In addition to immunoglobulins (IVIG), other commonly administered Western medicine therapies are intravenous Rho(D) immune globulin (RhIG) for Rh-positive patients. Are there any potential side effects or complications from these therapies? Is it necessary to suppress the immune system in ANA positive and anti-dsDNA antibody positive patients? When should I suppress (drain)? When should I supplement? What factors should I consider in conducting pattern identification as the basis for determining treatment?

A: In my opinion, for idiopathic thrombocytopenic purpura (ITP) patients it is better to evaluate the complement levels. If antibody (i.e., ANA (+) and anti-dsDNA antibody (+)) levels are increased and complement levels (i.e., C3, C4) are decreased, then this can be identified as heat pattern. For patients with enduring, chronic conditions who have previously been administered corticosteroids and also have increased antibody levels, this is the time you should administer qi and blood-supplementing and yang-supplementing medicinals adding small doses of heat-abating medicinals as a counterbalance. These patients who are still being administered corticosteroids can be identified as spleen, kidney, or liver yang vacuity pattern, requiring administration of formulas such as Xiang Sha Liu Jun Zi Tang, Sheng Yu Tang, You Gui Wan, Shen Qi Wan, or Shi Quan Da Bu Tang adding "the Three Great Yang-Supplementers" (Gan Jiang, Fu Zi, and Yu Gui), Ren Shen (powder), Xi Lu Rong (powder), Tu Si Zi, Huang Qi, and Huang Qin.

Again, for these patients who have either previously been administered or are currently being administered corticosteroids that present with increased antibody levels and low complement levels (i.e., C3, C4); this is the time you should prescribe great yang-supplementing, qi and blood-supplementing, and spleen, kidney, or liver yang-supplementing medicinals! If antibodies are increased and complement levels (i.e., C3, C4) are normal, and the patient has "not" been administered corticosteroids, then this can be identified as heat pattern, requiring administration of formulas such as (Yu Sheng) Hyperactive Immune Formula, Xiao Chai Hu Tang, Di Gu Pi Yin, or Qin Lian Ru Mo Si Wu Tang adding Qin Hao, Zhi Mu, and Di Gu Pi along with Ce Bo Ye, Ou Jie, Qian Cao, Niu Xi, and Chuan Qi (powder). If antibodies are increased and complement levels (i.e., C3, C4) are normal, and the patient is presently being administered corticosteroids, then this can be identified as heat pattern with residual heat for which you should prescribe (Yu Sheng) Hyperactive Immune Formula to induce a rapid increase in PLT levels and a decrease in antibody levels. I hope this explanation about my treatment approach has answered your questions.

Remember! For patients receiving long-term administration of corticosteroids, once corticosteroids have been discontinued (or the effect wears off), PLT levels will inevitably drop, but the antibody levels will slightly increase and complement levels (i.e., C3, C4) will remain normal or only moderately low: it is for these types of patients with fluctuating levels due to stoppage and continuation of corticosteroid treatment whom you should add small doses of Gan Jiang, Fu Zi, and Yu Gui to your main formula – (Yu Sheng) Hyperactive Immune Formula! If you apply the yang-supplementing approach to decreasing antibody levels while gradually discontinuing administration of Westerm medicine drugs, there is no need to worry about the yang-supplmenting medicinals inducing a relapse. However, for rheumatoid arthritis (RA) patients the situation is different, as you must immediately subtract the yang-supplementing medicinals that were added to the (Yu Sheng) Hyperactive Immune Formula.

The purpose of receiving a splenectomy is to mainly eliminate platelet destruction (and antibody production to some extent). If the procedure is performed and PLT levels remain low, then this indicates that the source of the problem was in fact "not" the spleen but another mechanism (e.g., liver). In this situation, you can prescribe either Xiang Sha Liu Jun Zi Tang, Gui Pi Tang, Bu Zhong Yi Qi Tang, Shi Quan Da Bu Tang, Ren Shen Yang Rong Tang, or Sheng Yu Tang adding Gan Jiang, Fu Zi, Yu Gui, Huang Qin, Huang Qi, and Tu Si Zi. This approach will be effective in increasing and sustaining PLT levels.

Case Study #8: Familial (Inherited) ITP – It's Worth Following Up!

Q: I have an idiopathic thrombocytopenic purpura (ITP) patient whom has already discontinued corticosteroids. Previously, I had prescribed (Yu Sheng) Sheng Yu Tang for 3 1/2 months and observed his PLT count increase from 3000 up to 168000. This patient's younger brother also has ITP and has been battling the disease for more than 20 years. He has tried corticosteroids in the past without successful results, and has suffered cerebral hemorrhage on 3 occasions (presently he is normal). He has received treatment regimens prescribed by South Korea's most renowned traditional Korean medicine (TKM) physicians for over 2 years. Now his PLT is 3000, and he said that the treatment was not at all effective (patient just remembers the formula contained Lu Rong among other medicinals). What's your opinion on this case?

A: This case of familial (inherited) ITP is worthy of keeping tabs on and following up. I recommend you contact the chairperson of the hematological oncology foundation to see if you can collaborate in efforts to investigate the blood or marrow of these two patients (brothers) with familial (inherited) ITP and compare the results with their parents to determine if any genetic precursors exist. This is really an fascinating case!

Case Study #9: ITP Prevalence Increasing in South Korea – Patients Seek TCM Treatment

Q: I never imagined there were so many idiopathic thrombocytopenic purpura (ITP) patients. In the past, the general public didn't believe TCM could effectively treat ITP. Right now I am treating two ITP patients. One of them has already had PLT levels increase to 160000, and the other took my TCM prescription for 1 week with PLT increasing from 5000 to 22,000 and then up to 25000 after week 2. (I prescribed relatively large doses of Gan Jiang, Fu Zi, and Yu Gui (4 qian each)). Can you offer more insights from your experience treating this pathocondition?

A: Ah! It is obvious you are gaining more confidence and experience treating ITP patients. Remember! (Yu Sheng) Sheng Yu Tang variant is only suitable for liver blood vacuity pattern. If increased PLT destruction occurs in the spleen or splenomegaly (platelet sequestration) presents, then you can prescribe either Gui Pi Tang or Jia Wei Gui Pi Tang variants; and if "mother-of-malaria" presents, then prescribe Bie Jia Jian variant. If liver damage presents from chemotherapy or poisoning (Western medicine drugs or food) causing spontaneous bleeding of the flesh (petechiae or purpura), then prescribe either (Yu Sheng) Sheng Yu Tang, Xiang Sha Liu Jun Zi Tang, (Yu Sheng) Xue Ku Fang, Qi Bao Mei Ran Dan, You Gui Wan, Shen Qi Wan, Shi Bu Da Quan Tang, or Ren Shen Yang Rong Tang variants.

Liver damage due to poisoning can be identified as stasis heat pattern, requiring the administration of heat-clearing and toxin resolving medicinals; however, if high-dose platelet transfusions and corticosteroids have been administered, but the PLT count still doesn't increase, then (Yu Sheng) Sheng Yu Tang variant is more suitable for this condition. External contraction (e.g., dengue fever) can be identified as frenetic movement of hot blood and Shao Yang heat pattern, requiring the administration of either Di Gu Pi Yin, Xi Jiao Di Huang Tang, or Xiao Chai Hu Tang adding Mu Dan Pi, Zhi Zi, Qing Hao, Zhi Mu, and Di Gu Pi.

When renal production of thrombopoietin is insufficient, then this can be identified as kidney cold stasis pattern, requiring the administration of You Gui Wan or Shen Qi Wan adding Ren Shen (powder), Xi Lu Rong (powder), and Chuan Qi (powder) (or subtract Chuan Qi (powder) replacing it with wine-soaked Zhu Qi). If the patient presents with a hisotology of hypoplasia and fibrosis inducing suppression of hematopoietic function in the bone marrow, then you should prescribe You Gui Wan or Shen Qi Wan adding Ren Shen (powder), Chuan Qi (powder), Xi Lu Rong (powder), and Er Xian Miao.

Acute myelogenous leukemia (AML) patients with hematopoietic disorders can be identified as steaming bone taxation heat (fever) pattern, requiring administration of either Zhi Bo Di Huang Tang, Xiao Chai Hu Tang, Di Gu Pi Yin, or Xi Jiao Di Huang Tang adding Qing Hao, Zhi Mu, Di Gu Pi, Ce Bo Ye, and Ou Jie. Remember! You must carefully differentiate each individual case. From my experience, the most difficult patients to treat are those incurring graft failure following allogeneic bone marrow transplant (aka stem cell transplant) and the resulting insufficiency of platelet, RBC, and WBC production. This condition demands a lot of patience. You must first verify whether there are abnormal cells in the marrow aspiration and biopsy; if there are, then it can be identified as steaming bone pattern; and if not, then it can be identified as kidney yang vacuity with cold stasis.

Multiple myeloma patients can be identified as steaming bone and stasis heat pattern, requiring administration of (Yu Sheng) Tong Jing Fang or (Yu Sheng) Ru Mo Si Wu Tang adding Qing Hao, Zhi Mu, and Di Gu Pi.

Case Study #10: Other Heat Pattern Conditions Complicated By Idiopathic Thrombocytopenic Purpura (ITP)

Q: I have a 42 y/o female ITP patient. One week ago she discovered tiny pinpoint lesions (petichiae) spread over the medial aspect of both lower legs and medial aspect of both elbows. These spots varied in color from red, purple and brown, did not itch, and were not painful. I prescribed Gui Pi Tang variant. Please offer you advice and guidance on this patient's condition.

A: Has the patient been definitively diagnosed with ITP (e.g., CBC, bone marrow aspiration, presenting symptoms, history)? If not, you must not rule out the possibility of febrile disease complicated by wind heat rash (macules and papules), requiring the administration of Yin Qiao San or Di Gu Pi Yin variants, and "not" Gui Pi Tang. Remember! Gui Pi Tang and Sheng Yu Tang variants are administered for patients with low PLT counts, while blood heat and wind heat rash (macules and papules) may or may not be associated with low PLT count. As you know, external contraction (microbial infection) can also cause platelet destruction, which at the onset can be identified as Shao Yang heat, exterior wind, and blood heat pattern. If the administration of these types of medicinals doesn't lower PLT levels, then you can switch to Gui Pi Tang and Sheng Yu Tang variants, and unless you are certain the patient has already been administered high doses of corticosteroids and/or received platelet transfusions, then you should also add Mu Dan Pi and Zhi Zi, which forms Jia Wei Gui Pi Tang variant. If you know for sure high doses of corticosteroids were administered, then add Gan Jiang, Fu Zi, Yu Gui, Ren Shen (powder), Xi Lu Rong (powder), and Zhu Jie Qi.

ITP is relatively rare in Taiwan and I didn't realize there were so many patients with this condition in South Korea. It's possible that patients' patterns (e.g., cold, heat, vacuity, repletion) are not being accurately identified, as Western medicine doctors are repeatedly administering corticosteroids whose actions may suppress and disguise the underlying condition. Thus, I think the more likely scenario is that many of these cases are simply maculopapular eruptions and not actually ITP. It's just that accurate pattern identification is not being made over and over again resulting in errant diagnosis one after the other!

Case Study #11: She Also Has Evans Syndrome

Q: I have a 38 y/o female patient who experienced postpartum hemorrhage (epitaxis and menorrhagia) and went to the hospital for examination, during which a PLT count below 10000 was revealed. She was diagnosed with idiopathic thrombocytopenic purpura (ITP) and since the hemorrhage was intractable her doctors recommended uterectomy. Following treatment the patient's PLT levels remained at between 20000~30000, and after administration of intravenous immune globulin (IVIG) PLT levels dropped further down to 5000 with the presentation of nosebleeds and bleeding gums. Current lab test results are as follows: Hb 7 and PLT 38000. Her doctors have diagnosed her with Evans syndrome. What's the best treatment approach for patients with this condition?

A: In my opinion, you can consider prescribing either Sheng Yu Tang, You Gui Yin, or Shen Qi Wan adding yang-supplementing medicinals, Ren Shen (powder), Zu Qi, Xi Lu Rong (powder), and Ai Cao (or Ce Bo Ye). If immune system hyperactivity presents, then add Qing Hao, Zhi Mu, Di Gu Pi, and Mu Dan Pi. Additionally, you can advise the patient to eat plenty of raw lotus root and drink fresh lotus root juice, or also add Lian Ou Jie into the formula. This should be helpful in remedying the patient's condition.

Section 4: Behcet's Disease

Case Study #1: My First Behcet's Disease Patient

Q: I consulted and provided treatment for my first Behcet's disease (BD) patient recently. The patient explained that 10 years ago she began having recurrent oral ulcers (aphthous stomatitis) in her mouth and frequently caught common colds. These symptoms endured for a long period of time with treatment efforts proving ineffective and prompting her to undergo examination at a hospital. Doctors diagnosed her with Behcet's disease and she began receiving treatment with Western medicine drugs. The medication didn't offer any noticeable improvement in her condition so she decided to seek TCM consultation and treatment.

Since her only presenting symptoms were recurring oral ulcers and susceptibility to catching common colds (external contraction), typically aversion to cold with heat pattern type, I prescribed Da Qing Long Tang adding Huang Qin and Sheng Pu Huang. Do you think this is a good approach? How about a long-term treatment approach?

A: Behcet's disease (aka "fox-creeper" in classical TCM pathological terminology) patients simply presenting with oral ulcers and susceptibility to external contraction can be identified as exterior pattern with residual heat. In this case, yes, Da Qing Long Tang adding Huang Qin and Sheng Pu Huang is a good choice, and you can also consider adding Huang Bo and Huang Lian. This formula can be prescribed long-term. TCM physicians in Japan commonly prescribe Wen Qing Yin, which is comrpised of Si Wu Tang combining Huang Lian Jie Du Tang. If it's really been that long since the patient received Western medicine drug treatment, then the physiological side effects should have already spontaneously metabolized by now, so you don't need to consider adding yang-supplementing medicinals to Da Qing Long Tang variant. In periods of remission, you can prescribe Xie Xin Tang (composed of Da Huang, Huang Lian, and Huang Qin) adding Pu Huang or just simply prescribe Pu Huang, instructing the patient to decoct these medicinals and drink the solution like a beverage.

Case Study #2: Behcet's Requires Long-term Administration of TCM Medicinals

Q: I have a 43 y/o female patient presenting as follows: painful sores (ulcerations) on tongue and mouth cavity and swollen, inflamed sores on external genitalia that flare up and then spontaneously resolve, and mild pain in both knee joints. The patient explained that she has been suffering from this condition for 11 years and had been on long-term administration of Western medicine drugs without effectiveness. She decided to try TCM and came to see me for consultation. Upon inspection I observed she had white thick tongue fir, aphthous ulcerations on her tongue and mouth cavity, and mild pain in both her knee joints without swelling. Her appetite, urine, and stool were all normal, and she didn't have a fever. I suspect this is Behcet's disease ("fox-creeper") and thus prescribed Wen Qing Yin adding Sheng Pu Huang. Do you think this was the correct diagnosis and treatment approach? Please offer your advice about the treatment course and prognosis.

A: References to Behcet's disease can be found in *On Cold Damage and Miscellaneous Diseases* under Fox-Creeper. Actually, for most patients this condition is not particularly difficult to treat. The key for treatment is long-term administration of a formula that contains "the Three Yellows" and Pu Huang (large doses of each), Mu Dan Pi, Qing Hao, Di Gu Pi, and Zhi Mu. And if joint pain presents, then add Huo Luo Dan; if erosions of the genitals present, then add Long Dan Cao; if erosion of the anus presents, then add Bai Zhi, Huai Hua, Di Yu, Fang Feng, and Bai Zhi; and if red and inflamed eyes present, then add Ru Xiang, Mo Yao, Chuan Qi (powder), and Tao Hong Hua.

The formula you prescribed is accurately based on the patient's presenting pattern identification. Remember! TCM treatment of this disease requires long-term administration of medicinals. The patient should have lab tests periodically performed so you can assess ESR and CRP levels. Once these levels are normal, you should change the formula to either Xian Fang Huo Ming Yin, Sheng Yu Tang, or Bu Yang Huan Wu Tang adding "the Three Yellows."

Case Study #3: Once Western Medicine Drugs Have Been

Discontinued – (Yu Sheng) Hyperactive Immune Formula

Q1: A 38 y/o female patient has suffered from oral cavity aphthous ulcerations (tongue and mouth) for more than 20 years. She explained that at the age of 9 she began having pain in both knees, prompting her to undergo examination which revealed rheumatoid factor (RF) positive. She was administered Western medicine drugs at the time and her symptoms were partially relieved, but ever since then she has felt malaise and tidal heat. Recently, a severe flare up in both wrist joints prompted her to spend five months in the hospital before resolving, and she worried that her illness would relapse again. Past administration of immunosuppressant medication caused allergic reactions so she doesn't want to take them anymore. Now, she wants to try TCM treatment. After taking history and examining this patient (even though she doesn't have the telltale genital ulcerations), I suspect she has Behcet's disease. Please offer your advice and guidance.

A1: Behcet's does commonly present in women and based on your description it does suggest she has fox-creeper (aka Behcet's disease (BD)). Remember! If your patient has not been administered corticosteroids, MTX, chemotherapeutic agents, or Cyclosporin A (immunosuppressant), but simply took analgesics, then this can be identified as heat pattern. Blood test results will not necessarily reveal abnormalities in C3/C4, ANA, and anti-dsDNA, but abnormal levels of Ig, ESR, CRP, and RF can all be identified as heat pattern, requiring the administration of Hyperactive Immune Formula (including large doses of "the Three Yellows") adding Sheng Pu Huang. If swollen and painful joints present, then add Ma Huang, Niu Qi, and Sheng Du Zhong (if in lower extremities); and if loose stools present, then add Cang Zhu, Fu Ling, and Ze Xie. The administration of TCM medicinals in patients whom have not been administered Western medicine drugs is the optimal scenario providing the most effective treatment. For patients who have already received long-term administration of Western medicine drugs, you should evaluate Hb and C3/C4 as the basis for pattern identification and treatment. If levels are low, then supplement qi, blood, and yang. If completment levels are normal, then advise the patient to gradually discontinue Western medicine drugs. Once

Western medicine drugs are fully discontinued and there have been no sudden exacerbations in symptoms over an extended period of time, then you can change the formula to (Yu Sheng) Hyperactive Immune Formula variant. Administration of this formula will ensure the patient's condition remains symptom free, and eventually administration of this formula can be gradually reduced and discontinued.

Q2: Sorry to trouble you again! Since she began taking (Yu Sheng) Hyperactive Immune Formula adding Sheng Pu Huang and Lian Qiao, the patient has had loose stools (5~10 times/day), cold hands and feet, chest distention and heaviness, and her oral ulcerations have worsened. I want to change formulas to Xiang Sha Liu Jun Zi Tang combining Huang Lian Jie Du Tang adding Lian Qiao, Pu Gong Ying, Wu Zhu Yu, Dang Gui, and Xi Xin. Do you think this is a good approach?

A2: If you are sure she has Behcet's disease, then the original formula is still best. Again, if the patient presents with loose stools, then either add Cang Zhu and Ze Xie to the main formula (Hyperactive Immune Formula); reduce the medicinal doses; or change the formula to Huang Lian Jie Du Tang (subtracting Zhi Zi) adding Sheng Pu Huang and "the Four Ling's."

Cold hands and feet is a typical psychosomatic symptom of the autonomic nervous system, thus it's not necessary to add Dang Gui, Xi Xin, and Wu Zhu Yu. However, you could consider prescribing formula variants such as Qing Zao Jiu Fei Tang (dryness-clearing and lung-moistening action); Sheng Yang Yi Wei Tang (spleen and stomach-supplementing and yin fire-draining action); or Ping Wei San combining Huang Lian Jie Du Tang adding Sheng Pu Huang (dampness-drying and spleen-fortifying, qi-moving and stomach-harmonizing, and heat-clearing and toxin-resolving action). Though I rarely prescribe these types of formulas, for some people's body constitutions it may be necessary. For instance, it sounds like I have a similar type of body consitition as this patient, because whenever I take "the Three Yellows" it causes me to have loose stools as well; and when I get a common cold (external contraction) I must apply Li Dong-yuan's approach by adding spleen and stomach-supplementing medicinals to the formula.

Q3: Thanks for your advice and guidance. After changing the formula to Xiang Sha Liu Jun Zi Tang adding Qing Hao and Zhi Mu (8 qian each); Lian Qiao, Pu Gong Ying, and Dang Shen (5 qian each); Jin Yin Hua (the patient has conjunctivitis); and Huo Luo Dan (swollen and painful knees); the patient's condition has improved dramatically. Not only have her bowel movements, cold hands and feet, and chest heaviness normalized, but the oral ulcerations, joint pain, and eye inflammation are getting much better.

A3: Behcet's disease (BD) can be identified as a true heat pattern. Congratulations on the accurate pattern identification and treatment. This makes both the patient and doctor happy!

Case Study #4: Painful Oral Ulcerations on the Tongue and Mouth – It Could Be Behcet's Disease

Q: A 6 y/o female patient went for a medical examination 3 years ago due to oral ulcerations on the side of her tongue and mouth (so painful she couldn't eat or drink hot or spicy foods) and excessive tearing (epiphora). At the time, blood tests were normal; and neither the medication (for ulcerations) nor the surgical procedure (for epiphora) were effective. To this day, she is still troubled with the recurring painful tongue and mouth ulcerations, prompting her mother to bring her in for consultation.

Despite the aphthous ulcerations on her tongue and oral cavity suggesting the patient has Behcet's disease, I think her condition looks more like Sjogren's syndrome (SS). Thus, I prescribed Hyperactive Immune Formula adding Sheng Pu Huang and Mai Men Dong. Administration of this formula resulted in rapid improvement in the patient's symptoms. Do you think I have accurately identified the pattern and provided an appropriate treatment?

A: According to TCM theory a painful tongue can be idenfitied as effulgent heart fire pattern and ulcerations on the side of the tongue and mouth cavity can be idenfitied as stomach heat pattern. The diagnosis of fox-creeper (aka Behcet's disease) is correct; it's not

Sjogren's syndrome (SS). However, your prescription of Hyperactive Immune Formula adding Sheng Pu Huang and Mai Men Dong is still based on accurate TCM pattern identification, so naturally you will have effective results!

Case Study #5: Sjogren's Syndrome – It's More Than Sicca Syndrome

Q: I have a 62 y/o female patient whom presented with dry mouth (xerostomia), painful gums, dry-fissured tongue, and swollen parotid glands. She explained that 1 year ago the same symptoms occurred, but test results couldn't isolate a definitive diagnosis. She takes Western medicine drugs, which is sometimes effective in remedying symptoms for 2~3 days before recurring again. Recently, her dry mouth has been so severe that when eating food she has a "burning" sensation, so she decided to visit my clinic. What are your thoughts on the diagnosis and treatment of this pathocondition?

A: Your description of this patient's sicca syndrome symptoms strongly suggests the diagnosis of Sjogren's syndrome (SS), but technically this diagnosis is not made unless there is laboratory evidence of autoimmune disease present. Regardless of the Western medicine diagnosis, for this condition you can consider prescribing formula variations such as Hyperactive Immune Formula; Huang Lian Jie Du Tang adding Si Wu Tang (aka Wen Qing Yin); or Wen Dan Tang (adding Huang Bo and Huang Lian) along with combinations of medicinals such as Qing Hao, Zhi Mu, Di Gu Pi, Tian Men Dong, Mai Men Dong, Tian Hua, Yuan Shen, or Sheng Pu Huang. You can determine which medicinals to add based on the patient's presenting signs, symptoms, and pattern identification. The "burning" sensation your patient feels when she eats is phantom pain or phantom heat, and for this you can add Quan Xie, Bai Jiang Can, Wu Gong, and Yu Sheng Wan.

Case Study #6: Viscous Saliva May Indicate Sjogren's

Syndrome

Q: A 70 y/o female patient began experiencing severely dry mouth (salivary gland hypofunction) and viscous saliva. In the past, she had taken Western medicine drugs but treatment attempts were not effective; and now, she has sought my consultation to treat this condition. What is the best approach for treating this patient?

A: Dry mouth, viscous saliva (sicca syndrome), and dry eyes (xerophthalmia) are the most commonly presenting symptoms in patients with the autoimmune disorder Sjogren's syndrome (SS). You should prescribe Hyperactive Immune Formula (including large doses of each medicinal (especially "the Three Yellows")) adding Sheng Pu Huang. This formula should effectively remedy this patient's condition.

Case Study #7: Exposure to Water Induces Skin Rash (Papules)

Q: A 49 y/o female patient complained of a skin rash with reddish, slightly raised papules on her arms and legs. She explained that this condition began presenting 3 days ago when "every time my arms and legs touched water a rash would appear on my skin." During her clinic visit, I saw this rash (tiny papules) appear myself when I sprinkled water on her arm as a test. Have you ever heard of this type of reaction before?

A: Exposure to water inducing skin rash with red papules can be identified as "reversal cold" and strongly suggests Raynaud's disease, which occurs when the amount of cryoglobulin (CR) in the blood is too high (cryoglobulinemia). TCM treatment of reversal cold typically calls for either Dang Gui Si Ni Tang or Dang Gui Si Ni Tang combining Wu Zhu Yu Gan Jiang Tang adding Huang Qin, Fu Zi, and Huang Qi.

Case Study #8: Reversal Cold Inducing Red Rash – Raynaud's Disease

Q: I have a 48 y/o female patient who is allergic to cold. Exposure to cold objects (e.g., cold water, ice) will initially induce itchiness (urticaria) and reddish painful swelling (angioedema), and then progress to a generalized rash (papules) over the entire body. She is so sensitive to cold that even air conditioning and raindrops will cause a rash (papules) to present. Her latest allergic reaction began about 3 weeks ago. How would you treat this condition?

A: Allergic reaction upon exposure to cold indicates the "reversal cold" of Raynaud's disease (RD), which is caused by increased levels of cryoglobulin (CR) in the blood (cryoglobulinemia) and resulting in cutaneous ischemia. Remember! This condition must "not" be identified as exterior wind-cold pattern. In the winter, these patients are susceptible to "sloughing flat-abscess" (gangrene) in which severe peripheral vasculature ischemia leads to necrosis. In Taiwan, we call this "black hand disease" and "black-foot disease." In the past, frostbite inducing gangrene was much more prevalent among people who worked outdoors (e.g., farmers, laborers) during the cold weather months. Nowadays, with the development of effective cold weather gear, improvement of labor conditions, and healthier nutritional intake, this condition is much less common. In your mother and father's (definitely grandmother and grandfather's) generation, the cracked skin and purulent erosions of "sloughing flat-abscess" (gangrene) were a much more common (though unpleasant!) sight.

To treat this condition, if a "painful" rash (papules) presents, then prescribe either Xue Ku Fang adding Gan Jiang, Fu Zi, Yu Gui, Wu Zhu Yu, and Huang Qin; or Dang Gui Si Ni Tang combining Wu Zhu Yu Gan Jiang Tang adding Fu Zi, Huang Qin, Chuan Qi (powder), and Ren Shen (powder).

Case Study #9: Irritable Bowel Disease (IBD) – Ulcerative Colitis (UC) and Crohn's disease (CD)

Q: I have a 40 y/o female patient whom has endured 10~20 stools (often with small amounts of fresh blood) per day for the past 30 years. Recently, her condition has worsened prompting her to go to the hospital for an examination. Colonoscopy revealed continuous areas of inflammation and ulcerations in the lining of the colon and rectum. Her doctors prescribed corticosteroids which have proven to be very effective. However, she can only take this medication for 2 months and she is worried about the condition recurring, so she decided to try TCM treatment. I diagnosed her condition as irritable bowel disease (IBD), and specifically chronic ulcerative colitis (UC), based on the location, distribution, and depth of the lesions. Please offer your advice and guidance on this patient's condition.

A: Colorectal ulcerations and Behcet's disease (BD) both correlate with the classical TCM pathological term "fox-creeper." In the early days of Western medicine morphine was prescribed to treat this condition and now corticosteroids are administered. Ulcerative colitis (UC) and Crohn's disease (CD) are the two main types of irritable bowel disease (IBD) in which the immune system attacks the mucous membrane lining of the intestinal walls (CD and UC) and other parts of the digestive tract and body (only CD).

In TCM, regardless if corticosteroids have been administered or not, this pathocondition can be identified as great heat pattern or possibly great heat with Shao Yang heat pattern. To treat this condition, I typically prescribe (Yu Sheng) Hyperactive Immune Formula (composed of Huang Lian Jie Du Tang subtracting Zhi Zi and adding Qing Hao, Zhi Mu, and Di Gu Pi) adding "the Four Ling's."

Case Study #10: Aphthous Tongue Ulcers – Heat Pattern of "Fox-Creeper"

Q: A 52 y/o male patient suddenly began having raised lesions and painful ulcers on his tongue. He was administered treatment with Western medicine drugs, which were not effective. Do you think this could be Sjogren's syndrome (SS)?

A: Raised lesions and painful ulcers on the tongue can be identified as heat pattern and can be classified as "fox-creeper"; it's not Sjogren's syndrome (SS). You can prescribe Hyperactive Immune Formula (including large doses of "the Three Yellows," Qing Hao, Zhi Mu, and Di Gu Pi) adding Sheng Pu Huang. You should instruct the patient to drink this decocted formula as follows: make sure the decoction has cooled to at least room temperature, drink the decoction like a beverage in small amounts over a 24-hour period, and thoroughly rinse the entire mouth slowly letting the liquid soak into the mucous membrane of the oral cavity prior to swallowing.

Sjogren's syndrome (SS) typically presents with the sicca syndrome symptoms of dryness of the exocrine glands, particularly the eyes (xerophthlamia) and mouth (xerostomia). It's possible for patients with SS to also have Behcet's disease (BD) and thus present with aphthous ulcerations, but up to now I have not witnessed this type of case in my clinical practice. If the sores and ulcerations appear bright red colored, then you can consider adding Pu Gong Ying, Yu Sheng Wan, and Wan Ling Dan. Remember! Both BD and SS can be idenfitied as heat pattern and thus the treatment is the same.

Case Study #11: Autoimmune Diseases – Amyloidosis Predisposition

Q: A 50 y/o female patient began suffering symptoms 2 years ago in June, prompting a hospital examination and resulting diagnosis of ulcerative colitis (UC). The patient was treated with hydrocotrisone rectal suspension for 3 months, which produced effective results. One year later in early July she began experiencing difficulty breathing (when walking upstairs) and dry cough, for which she took Western medicine drugs without effective results. After hospital examination she was diagnosed with bronchiolitis obliterans organizing pneumonia (BOOP) and was treated with large doses of corticosteroids. Blood oxygen levels were normal and aside from the breathing difficulty, dry cough, and loose stools, all other test results were normal and the symptoms were not severe.

The patient's husband is the editor-in-chief of South Korea's largest newspaper. They have several Western medicine doctors in their family and don't have much faith in TCM. However, after ineffective Western medicine treatment, the director of the radiology oncology department (also my academic advisor) at my university's hospital personally introduced me to this patient. I have a lot of pressure on this case. Please offer your much appreciated advice and guidance.

A: Ulcerative colitis (UC) and Crohn's disease (CD) are two closely related types of irritable bowel disease (IBD) caused by the immune system attacking the lining of the GI tract and other mucous membranes (only in the case of CD). Both UC and CD can be classified under the TCM condition called fox-creeper (aka Behcet's disease). If large doses of methylprednisolone pulse therapy, anticancer agents, and immunosuppressants (MTX) have been administered, which interferes with hematopoiesis and immnue functions, then this can be identified as kidney yang vacuity. In all other cases, these pathologies are heat conditions manifesting in either yang hyperactivity, yang hyperactivity of the Shao Yang channel, yin vacuity, or steaming bone with taxation heat pattern. For yang vacuity pattern, if blood test results are normal after 3~6 months prior to discontinuing Western medicine drugs, then this pathocondition has returned to its "essential state" of either yin vacuity wtih yang hyperactivity pattern or hyperactivity of the three yang channels pattern. Once the condition returns to its "essential heat pattern state," you should prescribe Hyperactive Immune Formula (containing the "the Three Yellows," Qing Hao, Zhi Mu, Di Gu Pi, and Cang Zhu).

People with autoimmune disease are predisposed to amyloid deposits forming in the tissues and capillary membranes of organs (e.g., heart, lungs, eyes, brain) thus interfering with normal function. The presentation of difficulty breathing and dry cough suggests this type of secondary amyloidosis. For this condition you should prescribe (Yu Sheng) Hyperactive Immune Formula adding Ma Huang, Xing Ren, Ting Li Zi, Fu Ling, and Ze Xie; Chuan Qiong, Chi Shao, Dan Shen, Yin Xing Ye, Ma Huang, and Xing Ren; Tian Men Dong, Mai Men Dong, Sha Shen, and Yuan Shen (lung yin-nourishing action); and if necessary Ci Yuan, Kuan Dong Hua, Wu Wei Zi, and Bai Bu (watery phlegm-dispelling action). These medicinals will effectively treat pathoconditions involving water amassment, stasis heat, lung yin vacuity, and lung cold phlegm shooting into the lung. Carefully assess the patient's condition to identify the pattern and determine the best medicinals for treatment.

Remember! The key factors during diagnosis are to differentiate between dry cough and watery phlegm, the presence of pleural effusion, edema of the upper and lower limbs, and night cough. Some telltale signs of pleural effusion are the following: the patient will begin to cough after sitting for a while, but when lying down they won't cough; or possibly cough for a brief period of time after lying down and then stop coughing; or cough once they turn over.

Case Study #12: Adult-onset Still's Disease (AOSD)

Q: A 30 y/o female patient began experiencing symptoms of generalized joint pain and swelling about 3 years ago prompting her to undergo hospital examination. Doctors suspected rheumatoid arthritis (RA) and did a workup only to find RF (-), ESR normal, and CRP slightly elevated. Based on these results, her doctors suspected adult-onset Still's disease (AOSD). Ever since then she has been receiving corticosteroids (her distinctive "moonface" will attest to that) to relieve the symptoms, but this approach has not offered lasting results. What is your opinion about this patient's condition?

A: Adult-onset Still's disease (AOSD) is an immune hyperactivity pathocondition that causes an inflammatory type of arthritis similar to rheumatoid arthritis (RA). Does the patient have any other symptoms such as tidal fever or sore throat? Also, you should advise the patient to have the following tested: C3/C4, ANA, anti-dsDNA, BUN, and Cr. Western medicine doctors will typically administer prednisone, immunosuppressants, and biologic response modifiers for the treatment of this pathocondition. Regardless of the Western medicine drugs prescribed, in TCM this pathocondition can be identified as yin vacuity heat pattern and treatment is the same as for dermatomyositis or rheumatoid arthritis (RA). Thus, I would prescribe (Yu Sheng) Hyperactive Immune Formula possibly adding Jian Ling Tang and Wan Ling Dan; bleed Da Zhui (DU14) (above, at, below), Wei Zhong (UB40), Tai Yuan (LU9), and the well points of the pericardium, liver, spleen, and stomach channels; and perform acupuncture on the acupoints of the Shao Yang channel (applying the draining technique). This approach should provide effective results in a relatively short period of time.

EPILOGUE

Our aim was to provide the reader with an insider's perspective on this subject matter through the compilation of these Q&A format case studies. We sincerely hope that TCM students, scholars, practitioners, physicians, and the interested layperson alike have gleaned valuable information on both the clinical application of TCM in primary and secondary care and as a first-line therapeutic option, as well as the integrative role TCM offers in neoadjuvant, adjuvant, complementary, and palliative therapy. This fluid introduction of a broad spectrum of pathologies is intended to inspire the reader to pursue further research and explore the vast potential for broader clinical applications. We recognize that the development and expansion of TCM clinical applications is in part influenced by prevailing cultural factors and institutional barriers existing within each respective society and nation. Amidst these dynamics, TCM's increasingly manifest scientific basis and overwhelming efficacy continues propelling this 3,000 year-old medical system to the forefront of inquiry and discovery into its promising possibilities. We anticipate that *Clinical Applications: Integrated Traditional Chinese Medicine (TCM) and Western Medicine (I)* has piqued your interests for learning more and encourage you to continue reading our upcoming volumes in the near future.

APPENDIX

Dr. Lee's Pharmacopeia

This section introduces the medicinals Dr. Lee most commonly prescribes and includes details on processing, dosage, and action. At times classical references will be included that provide insight into the foundations for Dr. Lee's application of these medicinals. Certain medicinals that are frequently administered together in pairs and combinations are introduced with a description of their actions and "grouped names." It is important to reiterate that these profiles are intended to highlight and clarify some of the distinctive properties, actions, and functions of Dr. Lee's commonly prescribed medicinals and does not attempt to present a complete listing of every medicinal Dr. Lee applies in clinical practice.

***Disclaimer**: The medicinal doses provided in Dr. Lee's commonly prescribed pharmacopeia listed below and throughout this entire book are "for reference purposes only" and are "not" intended for indiscriminate administration by other individuals or parties. Prescription of these medicinals should only be administered by a licensed traditional Chinese medicine (TCM) physician or practitioner whom has carefully evaluated the patient's history, signs, and symptoms and then conducted pattern identification as the basis for determining treatment. Licensed TCM physicians or practitioners must be aware that these medicinals and medicinal doses are "for reference purposes only" and are "solely" intended for administration by Dr. Lee in his own clinical practice.

Da Huang (大黃) – This medicinal should be first steeped in rice wine over a period of 10 days (in warm weather) to 2 weeks (in cold weather), oven-dried, and then cut to be used as raw decocting pieces or pulverized into a powder for topical application. This medicinal is administered for patients with a wide range of pathoconditions from gastrointestinal disorders (e.g. constipation, gallstones) to elevated intracranial pressure. Its heat-clearing and draining precipitation, fire-draining and accumulation-attacking, and blood-quickening and stasis-transforming actions promote the removal of metabolic waste byproducts resulting from nerve cell damage and static blood; break down bile; reduce pressure of the portal vein and relax the diaphragm muscles; stimulate intestinal motility; and eliminate endothelial hyperplasia (e.g., inflammation from autoimmune disease, viral infection). For the treatment of increased intracranial pressure (ICP), initially small amounts are prescribed increasing incrementally in 5 fen doses up to 7~8 qian until the desired draining precipitation action is achieved, which is typically 2~3 stools per day (sometimes as much as 5 stools per day depending on the pathocondition). In addition to oral administration, **Da Huang (powder) (大黃粉)** can also be topically applied on open sores as an antimicrobial and to stanch bleeding. It dries and forms a protective barrier that prevents infectious agents from entering the wound and also fights infection within the lesion. Da Huang can also be blended into either a petrolatum or an emulsifying hydrophilic ointment base for inflammatory skin pathoconditions (e.g., streptococcal, stapholococcal).

"The Three Great Yang-Supplementers" ("三大補陽") – The medicinal combination of **Gan Jiang (乾薑)**, **Fu Zi (附子)**, and **Yu Gui (玉桂)** comprise one of the pillars of Dr. Lee's treatment approaches. These great heat spleen and kidney yang-supplementing medicinals are prescribed for yang vacuity and cold stasis conditions in the post-acute and chronic stages or following surgery and radiotherapy or administration of Western medicine drugs such as immunosuppressants (e.g., corticosteroids, monoclonal antibodies, cyclosporine) and chemotherapeutic agents. Dr. Lee also prescribes this medicinal combination when the treatment regimen has reached a point where only marginal or no further improvement is being made. These great heat kidney yang-supplementing medicinals boost the metabolism by innervating the nervous system (central nervous system (CNS), peripheral nervous system (PNS), and autonomic nervous system (ANS) and engage a cascade of endocrine and hormonal factors. And when **Ren Shen (人參)**, **Huang Qi (黃耆),** and **Lu Rong (鹿茸)** are prescribed together in a formula that includes "the Three Great Yang-Supplementers" this combination stimulates the body's capacity for self-repair, regeneration (e.g., nerves, skin, tissue, bone), and hematopoiesis. An initial dose of 2~3 qian for each medicinal will be prescribed increasing incrementally up to 5~8 qian each. Once the combined dose reaches 10~12 qian, then 3~5 qian of either Huang Qin (黃芩), Huang Bo (黃柏), or Huang Lian (黃連) are added to counteract the potential of adverse effects (e.g., excessive cerebral vascular blood perfusion that might lead to rupture and hemorrhage).

Fu Zi (附子) – In this book the medicinal referred to as Fu Zi is actually **Tian Xiong (天雄)**, which is the root tuber of this plant without the daughter (accessory) roots. Processing of this medicinal entails steeping in a solution of magnesium chloride ($MgCl_2$), sodium chloride (NaCl), and water and then it is dried and sliced into small pieces. Classical literature on pharmacopeia describes the parts of the aconite plant as follows: "The mother [root] is **Wu Tou (烏頭)**, the [peripheral] accessory roots are **Fu Zi (附子)**, the [peripheral] extensions [of the accessory roots] are **Ce Zi (側子)**, and the long slender part [extending from the mother root] is **Tian Xiong (天雄)**." In classical literature on pharmacopeia **Fu Zi** is described as having "...great drying and yang returning, supplementing kidney and life fire, and expeling wind-cold-damp [actions]" and the capacity to "...free the twelve channels [with] no limits beyond its reach."

Yu Gui (玉桂) – (also known as **Rou Gui (肉桂)**, **Guang Gui (官桂)**, and **Gui Xin (桂心)**) The majority of formulas Dr. Lee prescribes are "classic" formulas derived from *On Cold Damage and Miscellaneous Diseases* (subsequently divided into two books called *On Cold Damage* and *Essential Prescriptions of the Golden Coffer*). Based on the instructions to "remove the skin" from **Gui Zhi (桂枝)** in these texts, which is tantamount to removing its main constituents and nullifying its medicinal actions, Dr. Lee believes that a clerical error was made in recording **Gui Zhi** and that **Yu Gui** was actually the intended medicinal prescribed. **Gui Zhi** was simply a less expensive, but inferior, alternative for **Yu Gui (Rou Gui)** and with the exception of some cases requiring mild exterior-resolving actions **Yu Gui (Rou Gui)** was prescribed instead. **Yu Gui**'s actions encompass those of **Gui Zhi** (i.e., exterior-resolving, spleen-fortifying, pain-relieving, antimicrobial) and also contains vasodilation actions that more effectively promote blood circulation. In fact, Dr. Lee even substitutes **Gui Zhi** with **Yu Gui** in exterior-resolving formulas such as Gui Zhi Tang (桂枝湯) and with the exception of Chai Ling Tang (柴玲湯) the only other time he prescribes **Gui Zhi** is for its function as an upper extremity channel-conducting medicinal. In classical literature on pharmacopeia **Yu Gui**'s action of freeing the channels and blood vessels is described as having the capacity to "free the twelve channels" and "conduct the hundred medicinals," which is further expressed here: "**Rou Gui [Yu Gui]** conducts medicinals throughout [the entire body]; there are no limits beyond its reach."

Gan Jiang (乾薑) – **Sheng Jiang (生薑)** is processed by steaming with sulfur to produce this medicinal. It has the actions of warming the center and dissipating cold. In classical literature on pharmacopeia it is described as having "drying, yang-returning, diffusing, and vessel-freeing [actions]" and the complementary relationship between **Fu Zi (附子)** and **Gan Jiang** is expressed as follows: "**Fu Zi** is mobile [extends throughout body] and **Gan Jiang** is both mobile and static [long-lasting effect]."

"The Three Yellows" ("三黃") – This term refers to the combination of **Huang Qin (黃芩)**, **Huang Bo (黃柏)**, and **Huang Lian (黃連)**. The heat-clearing and toxin-resolving (antimicrobial and anti-inflammatory) actions of these medicinals make them among the most important and commonly used medicinals in Dr. Lee's pharmacopeia and comprise one of the pillars of Dr. Lee's treatment approaches. They provide exceptional efficacy for the treatment of all kinds of infections and inflammation whether it be nasal, upper respiratory tract, gastrointestinal, hepatic, renal, autoimmune, etc.; and are also used in Yu Sheng formulas to counteract great heat of **"the Great Heat Yang-Supplementers"** – **Gan Jiang (乾薑)**, **Fu Zi (附子)**, and **Yu Gui (玉桂)**. Classical literature on pharmacopeia differentiates the specific actions of these three medicinals as follows: "...**Huang Lian** drains heart fire and middle burner fire, **Huang Qin** drains upper burner fire, **Huang Bo** drains lower burner fire...." Dr. Lee also acknowledges these differentiations using **Huang Lian** for the gastrointestinal tract, **Huang Qin** for the upper respiratory tract, and **Huang Bo** for the kidneys and urinary tract. However, from his clinical experience these specific distinctions aren't vital to achieve efficacy and when evil qi (i.e., microbial infection) is being treated the combination of **"the Three Yellows"** provides effective broad spectrum antimicrobial action.

Huang Qin (黃芩) – In classical literature on pharmacopeia it is described as follows: "**Huang Qin** has a bitter [flavor] and cold [nature], bitter drains liver fire, drains middle burner repletion fire, and eliminates spleen [family] damp heat"; "Bitter [flavor] enters the heart [and] cold [nature] overcomes heat to drain the middle burner fire [and] eliminate spleen family damp heat"; "**Huang Qin** downbears phlegm and [along with it] downbears fire"; and "**Huang Qin** is an upper and middle burner medicinal." In contemporary texts this medicinal is described as having a cold nature and bitter flavor; entering the lung, stomach, gallbladder, and large intestine channels; and having heat-clearing and dampness-drying, fire-draining and toxin-resolving, blood-cooling and blood-stanching, and heat elminating and fetus-quieting actions.

Huang Bo (黃柏) – In classical literature on pharmacopeia it is described as "Draining ministerial fire [and] supplementing kidney water"; "**Huang Bo** has a bitter [flavor] and cold [nature] and drains fire and nourishes yin [for the treatment of] steaming bone and damp-heat and precipitation of blood"; a "Foot Tai Yang channel conductor medicinal"; and "Combined with **Cang Zhu (蒼朮)** it is called Er Miao San (二妙散) (aka Mysterious Two Powder), which is an essential medicinal for treating wilting [pattern]." In contemporary texts this medicinal is described as having heat-clearing and dampness-drying, fire-draining and toxin-resolving, and heat-abating and steam-eliminating actions.

Huang Lian (黃連) – In classical literature on pharmacopeia it is described as "**Huang Lian** has a bitter flavor [and the actions of] draining the heart and eliminating impediment, draining heat and resolving toxin, and thickening the intestines and checking diarrhea" and "It has six actions: one is draining heart fire, two is eliminating middle burner heat, three is essential [medicinal] for all sore [pathoconditions], four is eliminates wind-damp, five is treats fulminant fire eye, and six is checks blood in the stool." In comtemporary texts this medicinal is described as having a cold nature and bitter flavor that enters the heart, liver, stomach, and large intestine channels with heat-clearing and dampness-drying and fire-draining and toxin-resolving actions. The market price of this medicinal frequently fluctuates and its higher price compared to the other of **"the Three Yellows"** means that smaller doses either reserved for more severe heat conditions or specific pathoconditions such as vasculitis and gastrointestinal ulcers.

"the Four Ling's" ("四苓") – This term derives from Si Ling Tang (四苓湯) recorded in the *Teachings of Dan Xi* (丹溪心法) (aka Dan Xi Xin Fa) and is composed of **Fu Ling (茯苓)**, **Ze Xie (澤瀉)**, **Zhu Ling (豬苓)**, and **Bai Zhu (白朮)**. This combination of medicinals fortifies the spleen, disinhibits water, and percolates dampness for the treatment of water-damp collecting internally, inhibited urination, diarrhea, swelling (edema), and bloody urine. **Fu Ling**, **Ze Xie**, and **Zhu Ling** all have similar flavor and nature (sweet, bland, and balanced); enter the kidney and urinary bladder channels; and share the complementary actions of disinhibiting water, percolating dampness, fortifying the spleen, and discharging heat. **Bai Zhu** has a bitter and sweet flavor and warm nature; enters the spleen and stomach channels; and supplements qi, fortifies the spleen, dries dampness, and disinhibits water.

These medicinals form one of the pillars of Dr. Lee's treatment approaches administered for a broad scope of pathoconditions involving water amassment or water-rheum collecting internally that causes obstruction or stagnation and leads to disruption of physiological mechanisms and pathological disorders. The resulting homeostatic imbalance may manifest in pathoconditions such as generalized edema, ascites, pericardial effusion, pleural effusion, and increased intracranial pressure (e.g., traumatic injury, hemorrhage, herniation, hypertensive cerebrovascular disease, obstruction of cerebrospinal fluid). Dr. Lee typically prescribes these medicinals in Wu Ling San (五苓散) as the main formula or adds them into another forumula based on presenting symptoms, signs, and pattern identification. For pathoconditions such as diarrhea, ascites, and increased intracranial pressure, Dr. Lee commonly includes **Da Huang (大黃)** to enhance the draining precipitation action and adds **Ren Shen (powder) (人參粉)** and **Cang Zhu (蒼朮)** as a counterbalance that aides the reabsoprtion of nutrients and electrolytes. Depending on the specific pathocondition, Dr. Lee may prescribe large doses of up to 8 qian~1 liang of each medicinal to ensure an adequate level of water disinhibition is achieved. .

Fu Ling (茯苓) – In classical literature on pharmacopeia it is described as follows: "**Fu Ling** has a sweet [flavor] and warm [nature], engenders liquid and checks thirst, abates heat and quiets the fetus, and boostst the spleen and aides yang" and "...[it] percolates dampness and disinhibits the orifices and eliminates dampness...." In contempary texts it is described as having a sweet, bland, balanced nature; enters the heart, spleen, and kidney channels;

and disinhibits water and percolates dampness and fortifies the spleen and quiets the spirit. It is experimentally proven to increases the urinary excretion of electrolytes such as potassium, sodium, and chloride, lowers blood sugar, and has sedative actions. Dr. Lee commonly pairs this medicinal with **Ze Xie (澤瀉)** to enhance water-inhibiting actions.

Ze Xie (澤瀉) – In classical literature on pharmacopeia it is described as follows: "[**Ze Xie**] enters the urinary bladder [channel], disinhibits urine, drains fire evil in the kidney channel, and specializes in disinhibiting dampness and moving water." In contemporary texts it is described as having a sweet and bland flavor and cold nature; enters the kidney and urinary bladder channels; disinhibits water, percolates dampness, and discharge heat. It is experimentally proven to increases urine output along with the excretion of urea and chloride, lower blood pressure, and lower blood sugar levels. As a rule, if large doses of this medicinal are prescribed (≥ 8 qian), Dr. Lee always includes a comparable dose of **Fu Ling (茯苓)**.

Zhu Ling (豬苓) – In classical literature on pharmacopeia it is decribed as the following: "[**Zhu Ling**'s] bitter [flavor] drains stagnation, bland [flavor] disinhibits the orifices, sweet [flavor] aides yang. [It] enters the urinary bladder kidney channel, [both] upraises and downbears, opens the interstices and promotes sweating, disinhibits urine and moves water, and has similar actions as **Fu Ling (茯苓)** except that it doesn't supplement." In contemporary texts it is described as having a sweet and bland flavor and balanced nature; enters the kidney and urinary bladder channels; and disinhibits water and percolates dampness. **Zhu Ling** has stronger water-disinhibiting action compared to Fu Ling, but not as strong of a supplementing action. The physiological mechanism of its urine-disinhibiting (diurectic) action primarily involves inhibiting the reabsorption of water and electrolytes (specifically potassium, sodium, and chloride) in the renal tubules of the nephron.

Bai Zhu (白朮) – In classical literature on pharmacopeia it is described as the following: "**Bai Zhu** is an essential medicinal for fortifying the spleen and stomach, expelling dampness, eliminating impediment, and dispersing food." In contemporary text is described as having a bitter and sweet flavor and warm nature; enters the spleen and stomach channels; and supplements qi and fortifies the spleen, dries dampness and disinhibits water, checks sweating, and quiets the fetus. It's primary constituent is atractylone and it also contains esters and carbohydrates (e.g., mannose and fructose) that strengthen the constitution (e.g., promotes absorption of nutrients by the spleen), disinhibit urine, lower blood sugar levels, and has anticoagulant actions.

Cang Zhu (蒼朮) – In classical literature on pharmacopeia it is described as follows: "[**Cang Zhu**] dries the stomach and strengthens the spleen, promotes sweating and eliminates dampness, and upbears and effuses yang qi in the stomach", "...[**Cang Zhu**] resolves the six depressions: phlegm, fire, qi, blood, dampness, and food," and "...an essential medicinal for dissipitating wind-cold-dampness in the treatment of wilting [pattern]." In contemporary texts it is described as having an acrid and bitter flavor and warm nature; enters the spleen and stomach channels; and fortifies the spleen, dries dampness, dispels wind-damp, promotes sweating, and remedies miasmic (damp, humid, heat environment with pestilent qi prevalent) epidemic. **Cang Zhu** has the spleen-fortifying action of **Bai Zhu (白朮)** along with the advantages of drying stomach dampness and antimicrobial actions for gastrointestinal disorders resulting in loose stools or diarrhea and various infectious diseases. Thus, this medicinal is ideal for Taiwan's hot, damp, and humid climate. Dr. Lee also includes **Cang Zhu** in many Yu Sheng formulas, either added into the formula or substituted in place of **Bai Zhu** (unless the patient presents with qi vacuity). The spleen-fortifying and dampness-drying action of **Cang Zhu** also counteracts the potential for digestion impairment and sloppy stools some patients experience when administered formulas containing large doses of medicinals (e.g., heat-clearing and toxin-resolving, yin-nourishing and blood-supplementing, blood-quickening and stasis-transforming, kidney yang supplementing), which may be impair digestion and cause some people to have "sloppy stools." Dr. Lee also prescribes this medicinal for the treatment of damp-heat pattern myasthenia gravis, which can be classified as wilting pattern. The physiological mechanism of its dampness-drying action primarily involves its capacity to promote increased interstitial permeability of water between membranes throughout the body.

Ren Shen (人參) – In classical literature on pharmacopeia **Ren Shen** is described as follows: "... [**Ren Shen**] has great supplementing original qi, fire-draining, checking thirst and engendering fluid, boosting earth, endendering the lungs, sharpening the wits, and regulating construction and nourishing defense actions." In contemporary texts it is described as having a sweet and mildly bitter flavor and mildly warm nature; enters the heart, lung, and spleen channels; and greatly supplements original qi, supplements the spleen and boosts the lung, engenders liquid, and quiets the spirit. In the vast majority of cases, Dr. Lee prefers to prescribe the pulverized powder (**Ren Shen (powder) (人參粉)**) of this raw medicinal, either adding directly into the formula after decocting and cooling or taken separately along with the decoction. **Ren Shen** is an expensive medicinal and administering it as a powder obviates the need for decoction (a process that diminishes potency) and thus maximizes efficacy. This medicinal is often paired with **Chuan Qi (powder) (川七粉)** to form one of the pillars of Dr. Lee's treatment approaches. Dr. Lee explains in a more modern biomedical perspective: "As an adaptogenic medicinal **Ren Shen** has the capacity to regulate cell metabolism down-regulating and up-regulating whenever it is necessary and offers exceptional efficacy in repairing and maintaining physiological functioning of spinal nerves."

Chuan Qi (川七) – (also known as **San Qi (三七)** or **Shan Qi (山七)**) In classical literature on pharmacopeia this medicinal is described as "...an essential medicinal for knife, club, and incised wounds, fractures" and prescribed for the treatment of "blood ejection and spontaneous external bleeding, blood dysentery and flooding..." and "...following [treatment] and recovery [**Chuan Qi**] doesn't leave behind statis blood in the channels and network vessels...and transforms blood stasis without compromising the engendering of new blood [making it] recognized as an exceptional blood-rectifying medicinal." In contemporary texts it is described as having a sweet and mildly bitter flavor and warm nature; enters the liver and stomach channels; and transforms stasis and stanches bleeding and quickens the blood and settles pain. **Chuan Qi** is clinically recognized as an essential medicinal for stanching blood and transforming stasis and also has blood-quickening and pain relieving actions for the treatment of conditions such as coronary artery disease (CAD) with angina, ischemic cerebrovascular disease, sequela of cerebral hemorrhage, and a wide range of other pathoconditions involving blood stasis. **Chuan Qi** is an expensive medicinal and administering it as a powder obviates the need for decoction (a process that diminishes potency) and thus maximizes efficacy. This medicinal is often paired with **Ren Shen (powder) (人參粉)** to form one of the pillars of Dr. Lee's treatment approaches. Since pulverized powder is typically prescribed instead of decocting pieces, listings of Yu Sheng formulas will not include **Chuan Qi**.

Ren Shen (powder) (人參粉) and Chuan Qi (powder) (川七粉) paired

– This medicinal pair forms one of the pillars of Dr. Lee's treatment approaches. Paired together these two medicinals have the qi-boosting and bleeding-stanching and origin-supporting and desertion-stemming actions for the treatment of vacuity taxation cough, enduring illness, all types of persistent bleeding, sweating on the verge of desertion, and angina of coronary artery disease. **Ren Shen** greatly supplements original qi, supplements the lung and boosts the spleen, and engenders liquid and checks sweating. **Chuan Qi** stanches bleeding and dispels stasis, disperses swelling and relieves pain, and is considered an essential medicinal for blood family pathoconditions. This medicinal combination exemplify the TCM classical theory of "qi is the commander of the blood and blood is the mother of qi," complementing and enhancing each other with the capacity to boost qi and settle pain, support the origin and stem desertion, stanch bleeding, and transform stasis. The pulverized powder (fěn 粉) of these medicinals are mixed together and placed in ziplock packets with a typical dosage of 7g/3x/day (a total of 21 g/day). For severe blood stasis, **Dan Shen (丹參)** decocting pieces are commonly prescribed along with this medicinal pair to further enhance the blood-quickening and stasis-transforming actions. The administration of medicinals with blood-quickening and stasis-transforming actions in chronic pathoconditions is based on the TCM classical theory of "enduring illness results in stasis."

"the Three Insects" ("三蟲") – This term refers to the combination of **Quan Xie (全蠍)**, **Wu Gong (蜈蚣)**, and **Bai Jiang Can (白僵蠶)**. These arthropods have evolutionary ancestry dating back nearly 500 million years and are composed of relatively smaller, more basic fundamental protein archetypes offering exceptional efficacy at regulating the transmission of neurotransmitters across chemical synapses. These three medicinals all enter the liver channel and share common actions of extinguishing wind and checking tetany with **Quan Xie (全蠍)** and **Wu Gong (蜈蚣)** attacking toxin and dissipating binds and freeing the network vessels and relieving pain, and **Bai Jiang Can (白僵蠶)** dispeling wind and relieving pain and transforming phelgm and dissipitating binds.

Dr. Lee typically administers **"the Three Insects"** along along with a main formula determined by pattern identification for the treatment of neuropathic pain (e.g., trigeminal neuralgia) and migraine headache. Modern pathophysiology postulates vascular compression resulting in focal demyelination as a potential cause of trigeminal neuralgia. This nerve damage produces inflammatory responses and metabolic waste resulting in stagnation and obstruction of the channels and causes pain. The predominating pathophysiological explanations for migraine headache (e.g., vascular theory, neuravascular theory, cortical spreading depression) also result in stagnation and obstruction of the channels and causes pain.

Quan Xie (全蠍) – In classical literature on pharmacopeia this medicinal is described as follows: "[**Quan Xie**] treats all wind with shaking and dizzy vision, fright epilepsy and pulling, deviated eyes and mouth...reverting yin wind and wood pathoconditions." In contemporary texts it is described as having an acrid flavor, balanced nature, and toxicity; enters the liver channel; and extinguishes wind and checks tetany, attacks toxin and disperses binds, and frees the network vessels and relieves pain. Traditionally, it is commonly paired with **Wu Gong (蜈蚣)** for the treatment of pathoconditions involving spasm and convulsion such as acute and chronic fright wind, tetanus, and wind striking the channels and network vessels with devitated eyes and mouth; and **Wu Gong (蜈蚣)** and **Bai Jiang Can (白僵蚕)** for the treatment of intractable headache and migraine headache (medial and hemilateral headache).

Wu Gong (蜈蚣) – In classical literature on pharmacopeia this medicinal is described as follows: "[**Wu Gong**] treats child fright epilepsy wind convulsion, infantile umbilical wind clinched jaw...." In contemporary texts it is described as having an acrid flavor, a warm, mobile and penetrating nature able to reach the interior and exterior, and toxicity; enters the liver channel; extinguishes wind and checks tetany, attacks toxin and dissipates binds, frees the network vessels and relieves pain. Traditionally, it is commonly paired with **Quan Xie (全蝎)** for the treatment of pathoconditions involving spasm and convulsion such as acute and chronic fright wind, tetanus, and wind striking the channels and network vessels with devitated eyes and mouth; and **Quan Xie (全蝎)** and **Bai Jiang Can (白僵蚕)** for the treatment of intractable headache and migraine headache (medial and hemilateral headache). Due to this medicinal's high market price, Dr. Lee typically only prescribes it in cases where the patient's pain is "unbearable."

Bai Jiang Can (白僵蚕) – In classical literature on pharmacopeia this medicinal is described as follows: "[**Bai**] **Jiang** [**Can**] doesn't putrify [and] upon exposure to clearing and transforming qi [it] has the capacity to treat wind and transform phlegm, dissipate binds and move the channels." In contemporary texts it is described as having a salty and acrid flavor and balanced nature; enters the liver and lung channels; and extinguishes wind and checks tetany, dispels wind and relieves pain, and transforms phlegm and dissipates binds. It is recognized as being particularly suitable for pathoconditions involving fright wind and epilepsy with phlegm heat. Traditionally, it is administered for the treatment of infantile phlegm-heat acute fright adding **Quan Xie (全蠍)** and other heat-clearing and phlegm-transforming and wind-extinguishing and tetany-checking medicinals. It can be combined with **Quan Xie** and **Wu Gong (蜈蚣)** for the treatment of tetanus, spasm, and convulsion and arch-backed rigidity; and **Wu Gong** and **Quan Xie** for the treatment of intractable headache and migraine headache (medial and hemilateral headache)

Tian Ma (天麻) – In classical literature on pharmacopeia this medicinal is described as follows: "**Tian Ma** is acrid [flavor] and warm [nature] and can treat dizzy head, infantile fright epilepsy, and hypertonicity and paralysis"; has the actions of "boosting qi and strenthening yin, freeing the blood vessels, strengthening the sinews, and coursing phlegm qi"; and "Treats head wind, headache, dizzy head and vacuity spinning, epilepsy and strong spasms, hypertonicity of the limbs...all [types of] wind stroke and wind phlegm." In contemporary texts it is described as having a sweet flavor and balanced nature; enters the liver channel; and extinguishes wind and checks tetany, represses the liver yang uprising, dispels wind and frees the network vessels. This medicinal shares many common properties with **"the Three Insects"** and Dr. Lee typically administers this medicinal either along with them or in combination with **Chuan Qiong (川芎)**, **Chai Hu (柴胡)**, **Ban Xia (半夏)**, and **Ge Gen (葛根)** for the treatment of dizziness, vertigo (e.g., Meniere's, benign paroxysmal positional vertigo (BPPV), idiopathic), and headache (e.g., migraine, cluster). Dr. Lee also prescribes this medicinal for the treatment of neurogenic hypertension caused by brainstem dysfunction. Depending on the severity of the patient's symptoms and signs, Dr. Lee may prescribe large doses of up to 1 liang.

Ren Dong Teng (忍冬藤) – Traditionally this medicinal is prescribed for its heat-clearing, toxin-resolving, and network vessel-freeing actions. In Dr. Lee's pharmacopeia it is an essential medicinal for inhibiting the synthesis of BUN and creatinine for the treatment of pathological conditions that result from hypoperfusion of blood through functionally normal kidneys (prerenal), structural damage to the renal parenchyma (intrinsic renal), and urinary tract obstruction (postrenal). Dr. Lee commonly pairs **Ding Shu Xiu (丁豎朽)** with this medicinal adding them into the main formula composition.

Ding Shu Xiu (丁豎朽) – This medicinal has urine-disinhibiting, toxin-resolving, and swelling-dispersing actions. In Dr. Lee's pharmacopeia it is an essential medicinal for inhibiting the synthesis of BUN and creatinine for the treatment of pathological conditions that result from hypoperfusion of blood through functionally normal kidneys (prerenal), structural damage to the renal parenchyma (intrinsic renal), and urinary tract obstruction (postrenal). Dr. Lee commonly pairs **Ren Dong Teng (忍冬藤)** with this medicinal adding them into the main formula composition.

Chi Shao (赤芍) – This medicinal has a bitter flavor and slightly cold nature; enters the liver channel; and clears heat and cools blood and dissipates stasis and relieves pain. **Bai Shao (白芍)** has a bitter, sour, and sweet flavor and slightly cold nature; enters the liver and spleen channel; and nourishes yin and regulates menstruation, calms the liver and relieves pain, and consolidates yin and checks sweating. In classical literature on pharmacopeia the attributes of **Chi Shao** and **Bai Shao** are described as follows: "**Bai Shao** supplements and contracts and **Chi Shao** drains and dissipates. **Bai** [**Shao**] benefits the spleen and drains water from earth [spleen]; **Chi** [**Shao**] dissipates evil and moves stagnation in the blood." In contemporary texts the differences are explained as follows: "**Chi Shao** excels at quickening the blood and dissipating stasis and **Bai Shao** is better at tranquilizing and relieving pain; both have supplementing actions with Bai Shao superior at supplementing blood and nourishing yin and **Chi Shao** superior at cooling the blood and expeling stasis." Dr.

Lee explains that most traditional formulas designed in times of antiquity originally included **Bai Shao** because the clinical presentation of dual qi and blood vacuity was far more prevalent back then thus warranting the emphasis of this medicinal's blood-nourishing actions. The lifestyle, diet, and living environs of today have altered people's body constitutions with blood stasis and stagnation and a predilection towards blood heat predominant. **Chi Shao** and its actions of cooling the blood and expeling stasis are more suitable for patients in our modern world who commonly present with blood stagnation and phlegm heat. Thus, in Yu Sheng formula compsositions and variations **Chi Shao** is always substituted for **Bai Shao**. Dr. Lee also adds large doses of this medicinal into formulas during certain stages of cancer treatment to inhibit tumor angionesis (neovascularization).

Huang Qi (黃耆) – Dr. Lee only administers premium quality **raw northern Huang Qi (生北黃耆)**, which is distinguishable by its reddish phloem that encircles the xylem of the vascular tissue. In classical literature this medicinal is described as follows: "**Raw [Huang Qi]** secures the exterior and in the absence of sweating it effuses, warms the seam of the flesh and fortifies the interstices of the flesh, drains yin fire, and resolves flesh heat. **Mix-fried [Huang Qi]** supplements the center and boosts original qi, warms the triple burner, and strengthens the spleen and stomach, engenders blood and flesh, expels pus and internal drawing, and [is classified as] a sore and welling-abscess sage medicinal." In contemporary texts this medicinal is described as having a sweet flavor and slightly warm nature; entering the spleen and lung channels; and supplementing qi and upbearing yang, disinhibiting water and dispersing swelling, and expressing sores and engendering flesh. For qi vacuity conditions Dr. Lee typically starts out with a dose of 1 liang and incrementally increases this dose by 5 qian every 1~2 weeks depending on the patient's condition and piques at a maximum dose of 2.5 liang (3 liang maximum). Excessive doses of beyond 3~5 liang may cause compromised blood vessels to rupture or paroxysmal increases in intracranial pressure in the presence of arteriosclerosis, atheroclerosis, hematoma, or adhesions in the subarachnoid space of the meninges.

Dr. Lee explains that **Huang Qi** promotes accelerated exchanges across membranes throughout the body and regulates the permeability of the glomerular membrane inhibiting protein loss. This medicinal has been experimentally and clincally proven to eliminate nephritic proteinuria, increase myocardial contractility, contains estrogen-like effects, and provides broad spectrum antimicrobial efficacy. Among its constituents astragalus saponins lowers blood pressure, promotes erythrocyte membrane stability, increases c-AMP content of blood plasma and tissues, boosts immune function, and promote the regeneration of liver DNA synthesis; and astragalus polysaccharide enhances immune function, regulates blood sugar levels, protects the cardiovascular system, and accelerates regeneration of tissue growth in patients suffering from radiotherapy complications.

Dan Shen (丹參) – In classical literature on pharmacopeia it is described as having "heart-supplementing, blood engendering, stasis dispeling, clearing heat and eliminating vexation, accumulation-breaking and menses-regulating, fetus-calming, [and] welling- and flat-abscess-dispersing [actions]." In contemporary texts this medicinal is described as having a bitter flavor and slightly cold nature; entering the heart and liver channels; and quickening the blood and regulating menstruation, cooling the blood and dispersing welling-abscesses, and quieting the spirit actions. Traditionally, it is one of the most commonly used medicinals for gynecological and obstetric pathoconditions and is recognized as "an essential medicinal for gynecology" and "Dan Shen San [丹參散] alone [is] equivalent to Si Wu [四物] [Tang (湯)]." Dr. Lee commonly prescribes **Dan Shen** instead of **Ren Shen (人參)** in qi-supplementing, blood-supplementing, and stasis-dispeling formulas to improve cerebrovascular, cardiovascular, and peripheral vascular circulation and diffuse depressed heat. This substitution is founded in the the TCM classical theory of "enduring illness results in stasis," which is appropriate for Dr. Lee's patients with severe patterns and chronic pathoconditions. Depending on the presenting symptoms, signs, and pattern, Dr. Lee may prescribe **Ren Shen (powder) (人**

參粉) (or **Ren Shen (powder) and Chuan Qi (powder) paired**) and **Dan Shen** together with their respective qi-supplementing and blood-supplementing actions forming a complementary pair that adheres to the classical theory of "qi is the commander of the blood and blood is the mother of qi."

Dang Gui (當歸) – This medicinal is processed in-house in Dr. Lee's own medicinal processing and decoction facility. **Raw Dang Gui (生當歸)** (head, body, and tails) is first washed and cleaned and then placed in barrels where it is steeped in cooking rice wine until the roots are fully saturated (anywhere from 10 days (hot weather) up to 2 weeks (cold weather)). The saturated roots are then oven-dried at low temperatures to preserve freshness and longer storage life. In classical literature on pharmacopeia this medicinal is described as the following: "[**Dang Gui**] supplements blood, moistens dryness, and lubricates the intestines"; "**Dang Gui** is sweet [in flavor] and warm [in nature], engenders blood and supplements the heart, supports vacuity and boosts detriment, and expels stasis and engenders the new"; and "**Dang Gui** has a sweet and heavy flavor and specializes in supplementing blood; its qi is light and acrid thus it also moves blood. Movement in the supplementation and supplementation in movement, indeed, it is a qi-in-blood medicinal and [classified] as a sage medicinal in the blood." In contemporary texts it is described as having a sweet and acrid in flavor and warm nature; entering the liver, heart, and spleen channels; and supplementing and activating the blood, regulating menstruation, checking pain, and moistening the intestines. Prescribed in small doses this medicinal nourishes blood and in large doses it has a blood-quickening and stasis-transforming action.

Ma Huang (麻黃) – In classical literature on pharmacopeia this medicinal is described as follows: "[**Ma Huang**] promotes sweating and resolves flesh, dispels cold evil at the construction [level] and wind-heat at the defense [level]. Regulates blood vessels, frees the nine orifices, and opens the pores." In contemporary texts it is described as having an acrid and slightly bitter flavor and warm nature; entering the lung and urinary bladder channels; and promoting sweating and resolving the exterior, diffusing the lung and calming panting, disinhibiting water and dispersing swelling, freeing the nasal orifices, outthrusting papules, and relieving itching. However, this medicinal takes on an even broader role in Dr. Lee's pharmacopeia. Dr. Lee interprets **Ma Huang**'s action of "opening the pores" broadly to mean it can "open up" and transport other medicinals across all membranes of the body down to the cellular levels thus making it an effective systemic channel conductor for all types of pathoconditions (e.g., dermatology, rheumatology, cardiology, neurology); and its action of "opening the nine orifices" as exciting the nervous system (i.e., CNS, PNS, ANS) prompting its application for neurologic pathologies of the brain and nervous system. Of course, Dr. Lee also utilizes the bronchodilation action for the treatment of respiratory system pathoconditions (e.g., sinusitis, bronchitis, COPD, pneumonia). As for dosage, it depends on the individual's constitution and particular season typically starting out with a small dose of .5 fen to 1.5 qian and increasing incrementally in doses of 5 fen up until the patient notices difficulty sleeping (a typical dose would be 1.5 qian~3 qian).

Di Long (地龍) – In classical literature on pharmacopeia this medicinal is described as the following: "[**Di Long**] is cold in nature and descends; cold nature resolves all types of heat pathoconditions and [its capacity to] descend disinhibits urine; and treats lower limb pathoconditions and frees the channels and network vessels." "...[treats] acute and chronic fright wind and joint-running wind pain." In contemporary texts it is described as having a salty flavor and cold nature; entering the liver, spleen, and urinary bladder channel; and having heat-clearing and wind-extinguishing, channel-freeing and network vessel-quickening, panting-calming, and urine-disinhibiting actions. Dr. Lee commonly pairs this medicinal with **Ma Huang** for pathoconditions affecting the respiratory and vasomotor centers in the brainstem (e.g., cerebral vasuclar accident (CVA), trauma, microbial infection) and for the treatment of wind-cold-damp impediment.

Sang Bai Pi (桑白皮) – In classical literature on pharmacopeia this medicinal is described as the following: "sweet and acrid in flavor and cold in nature" and "[**Sang Bai Pi**] drains fire evil in the lung, but not lung qi. Fire and original qi are incompatible, and once fire is eliminated then qi will be calm." In contemporary texts it is described as having sweet flavor and cold nature; entering the lung channel; and having lung-draining and panting-calming and water disinhibiting and swelling-dispersing actions. Dr. Lee describes this medicinal as having the capacity to "clean up the metabolic waste that clogs cell membranes throughout the entire body." This metabolic waste build up may derive from normal metabolic processes or inflammatory responses to disease (or possibly even in response to the build up of this metabolic waste clogging the cell membranes). This may inhibit (or further exacerbate) the normal function of cellular mechanisms and disrupt homeostasis thus leading to heat pattern pathoconditions such as diabetes. For this reason, **Sang Bai Pi** is an essential medicinal for the treatment of diabetes and it is also prescribed for other heat pattern pathoconditions of the respiratory tract (e.g., acute bronchitis, emphysema) and skin (e.g., atopic dermatitis).

Yin Xing Ye (銀杏葉) – This medicinal is the leaf of Ginkgo biloba L. and its seed is **Bai Guo (白果)**. **Yin Xing Ye** has the actions of lowering serum cholesterol, transforming phlegm, and quickens the blood to relieve pain. Dr. Lee explains that one of its main physiological mechanisms involves increasing exchanges across blood vessel membranes. This is a commonly prescribed medicinal in Dr. Lee's pharmacopeia and is used for the treatment of such conditions as coronary artery disease (CAD), angina pectoris, hyperlipidemia, atherosclerosis, hypertension, cerebral vasospasm, and aneurysms. It is also an essential medicinal in the Yu Sheng version of Bu Yang Huan Wu Tang (補陽還五湯), which is typically prescribed for stroke patients with sequelae, Parkinson's disease (PD), Alzheimer's disease (AD), and other cerebrovascular and neurodegenerative pathoconditions.

Ji Nei Jin (雞內金) – This medicinal is sweet in flavor and neutral in nature; enters the spleen, stomach, small intestine, and urinary bladder channels; and has food-dispersing and stomach-strengthening actions. Dr. Lee commonly adds it into formulas that contain large doses of medicinals (e.g., heat-clearing and toxin-resolving, yin-nourishing and blood-supplementing, blood-quickening and stasis-transforming, kidney yang supplementing), which may impair digestion and cause some people to have "sloppy stools." In addition, Dr. Lee also adds **Ji Nei Jin** and **Xian Zha (仙楂)** into formula compositions for treating hyperlipidemia and hypertrigliceridemia. Due to the fluctuating price and scarce availability of good quality **Ji Nei Jin**, Dr. Lee may simply substitute this medicinal with **Xian Zha**.

Xian Zha (仙楂) (aka **Shan Zha (山楂)**) – In classical literature this medicinal is described as follows: "Sour, sweet, and salty in flavor and warm in nature." "[**Xian Zha**] strengthens the spleen and moves qi, dissipates stasis and transforms phlegm, disperses food and grinds accumulations... [and] relieves postpartum infant's pillow pain." In contemporary texts it is described as sour and sweet in flavor and slightly warm in nature; enters the spleen, stomach, and liver channels; and has food-dispersing and accumulation-transforming and qi-moving and stasis-dispersing actions. Dr. Lee commonly adds it into formulas that contain large doses of medicinals (e.g., heat-clearing and toxin-resolving, yin-nourishing and blood-supplementing, blood-quickening and stasis-transforming, kidney yang supplementing), which may impair digestion and cause some people to have "sloppy stools." In addition, Dr. Lee also prescribes this medicinal for treating hyperlipidemia and hypertrigliceridemia; and for static blood pattern pathconditions such as "postpartum infant's pillow pain" (postpartum abdominal pain) and coronary artery spasm.

Gan Di Huang (乾地黃) – This medicinal is sweet and bitter in flavor and cold in nature; enters the heart, liver, and lung channels; and has heat-clearing and blood-cooling and yin-nourishing and liquid engendering actions. **Shou Di Huang (熟地黃)** is sweet in flavor and slightly warm in nature; enters the liver and kidney channels; and has blood-supplementing and yin-enriching and essence-boosting and marrow-replenishing actions. The traditional processing method (involving steeping **Sheng Di Huang (生地黃)** in yellow wine mixed with S**ha Ren (砂仁)** and steaming and sun-drying repeatedly nine times) is extremely time-consuming and expensive, and thus seldom performed anymore. The modern method of processing **Shu Di Huang** results in inferior quality that differs in nature and property compared to its predecessor. Taking these factors into consideration, Dr. Lee will always uses **Gan Di Huang** as a substitute for **Shu Di Huang** in his set formula compositions and variants.

Lu Rong (鹿茸) – In classical literature this medicinal is described as follows: "sweet in flavor, warm in nature, and pure yang," "greatly supplements vacuity taxation," and "[**Lu Rong**] engenders essence and supplements marrow, nourishes blood and assists yang, [and] strengthens sinews and fortifies bone. "[**Lu Rong**] treats lumbar and kidney vacuity cold, aching and pain in the extremities, dizzy head and black eyes, flooding and vaginal discharge and seminal emission...." In contemporary texts this medicinal is described as having a sweet and salty flavor and warm nature; entering the kidney and liver channels; and having yang-invigorating, blood and essence-supplementing, sinew and bone-strengthening, thoroughfare and controlling vessel-harmonizing, and toxin and sore-expressing actions. **Lu Rong** is the whole cartilaginous antler in a pre-calcified stage with hair that looks and feels like velvet. It contains many growth factors (e.g., NT-3, NGF, IGF) and has been experimentally and clinically proven to increase hormone levels (e.g., testosterone, luteinizing hormone), stimulate adrenal cortical function, and promote hematopoiesis.

Xi Lu Rong (細鹿茸) – Dr. Lee uses premium quality **Lu Rong** (reaching 60% to 70% growth at peak hormone production levels) offering superior medicinal efficacy. Dr. Lee calls this **Xi Lu Rong (細鹿茸)** with the "fine" (細 xi) velvet sheen of the antler describing its texture and appearance. **Lu Rong** is a precious natural resource, very expensive, and typically only requires small doses to achieve efficacy. Due to these considerations, Dr. Lee administers this medicinal in pulverized powder form (**Lu Rong (powder)** (**鹿茸粉**)) making it convenient to administer in small doses (typically 5 fen/3x/day). This medicinal offers superior medicinal efficacy for pathoconditions that inhibit hematopoiesis (e.g., myeloproliferative disorders); myelosuppression resulting from chemotherapy, radiotherapy, and immunotherapy in patients with cancer and autoimmune disorders; and osteoporosis.

Cu Lu Rong (粗鹿茸) – Dr. Lee also uses another type of **Lu Rong** that is fully developed but not yet completely calcified (hormone level production low) called **Cu Lu Rong (粗鹿茸)** with the "coarse" (**粗** c▢) hairs covering the antler describing its texture and appearance. This medicinal is less expensive than **Xi Lu Rong (細鹿茸)** and requires larger doses to achieve efficacy, thus Dr. Lee administers this medicinal in decoction pieces making it convenient to prescribe large doses (typically 8 qian/day). **Cu Lu Rong** is inferior to **Xi Lu Rong (細鹿茸)** at increasing hormone levels and promoting hematopoiesis, but superior to **Lu Jiao (鹿角)** at quickening the blood and transforming stasis. This medicinal has been experimentally and clinically proven to inhibit tumor vasculature from generating hormones and thus functioning to inhibit tumor angionesis and tumerogenesis. Dr. Lee typically prescribes **Cu Lu Rong** for pathoconditions such as cancer patients at high risk of bone metastasis or established metastasis, bone cancers, spinal cord tumors, and fractures that fail to heal properly (e.g., delayed union or nonunion).

Lu Jiao (鹿角) refers to the completely calcified antler whose coarse hairs have shed and contains high calcium phosphate content. In classical literature this medicinal is described as follows: "salty in flavor and warm in nature" and "...dissipates heat and moves blood, disperses swelling and repels evil...." In contemporary texts this medicinal is described as having a salty flavor and warm nature and blood-quickening and stasis transforming actions for the treatment of all types of vacuity taxation and offers exceptional efficacy for flat-abscesses and cold-type pus sores. **Lu Jiao** can be processed into **Lu Jiao Shuang (鹿角霜) (degelatinated deer antler)** which Dr. Lee uses in powder form combined with Fu Zi and Gan Jiang for the treatment of chronic (dry) skin ulcerations (e.g., diabetic ulcers). **Lu Jiao** can also be processed into **Lu Jiao Jiao (鹿角膠)** combined with **Gui Ban Jiao (龜板膠) (tortoise plastron glue)** to make Gui Lu Er Xian Jiao (龜鹿二仙膠) (Tortoise Shell and Deerhorn Two Immortals Glue) which Dr. Lee typically includes in formulas treating pathoconditions such as true origin vacuity detriment, extreme (exhaustion) of essence, extreme (exhaustion) of bone (e.g., osteoporosis), emaciation and shortage of qi, and dim vision (e.g., presbyopia); or administered in small doses and eaten like "candy" (soft and chewey) as a method of regulating the constitution for the elderly.

Mang Xiao (芒硝) – This medicinal has the action of inhibiting the large intestine's capacity to absorb water and thus promotes the excretion of large amounts of water, but it must be prescribed prudently in small doses to prevent excessive watery diarrhea that may lead to malabsorption. Dr. Lee typically only prescribes this medicinal if large doses (5~7 qian) of Da Huang have already been administered for a period of time without efficacy in promoting defecation and maintaining 2~3 stools per day.

Tu Si Zi (菟絲子) – This medicinal is processed in-house in Dr. Lee's own medicinal processing and decoction facility. **Raw Tu Si Zi (生菟絲子)** is stir-fried on low flame until a faint crackling sounds can be heard and an aromatic scent arises at which time these seeds will be dark yellow to light brown in color. The purpose for processing in this way is to crack open the seed coat thus allowing the constituents to be easily extracted upon decoction.

Xiong Huang (雄黃) – This is an essential medicinal in Bao An Wan Ling Dan (保安萬靈丹) (aka Safeguard Unlimited Efficacy

Elixir). This medicinal contains the toxic property arsenic sulfide (As_2S_2). To mitigate the potential for harmful side effects and ensure safety, a time-consuming and rigorous traditional water grinding (elutriation) processing method must be performed (*calcination is strictly prohibited), and this processed pulverized powder form **Xiong Huang (powder) (雄黃粉)** is used for clinical application. It is experimentally and clinically proven to provide possess potent and effective toxin-resolving, worm-killing (e.g., antimicrobial), and anticancer actions (e.g., suppresses cell differentiation, induces apoptosis, and inhibits tumor growth and angiogenesis). Taken orally this can only be administered in minuscule doses and added within a well-balanced formula composition due to the potential risk of adverse effects if taken in excessive dosages (e.g., suppresses hematopoiesis). Dr. Lee also uses this as an external application for the treatment of herpes zoster skin rash.

Dang Shen (黨參) – In classical literature on pharmacopeia it is described as follows: "[**Dang Shen**] supplements the center and boosts qi, harmonizes the spleen and stomach, [and] eliminates vexation-heat. Use [this medicinal] to regulate and supplement [in cases of] center qi mild weakness, it's the most appropriate." In contemporary texts this medicinal is described as having a sweet flavor and slightly warm nature and center-suplementing and qi-boosting, spleen- and stomach-harmonizing, and metabolism-increasing actions. Considering the comparatively high cost of **Ren Shen (人參)** many TCM physicans will substitute **Dang Shen** for mild cases of center qi vacuity. However, Dr. Lee only rarely prescribes this medicinal because he hasn't found it be nearly as clinically effective as the more revered and expensive **Ren Shen**, particularly for the complex pathoconditions Dr. Lee commonly treats.

Dr. Lee's Formulas

This section introduces the formulas Dr. Lee most commonly prescribes and includes details about their composition, the doses of each medicinal, overall actions, and administration for specific conditions. Many of these formulas are variants on "classical formulas" from the Han Dynasty, some are variants on more contemporary formulas, and others are entirely new formulas designed by Dr. Lee. Throughout the text the name "(Yu Sheng)" may be included in front of the formula name to highlight that the formula is Dr. Lee's variant on an existing traditional formula or his own unique composition. In fact, all of the formulas Dr. Lee and Dr. Yang prescribe in this text refer to "(Yu Sheng)" formula variants except where specifically indicated. The term "Yu Sheng" simply refers to Yu Sheng Chinese Medicine Clinic for which Dr. Lee is the founder, director, and chief physician. To alleviate unnecessary repetition, the list of formula profiles provided below will not include "(Yu Sheng)" except for certain instances where emphasis is deemed necessary. The following formulas introduced here are set compositions designed to treat the extensive scope of pathoconditions that Dr. Lee has commonly incurred throughout his nearly 40 years of clinical practice. These decocting pieces formulas are either purchased already processed or processed and/or produced in-house, and then pre-weighed and pre-packaged into semiporous decocting packets (not yet sealed) for convenient storage and administration. Dr. Lee typically makes modifications to these formulas by adding or increasing the dose of medicinals based on each individual patient's signs, symptoms, and pattern identification, and then the packets will be sealed and ready for administration and decocting. However, this is not an exhaustive listing; when special cases present Dr. Lee will compose formulas designed for a specific case. As time evolves, social, environmental, and technological advancements impact the manifestation of maladies in the human body, mind and spirit. Dr. Lee continues searching for the best approaches to provide the most effective treatment in our modern world.

***Disclaimer**: The formula compositions and medicinal doses provided in Dr. Lee's commonly prescribed formulas listed below and throughout this entire book are "for reference purposes only" and are "not" intended for indiscriminate administration by other individuals or parties. Prescription of these formulas should only be administered by a licensed traditional Chinese medicine (TCM) physician or practitioner whom has carefully evaluated the patient's history, signs, and symptoms and then conducted pattern identification as the basis for determining treatment. Licensed TCM physicians or practitioners must be aware that these formula compositions and medicinal doses are "for reference purposes only" and are "solely" intended for administration by Dr. Lee in his own clinical practice.

*In this text doses of medicinals are given in Chinese units with their equivalencies in grams (g) as follows:

1 fen = 0.375 g
1 qian (10 fen) = 3.75 g
1 liang (10 qian) = 37.5 g
1 jin (16 liang) = 600 g

Ban Xia Tian Ma Bai Zhu San (半夏天麻白朮散)

Dang Gui (當歸) 2 qian, Ban Xia (半夏), Bai Zhu (白朮), Fu Ling (茯苓), Cang Zhu (蒼朮), Ze Xie (澤瀉), Chen Pi (陳皮), Shen Qu (神曲), Mai Ya (麥芽), Gan Jiang (乾薑), Huang Bo (黃柏) 3 qian each, Fu Zi (附子), Tian Ma (天麻) 5 qian each, Huang Qi (黃耆) 1 liang

The Yu Sheng version is virtually the same as the original formula except for the addition of Dang Gui (當歸) and Fu Zi (附子), and Ren Shen (powder) (人參粉) is taken separately or added into the formula after decoction. Dang Gui supplements and quickens the blood and Fu Zi returns yang, stems counterflow, reinforces yang, supplements fire, dissipates cold, and relieves pain. These additions complement this foot greater yin spleen channel formula's overall spleen and stomach-supplementing, phlegm-damp transforming, and wind-stabilizing actions. TCM classical pathophysiological explanations of this formula are as follows: "Phlegm reversal [indicates] phlegm-damp reversal ascending counterflow. Phlegm counterflow leads to upper body repletion causing headache, dizzy head, and seeing black [spots] [in field of vision]." This is among Dr. Lee's most commonly prescribed formulas administered for a wide range of pathoconditions including Meniere's disease, benign paroxysmal positional vertigo (BPPV), psychosomatic disorders (presenting with abdominal distention, malaise, and fatigue among other symptoms), migraine and cluster headaches, brain damage caused by trauma resulting in increased intracranial pressure, and benign brain tumors. It is also one of the commonly prescribed formulas in Dr. Lee's cancer treatment protocol specifically administered for malignant brain tumors.

Bao An Wan Ling Dan (保安萬靈丹) (aka Safeguard Unlimited Efficacy Elixir)

Tian Ma (天麻), Chuan Xiong (川芎), Chuan Wu (川烏), Wu Cao (草烏), Fang Feng (防風), Jing Jie (荊芥), Ma Huang (麻黃), Xi Xin (細辛), Qiang Huo (羌活), He Shou Wu (何首烏), Dang Gui (當歸), Shi Hu (石斛), Quan Xie (全蝎), Gan Cao (甘草) 1 liang

Cang Zhu (蒼朮) 8 liang, Xiong Huang (雄黃) 6 qian

Dr. Lee uses the *Orthodox Manual of External Medicine* version of this formula and commonly abbreviates the name calling it simply **Wan Ling Dan (萬靈丹)** (aka **Unlimited Efficacy Elixir**). It is composed of medicinals that dispel wind, eliminate dampness, dissipate cold, extinguish wind, quicken the blood, supplement the blood, check tetany, free the network vessels, open the orifices, resolve toxin, dissipate binds, and relieve pain. Xiong Huang (雄黃) is among the principal medicinals in this composition with its antimicrobial and anticancer actions (e.g., suppresses cell differentiation, induces apoptosis, and inhibits tumor growth and angiogenesis). As its name implies, this formula has been traditionally administered for the treatment of a broad spectrum of pathoconditions including welling- and flat-abscesses, deep pus sores, clove toxin, mouth-level nape flat abscess, jowel effusion, damp phlegm streaming sore, bone flat-abscesses, crane's-knee wind, wind-cold-damp impediment, paralysis, tetanus, and migraine headaches. Dr. Lee prescribes this formula for various types of acute, chronic, and intractable pathoconditions including innominate toxin swelling, tumors (benign), and paralysis (i.e., resulting from parasitic infection). It also constitutes one of the pillars of Dr. Lee's cancer treatment protocol prescribed as a part of the regimen for all types of solid tumors (e.g., carcinoma, sarcoma) and hematological cancers (i.e., leukemia, lymphoma, myeloma) and combined with other medicinal formulas has the capacity to induce partial or complete remission and lower the chances of recurrence and metastasis.

Bu Yang Huan Wu Tang (補陽還五湯)

Dang Gui (當歸), Chuan Qiong (川芎), Chi Shao (赤芍), Dan Shen (丹參), Yin Xing Ye (銀杏葉) 4 qian each, Huang Qi (黃耆) 2 liang

The Yu Sheng version is based on the original formula, but only contains 2 liang of Huang Qi (黃耆) as opposed to 4 liang, excludes Di Long (地龍), Tao Ren (桃仁), and Hong Hua (紅花), and adds Yin Xing Ye (銀杏葉) and Dan Shen (丹參). Ren Shen (powder) (人參粉) is included in this composition just as in the original formula and is often paired with Chuan Qi (powder) (川七粉) (Ren Shen (powder) and Chuan Qi (powder) paired), serving to complement the qi-supplementing action of Huang Qi and the blood-quickening action of Dan Shen. Excessive doses of Huang Qi may cause compromised blood vessels to rupture or sudden increases in intracranial pressure in the presence of arteriosclerosis, atheroclerosis, hematoma, or adhesions in the subarachnoid space of the meninges. Yin Xing Ye (銀杏葉) is an essential medicinal in this formula and Dr. Lee utilizes its capacity of increasing exchanges across blood vessel membranes (e.g., promotes lymphatic circulation) and phlegm transforming actions to reduce blood viscosity and eliminate plaque for patients with stroke sequelae, transient ischemic attacks (TIAs), Parkinson's disease (PD), Alzheimer's disease (AD), and other cerebrovascular and neurodegenerative pathoconditions. Tao Ren, Hong Hua, and Di Long are excluded because unlike stroke patients in the 18th and 19th centuries when this formula was designed, modern Western medicine has already intervened to accelerate reperfusion with drugs and surgical decompression during the acute stage obviating the need for these types of potent blood-quickening, stasis-dispeling, and network vessel-freeing medicinals. Nowadays, the primary role of TCM is to treat the neurological sequelae and prevent subsequent attacks. This requires the administration of dual supplementation of blood and qi, blood-quickening, and phlegm-transforming medicinals to reduce blood viscosity and maintain plaque-free vasculature and prevent the development of emboli or thrombi. Prescribed for the treatment of neurodegenerative diseases (e.g., AD, PD, Huntington's disease), this formula slows down the rate of degeneration, enhances quality of life, and extends life expectancy.

Bu Zhong Yi Qi Tang (補中益氣湯)

Huang Qi (黃耆) 1 liang, Dang Gui (當歸) 2 qian

Dan Shen (丹參), Cang Zhu (蒼朮), Chen Pi (陳皮), Gan Cao (甘草), Sheng Ma (升麻), Chai Hu (柴胡) 3 qian each

The Yu Sheng version is similar to the original formula except that Dan Shen (丹參) replaces Ren Shen (人參) for its blood-engendering and stasis-dispelling action and Cang Zhu (蒼朮) replaces Bai Zhu (白朮) for its spleen-fortifying and dampness-drying action which aides digestion and is more suitable for northern Taiwan's humid climate. Depending on the presenting symptoms, signs, and pattern, Dr. Lee may also add Ren Shen (powder) (人參粉) (or Ren Shen (powder) and Chuan Qi (powder) paired). Dr. Lee prescribes this qi-boosting, yang-upbearing and fall-raising, and spleen and stomach regulating and supplementing formula for pathoconditions such as anal prolapse, uterine prolapse, gastroptosis, nephroptosis, inguinal hernia, anal fissures, hemorrhoids, myasthenia gravis (qi vacuity pattern type), qi-vacuity pattern leukorrhea, and proteinuria (intrinsic renal disease) in pediatric patients. Additionally, this formula's exceptional efficacy at promoting tissue repair and mucous membrane healing makes it an essential formula for the treatment of post-surgical wounds and cancer patients whom have undergone (or are currently receiving) radiotherapy or chemotherapy.

Chai Ling Tang (柴苓湯)

Huang Qin (黃芩), Fu Ling (茯苓), Zhu Ling (豬苓), Ze Xie (澤瀉), Cang Zhu (蒼朮), Yuan Hu Suo (元胡索), Mu Xiang (木香), Gui Zhi (桂枝) 3 qian each, Dan Shen (丹參), Xia Ban (半夏), Gan Cao (甘草), Sheng Jiang (生薑) 5 qian each, Hong Zao (紅棗) 3 pieces, Chai Hu (柴胡) 6 qian

The Yu Sheng version is similar to the original formula with the addition of Yuan Hu Suo (元胡索), Mu Xiang (木香), and Dan shen (丹參); and Cang Zhu (蒼朮) replaces Bai Zhu (白朮); Ren Shen (powder) (人參粉) is used instead of decocting pieces; and unlike other Yu Sheng formulas Gui Zhi (桂枝) is not replaced by Yu Gui (玉桂). Yan Hu Suo and Mu Xiang relax smooth muscle and thus relieve pain. This is a compound formula that includes elements of **Xiao Chai Hu Tang (小柴胡湯)** and **Wu Ling San (Calculi Formula) (五苓散) (結石方)** and functions to dispel cold, eliminate heat, disinhibit water, and transform phlegm for pathoconditions involving cold damage with residual heat, chest and ribside distention and impediment, difficult urination, and vomiting and diarrhea upon drinking water. Dr. Lee typically prescribes this formula for patients presenting with portal hypertension and ascites resulting from advanced chronic liver disease (e.g., hepatitis, cirrhosis, hepatocellular carcinoma); fulminant hepatitis; hepatorenal syndrome (HRS); pleuritis; and cerebral edema and increased intracranial pressure resulting from encephalitis, trauma, or radiotherapy. It is also one of the commonly prescribed formulas in Dr. Lee's cancer treatment protocol specifically administered for lesser yang (Shao Yang) cancers, which are identified as membranous tissue cancers in organs such as the liver, kidney, and lung.

Dang Gui San (當歸散)

Dang Gui (當歸), Chuan Qiong (川芎), Sheng Bai Shao (生白芍), Sheng Di Huang (生地黃) Chao Bai Zhu (炒白朮), Xu Duan (續斷), Du Zhong (杜仲), Gan Cao (甘草) 3 qian each, Huai Shan (淮山), Ai Cao (艾草) 5 qian each, Huang Qin (黃芩) 2 qian

The Yu Sheng version is composed of the same essential medicinals as the original formula – Dang Gui (當歸), Chuan Qiong (川芎), Sheng Bai Shao (生白芍), Chao Bai Zhu (炒白朮), and Huang Qin (黃芩) – along with the addition of Huai Shan (淮山), Ai Ye (艾葉), Sheng Di Huang (生地黃), Xu Duan (續斷), Du Zhong (杜仲), and Gan Cao (甘草). Sheng Di Huang clears heat and cools the blood and nourishes yin and engenders liquid; Xu Duan quickens the blood, stanches bleeding, quiets the fetus, and supplements the liver and kidney; Du Zhong serves as channel conductors directing medicinals downwards to the lumbus and lower limbs, supplements the liver and kidney, and quiets the fetus; Ai Ye warms the channels and stanches bleeding, dissipates cold and regulates menstruation, and quiets the fetus; Huai Shan boosts qi and nourishes yin, supplements the spleen, lung, and kidney, and secures essence and checks vaginal discharge; and Gan Cao supplements the center and harmonizes the nature of medicinals. These additions enhance and complement the blood-nourishing and blood-harmonizing, stasis-moving and blood quickening, liver-emolliating and construction aspect harmonizing, heat-clearing and blood-cooling, and spleen-fortifying and dampness-drying actions of this formula's essential medicinals. This blood-nourishing and fetus-quieting formula promotes a healthy pregnancy and treats all types of prenatal and postpartum pathoconditions; and is traditionally prescribed for women with a history of habitual abortion and/or premature labor, stirring fetus, scant blood with heat, heat vexation and thirst, hysteria, and aching lumbus and abdominal pain. This is Dr. Lee's first-line formula administered for a broad spectrum of obstetric pathoconditions such as the prevention of spontaneous abortions due to poor implantation of the blastocyst embryo during the first two weeks of pregnancy, absence of cervical mucous, ovulation disorders (e.g., anovulation, poor ("weak") ovulation), thin endometrial lining, absence of cervical mucous, morning sickness, preeclampsia, and gestational diabetes; and also postpartum pathoconditions such as "baby blues" (depression), perenial pain, uterus infection, and mastitis.

Di Gu Pi Yin (地骨皮飲)

Dang Gui (當歸), Chuan Qiong (川芎), Chi Shao (赤芍), Gan Di Huang (乾地黃), Gan Cao (甘草), Huang Qin (黃芩) 3 qian each, Cang Zhu (蒼朮) 4 qian, Di Gu Pi (地骨皮), Mu Dan Pi (牡丹皮) 5 qian each

The Yu Sheng version is based on the *On Blood Pathoconditions* (血症論) formula. It is composed of a variant of **Si Wu Tang (四物湯)** (Dang Gui (當歸), Chuan Qiong (川芎), Chi Shao (赤芍), Gan Di Huang (乾地黃)) adding Di Gu Pi (地骨皮), Mu Dan Pi (牡丹皮), Huang Qin (黃芩), and Cang Zhu (蒼朮). **Si Wu Tang (四物湯)** supplements and quickens the blood; Di Gu Pi nourishes yin, cools the blood, downbears latent heat in the lung, and supplements right qi; Mu Dan Pi drains latent heat in the blood, and harmonizes, cools, and engenders blood; Huang Qin clears heat and dries dampness and drains fire and resolves toxin; and Cang Zhu fortifies the spleen and dries dampness to counteract the digestion impairment and loose stools some patients experience when administered blood-nourishing and yin-enriching medicinals. Dr. Lee typically prescribes this formula for pathoconditions involving thrombosis and vascular inflammation (e.g, thromboangiitis obliterans (aka Buerger disease), retinopathy).

Diao Fen (吊粉) (aka Suspension Powder)

Da Huang (大黃), Huang Bo (黃柏), Ru Xiang (乳香), Mo Yao (沒藥), Xu Duan (續斷), Gu Sui Bu (骨髓補), Chuan Wu (川烏), Cao Wu (草烏), Rice Wine (米酒)

These medicinals are pulverized into medicinal powder and then mixed with rice wine (20~30° (27°)) to form a medicinal paste that is topically applied in the acute stage of inflammation presenting with heat, pain, redness (or purplish), and swelling for traumatic injuries such as sprains, subluxation, and fractures. It has anesthetic and pain-relieving, inflammation-resolving and heat-dispersing, and blood-quickening and stasis-transforming actions. This medicinal paste is spread on fine burlap cloth, covered with gauze, and then sufficiently wrapped with bandage and secured with tubular elastic net dressing, applied just tight enough so that healthy circulation remains unaffected. For best efficacy, it is recommended that the medicinal paste be left on for 6~8 hours, but should be removed sooner in the rare cases where the patient feels itchiness, tingling, and discomfort due to a mild allergic reaction.

Er Chen Tang (二陳湯)

Huang Qin (黃芩) 3 qian, Chen Pi (陳皮), Ban Xia (半夏), Fu Ling (茯苓), Gan Cao (甘草) 4 qian each

The Yu Sheng version is similar to the original except for the substraction of Sheng Jiang (生薑) and Wu Mei (烏梅) and the addition of Huang Qin (黃芩), whose heat-clearing and dampness-drying actions are acclimated for the the humid climate in northern Taiwan and complements this formulas overall dampness-drying and phlegm-harmonizing and qi-normalizing and harmonizing the center actions. The derivatives of **Er Chen Tang – Wen Dan Tang (溫膽湯)** and **Ban Xia Tian Ma Bai Zhu San (半夏天麻白朮散)** – are frequently prescribed for a broad scope of pathoconditions ranging from external contraction (common cold) and psychosomatic disorders to infertility and brain tumors.

Feng Shi Fang (風濕方)

Ma huang (麻黃) 1.5 qian, Yu Gui (玉桂), Chi Shao (赤芍), Gan Cao (甘草), Gan Jiang (乾薑), Fu Zi (附子), Huang Qin (黃芩), Huang Bo (黃柏), Fu Ling (茯苓), Zhu Ling (豬苓), Ze Xie (澤瀉), Cang Zhu (蒼朮), Sheng Shi Gao (生石膏), Jin Yin Hua (金銀花), Wu Wei Zi (五味子), Yin Yang Huo (淫羊藿) 3 qian each, Hong Zao (紅棗) 5 pieces

This Yu Sheng original formula was designed by Dr. Lee early on in his clinical practice and was specifically administered for patients with rheumatic disorders (e.g., osteoarthritis (OA) and rheumatoid arthritis (RA)) whom are currently being (or have recently been) administered systemic corticosteroids. In year's past, Western medical doctors in Taiwan indiscriminately prescribed systemic corticosteroids for the treatment of all types of inflammatory pain, including rheumatic disorders, without any consideration given to the deleterious side effects. Nowadays, this practice has been largely abandoned and Dr. Lee typically prescribes the **(Yu Sheng) Hyperactive Immune Formula (免疫過方)** for these types of pathoconditions instead.

Gan Mai Da Zao Tang Combining Ban Xia Hou Po Tang (甘麥大棗湯合併 半夏厚朴湯)

Ban Xia (半夏), Hou Po (厚朴), Zi Su Zi (紫蘇子), Fu Ling (茯苓) 4 qian, Gan Cao (甘草) 5 qian, Hong Zao (紅棗) 10 pieces, Fu Xiao Mai (浮小麥) 1 liang

This a compound formula with a composition almost identical to the original formulas except for the subtraction of Sheng Jiang (生薑). **Gan Mai Da Zao Tang (甘麥大棗湯)** has the actions of harmonizing the center, relaxing tension, quieting the spirit, and calming agitation and is traditionally prescribed for the treatment of visceral agitation; and **Ban Xia Hou Po Tang (半夏厚朴湯)** has the actions of moving qi, dissipating stasis, downbearing counterflow, and transforming phlegm and is traditionally prescribed for the treatment of seven-affect binding depression (e.g., mood disorders such as anxiety, depression, hypomania), insomnia and palpitations, gastrointestinal neurosis, vocal cord nodules and polyps, plum-pit qi, and menopausal syndrome. Since the functions of these two formulas overlap and correlate Dr. Lee has combined them for the treatment of a broad spectrum of mood, psychosomatic, and neuropsychiatric disorders (e.g., mild cases of Tourette syndrome) including those mentioned above. Dr. Lee rarely prescribes this compound formula on its own, instead typically combining it with another formula such as Ban Xia Tian Ma Bai Zhu San.

Ge Gen Tang (葛根湯)

Ma Huang (麻黃) 1.5 liang, Huang Qin (黃芩), Cang Zhu (蒼朮) 3 qian each, Ge Gen (葛根), Chi Shao (赤芍), Gan Cao (甘草), Yu Gui (玉桂), Sheng Jiang (生薑) 5 qian each, Hong Zao (紅棗) 5

pieces

The Yu Sheng version is very similar to the original formula, which is a derivative of Gui Zhi Tang (桂枝湯), but as in Dr. Lee's other formulas Yu Gui (玉桂) replaces Gui Zhi (桂枝) and Chi Shao (赤芍) replaces Bai Shao (白芍), and Cang Zhu (蒼朮) and Huang Qin (黃芩) are added due to considerations for northern Taiwan's humid climate. This formula promotes sweating and resolves the exterior and upbears liquid and courses the channels. Dr. Lee commonly prescribes variants of this formula for external contraction with yang brightness (yang ming) headache and body ache, heat (fever) without sweating, aversion to cold, stretched stiffness of the nape and back, sinusitis, and crick in the neck. This formula is also prescribed for patients with acute stage facial palsy (caused by trauma, tumor, virus), Bell's palsy (caused by virus (most commonly herpes simplex virus (HSV)), and trigeminal neuralgia whom have not been administered corticosteroids. The inclusion of Huang Qin and Cang Zhu in the Yu Sheng version of this formula also makes it easily modified into **Ge Gen Huang Qin Huang Lian Tang (葛根黃芩黃連湯)** (i.e., adding Huang Lian (黃連)) for the treatment of heat evil entering the interior causing diarrhea or dysentery (gastroenteritis) and exterior evil not yet resolved.

Gui Qi Jian Zhong Tang (歸耆建中湯)

Dang Gui (當歸) 2 qian, Gan Jiang (乾薑), Huang Qin (黃芩), Cang Zhu (蒼朮) 3 qian each, Yu Gui (玉桂), Chi Shao (赤芍), Gan Cao (甘草), Fu Zi (附子) 5 qian each, Hong Zao (紅棗) 5 pieces Huang Qi (黃耆) 1 liang

This formula is derived from **Xiao Jian Zhong Tang (小建中湯)** adding Dang Gui (當歸) and Huang Qi (黃耆). The Yu Sheng version of this formula is similar to the original version, but includes large doses of Huang Qi (黃耆); replaces Bai Shao (白芍) with Chi Shao (赤芍), Sheng Jiang (生薑) with Gan Jiang (乾薑), and Gui Pi (桂皮) with large doses of Yu Gui (玉桂); and adds Cang Zhu (蒼朮), Hong Zao (紅棗), and a large dose of Fu Zi (附子). Huang Qin (黃芩) is also added for its heat-clearing and dampness-drying and fire-draining and toxin-resolving actions that counteract the great heat medicinals. Huang Qi functions as a channel conductor for the upper limbs and Yu Gui as a channel conductor for the four extremities (the limbs).

The additions to the Yu Sheng version of this formula enhance its qi-supplementing and center-fortifying, tension-relaxing and interior-harmonizing, and blood supplementing actions, while also equipping it with the capacity to treat vacuity cold pathoconditions of the upper body. Dr. Lee commonly prescribes this formula for cold impediment of the greater yang small intestine channel, neuropathy, frozen shoulder, and Raynaud's disease (and phenomenon); and for skin pathoconditions such as non-eruption of papules (acne) and menopausal skin changes.

Gui Zhi Jia Long Gu Mu Li Tang
(桂枝加龍骨牡蠣湯)

Cang Zhu (蒼朮) 4 qian, Yu Gui (玉桂), Chi Shao (赤芍), Gan Cao (甘草), Sheng Jiang (生薑), Sheng Long Gu (生龍骨), Sheng Mu Li (生牡蠣), Shan Yao (山藥), Dang Shen (黨參) 5 qian each Hong Zao (紅棗) 5 pieces.

The Yu Sheng version contains all of the essential medicinals of the original formula with the exception of Yu Gui (玉桂) replacing Gui Zhi (桂枝) and the addition of Dang Shen (黨參), Shan Yao (山藥), and Cang Zhu (蒼朮). The qi-boosting, spleen-fortifying, essence-securing, and dampness drying actions of these additional medicinals complement this formula's overall action of neutrally supplementing yin and yang, subduing and settling, and securing essence and containing urination. This formula is traditionally prescribed for pathoconditions such as vacuity taxation with dual yin and yang vacuity, dreaming with seminal emission, hypertonicity of the lesser abdomen, lower burner vacuity cold, stirring palpitations below the umbilicus resulting from urinary incontinence, and hysteria. In addition to these pathoconditions, Dr. Lee may prescribe this formula to treat juvenile acne, stress-related hair loss (e.g., alopecia areata, hair shedding (aka telogen effluvium), trichotillomania), and children with hyperactivity or impulsivity (e.g., attention deficit hyperactivity disorder (ADHD)). Early on in Dr. Lee's clinical practice he would prescribe this formula for obstretics pathoconditions, but in recent years he typically prescribes **Dang Gui San (當歸散)** variants instead.

Huang Lian Jie Du Tang (黃連解毒湯)

Huang Lian (黃連), Huang Qin (黃芩), Huang Bo (黃柏), Zhi Zi (梔子) 3 qian each, Cang Zhu (蒼朮) 4 qian, Gan Cao (甘草) 5 qian

The Yu Sheng version is virtually the same as the original formula except for the addition of Cang Zhu (蒼朮) and Gan Cao (甘草). Cang Zhu fortifies the spleen and dries dampness and Gan Cao supplements the center and harmonizes the nature of medicinals – a pair that combines to promote digestion and protect the stomach from the bitter cold bitter medicinals. It is important to note here that long-term administration (≥ 3 months) of Zhi Zi (梔子) may cause transient grayish yellow skin pigmentation in some patients and thus Dr. Lee only prescribes this formula proper over a short term. In cases where long-term administration is necessary Dr. Lee will typically prescribe **Hyperactive Immune Formula (免疫過方)** in place of **Huang Lian Jie Du Tang**. This formula contains "the Three Yellows" – Huang Qin (黃芩), Huang Bo (黃柏), and Huang

Lian (黃連) – which are among the most commonly prescribed medicinals in Dr. Lee's pharmacopeia and among the pillars of Dr. Lee's treatment approaches.

This is a commonly administered formula for triple burner heat toxin congestion. Huang Lian drains heart fire and middle burner fire, Huang Qin drains upper burner fire, Huang Bo drains lower burner fire, and Zhi Zi frees and drains heat in all three burners and abducts heat downward where the heat evil is excreted in the urine. In modern biomedical terms this formula can be classified as a "broad spectrum antimicrobial and anti-inflammatory." All of these medicinals contain powerful heat-clearing and toxin-resolving (antimicrobial and anti-inflammatory) actions which combined together into one formula provide exceptional efficacy for the treatment of all types of infections and inflammation (e.g., upper respiratory tract, gastrointestinal, hepatic, renal, autoimmune disorders).

Huo Luo Dan (活絡丹) (aka Network-Quickening Elixir)

Dang Gui (當歸), Ru Xiang (乳香), Mo Yao (沒藥), Dan Shen (丹參), Di Long (地龍), Chuan Wu (川烏), Wu Cao (草烏), Tian Nan Xing (天南星), Ma Huang (麻黃) 5 jin each

The Yu Sheng version is identical to the original formula, which is also known as **Xiao Huo Luo Dan (小活絡丹) (aka Minor Network-Quickening Elixir**), except for the addition of Dang Gui (當歸), Dan Shen (丹參), and Ma Huang (麻黃). Dang Gui supplements and quickens the blood; Dan Shen engenders blood, cools blood, and dispels stasis; and Ma Huang "opens up" and transports medicinals across all membranes. These additions complement and further enhance this formula's overall wind-dispeling, dampness-dispersing, network vessel-freeing, blood-quickening, stasis-dispelling, and pain-relieving actions. This formula is traditionally prescribed for the treatment of wind-cold-damp evil invading the channels and network vessels, contraction and pain of the sinews and vessels, inhibited bending and stretching of the joints, and wandering aches and pain; insensitivity of the limbs following stroke and phlegm-damp dead blood in the channels and network vessels; and knocks and falls (traumatic injury) and stasis obstruction in the channels and network vessels causing pain. Dr. Lee utilizes this pill's (elixir's) blood-quickening, stasis-dispeling, and channel and network vessel-freeing actions for its exceptional efficacy in relieving pain, particularly for wind-damp impediment and traumatic injuries involving the lumbus and lower limbs. This pill (elixir) is produced and processed in-house using a strictly controlled fermentation method and oven-roast process that safely ensures the potential toxicity of medicinal components are mitigated.

Hyperactive Immune Formula (免疫過抗方) (aka Mian Yi Guo Kang Fang)

Huang Lian (黃連), Huang Qin (黃芩), Huang Bo (黃柏), Cang Zhu (蒼朮), Qing Hao (青蒿), Zhi Mu (知母), Di Gu Pi (地骨皮) 5 each qian

This formula was designed relatively later in Dr. Lee's clinical practice specifically for treating patients with connective tissue and/or systemic inflammation either of autoimmune or degenerative origin whom have not yet been administered systemic corticosteroid therapy (or if administration has been for ≤ 1 week (approximately 3~4 days)). It is composed of the essential medicinals from **(Yu Sheng) Huang Lian Jie Du Tang (黃連解毒湯)** – Huang Lian (黃連), Huang Qin (黃芩), Huang Bo (黃柏), Cang Zhu (蒼朮) – along with the addition of Qing Hao (青蒿), Zhi Mu (知母), Di Gu Pi (地骨皮). These medicinals combine to form a potent combination of heat-clearing and toxin-resolving (anti-inflammatory), vacuity heat-clearing, steaming bone-eliminating, fire-draining, yin-enriching, dryness-moistening, and blood-cooling actions. As mentioned above in the **(Yu Sheng) Feng Shi Fang (風濕方)** profile, the changing practices of Taiwan's Western medicine institution has seen a trend away from indiscriminate administration of systemic corticosteroids. In response, Dr. Lee now commonly prescribes this formula for treating patients with a broad scope of pathoconditions involving acute stage inflammation and chronic autoimmune and degenerative diseases such as osteoarthritis (OA), rheumatoid arthritis (RA), ankylosing spondylitis (AS), systemic lupus erythematosis (SLE), polymositis, dermatomyositis, scleroderma, multiple sclerosis (MS), Behcet's disease, Sjogren's syndrome (SS), immune thrombocytopenic purpura (ITP), inflammatory bowel disease (IBS), and vasculitis. In addition to applying eight-principle and six-channel pattern identification methods, inflammatory indices (e.g., erythrocyte sedimentation rate (ESR), antinuclear antibody (ANA)) are invaluable diagnostic tools for determining the presence and severity of inflammation. This formula provides quick and lasting effectiveness in resolving inflammation and relieving symptoms (i.e., treating the tip), allowing the patient to proceed on to other TCM formulas that function to treat the root of disease.

Jian Ling Tang (健瓴湯)

Zi Shi (磁石) 3 qian, Bo Zi Ren (柏子仁) 4 qian

Niu Xi (牛膝), Chi Shao (赤芍), Sheng Long Gu (生龍骨), Sheng Mu Li (生牡蠣), Gan Di Huang (乾地黃), Shan Yao (山藥) 5 qian each, Dai Zhe Shi (代赭石) 8 qian

The Yu Sheng version is virtually the same as the original formula with the exception of Chi Shao (赤芍) replacing Bai Shao (白芍) and the addition of Zi Shi (磁石). As in many Yu Sheng formulas Chi Shao is selected for its superior blood-quickening and stasis-dispeling actions. The defining constituents of this spirit-quieting by heavy settling formula are Dai Zhe Shi (代赭石) – enters the blood aspect of the liver and heart channels, eliminates heat, calms the liver and subdues yang, and downbears counterflow by heavy settling; Zi Shi – governs the lung and kidney, settles fright and quiets the spirit, and calms the liver and subdues yang; enters the liver and kidney channels; Sheng Long Gu (生龍骨) – enters the heart, liver, and kidney channels, and subdues yang and quiets the spirit; and Sheng Mu Li (生牡蠣) – calms the liver and subdues yang, softens hardness and dissipates binds, and astringes and secures. It is important to note that raw (shēng (生)) Long Gu and Mu Li are used here preserving the properties of calcium ions (Ca^{2+}) for a calming action as opposed to calcined (duàn (煅)) which has an astringing action produced from the resulting magnesium ions (Mg^{2+}) properties. Dr. Lee typically reserves this formula for only the most severe cases of ascendent hyperactivity of yang manifesting in pathoconditions such as hyperglycemia (diabetes), hypertension, hyperthyroidism, insomnia, schizophrenia, and Tourett's syndrome. This includes cases in which Western medicine drug therapy has been administered without efficacy or with initial efficacy but is no longer able to effectively control the pathocondition.

Long Dan Xie Gan Tang (龍膽瀉肝湯)

Long Dan Cao (龍膽草), Huang Qin (黃芩), Zhi Zi (梔子), Dang Gui (當歸), Sheng Di Huang (生地黃), Mu Tong (木通), Chai Hu (柴胡), Che Qian Zi (車前子) 3qian, Cang Zhu (蒼朮), Ze Xie (澤瀉) 4 qian, Sheng Gan Cao (生甘草) 5 qian

The Yu Sheng version is identical to the original except for the addition of Cang Zhu (蒼朮) with its wind-damp dispelling actions further enchancing this formula's potent overall liver-clearing and dampness-disinhibiting actions as it drains liver and gallbladder repletion fire and clears lower burner damp-heat. Traditionally, this formula is prescribed for liver and gallbladder repletion fire flaming upward pattern pathoconditions presenting with rib-side pain (e.g., herpes zoster) and headache (e.g., acute hepatitis, acute cholecystitis), red eyes (e.g., acute conjunctivitis, keratitis) and bitter taste in mouth, and deafness and swelling of the ear (e.g., otitis media, sinusitis); and liver channel damp-heat pouring downward pattern presenting with urinary dribbling and stranguary-turbidity (e.g., urinary tract infection (UTI)), pudendal itch (e.g., acute pyelonitis) and genital swelling (e.g., acute epididymitis) and vaginal discharge (e.g., vaginitis). In addition to these pathoconditions, Dr. Lee also administers this formula for pain wind (gout and pseudogout).

Ma Xing Shi Gan Tang (麻杏甘石湯)

Ma Huang (麻黃) 1.5 qian, Cang Zhu (蒼朮) 3 qian, Xing Ren (杏仁) 4 qian, Gan Cao (甘草) 5 qian, Shi Gao (石膏) 1 liang

The Yu Sheng version is identical to the original formula except for the addition of Cang Zhu (蒼朮), which is included for its wind-damp dispelling and dampness-drying actions. This formula's lung-diffusing, heat-draining, cough-suppressing, and panting-calming actions are traditionally administered for the treatment of externally contracted wind-cold and exuberant lung heat, failure to resolve generalized heat (fever), and panting counterflow and rapid breathing. Dr. Lee typically prescribes this formula for the treatment of common colds (exterior wind-heat external contraction), acute bronchitis, and pneumonia. Additionally, Dr. Lee may also add Yi Yi Ren (薏苡仁) to form a variant of **Ma Xing Yi Gan Tang (麻杏薏甘湯)** with its exterior-resolving and dampness-eliminating and lung qi diffusing and disinhibiting actions administered for the treatment of wind-damp exterior pattern external medicine (dermatological) pathoconditions such as eczema, urticaria, and some types of seborrheic dermatitis.

Mai Men Dong Tang (麥門冬湯)

Ma Huang (麻黃) 1.5 qian, Xing Ren (杏仁), Cang Zhu (蒼朮) 4 qian, Mai Men Dong (麥門冬), Xuan Shen (玄參), Ban Xia (半夏), Gan Cao (甘草), Shan Yao (山藥), Sheng Jiang (生薑) 5 qian each,

Hong Zao (紅棗) 5 pieces

The Yu Sheng version is the same as the original formula except for the subtraction of Jing Mi (粳米); Ren Shen (powder) (人參粉) replacing decocting pieces; and the addition of Ma Huang (麻黃), Xing Ren (杏仁), Cang Zhu (蒼朮), Xuan Shen (玄參), Shan Yao (山藥), and Sheng Jiang (生薑). As in **Jia Wei Mai Men Dong Tang (加味麥門冬湯)** the qi-boosting and yin-enriching, spleen, lung, and kidney-supplementing, and essence-securing actions of Shan Yao replaces Jing Mi. Xuan Shen's heat-clearing and blood-cooling and yin-enriching and toxin-resolving actions complement the yin-nourishing, lung-moistening, and liquid-engendering actions of Mai Men Dong (麥門冬) and the liquid-engendering and spleen-supplementing and lung-boosting actions of Ren Shen. Ma Huang suppresses cough and counterflow qi and opens the nine orifices; Xing Ren downbears and drains lung qi and suppresses cough and calms panting; and Cang Zhu (蒼朮) has the action of drying dampness and fortifying the spleen. This formula is traditionally prescribed to clear heat, nourish the lung and stomach, downbear counterflow, and precipitate qi for the treatment of lung yin vacuity, lung wilting, upflaming vacuity fire, and qi counterflow panting and coughing. These types of pathoconditions result from microbial infections (i.e., bacteria, virus, fungus) damaging the mucous membranes (i.e., ciliated pseudostratified columnan epithelium) of the respiratory tract (e.g., larynx, trachea, bronchi) and inhibiting the secretion of epithelial lining fluid (ELF) which maintains epithelial moisture, traps particulate material and pathogens moving through the airway, and transports mucous (e.g., metabolic waste, pus, phlegm-rheum) upwards through the trachea towards the mouth where it is either coughed out or swallowed. This formula functions to promote healing of the mucous membranes and serves to restore normal regulation of fluid secretion in the respiratory tract. Dr. Lee classifies these types of pathoconditions as "yin vacuity cough" (aka dryness cough) in the lung channel and will also prescribe this formula for side effects resulting from radiotherapy (e.g., head and neck cancers) and chemotherapy such as dry mouth and throat and skin redness, blistering and peeling.

Paralysis Formulas (截癱方) (3 variants)

These three formulas were specially designed early on in Dr. Lee's clinical practice for the treatment of paresis and paralysis, which correlates with "wilting pattern" in classical pathological terminology, resulting from traumatic injury (including iatrogenic), microbial infection, and degenerative diseases of autoimmune and hereditary origin with each formula having a specific function throughout the various stages of the pathocondition. It is important to note that the determination of treatment is based on symptoms, signs, and pattern identification, thus in addition to this **Paralysis Formula (截癱方)** series Dr. Lee may also prescribe other formulas for the treatment of paresis, paralysis, and other neuropathies (i.e., CNS, PNS, ANS). For instance, in specific cases involving viral infection inducing paralysis, if the patient has not yet been administered corticosteroids and it is still in the acute stage (approximately ≤ 1 week), Dr. Lee will approach this as an external contraction wind-heat pattern prescribing a formula such as **Ge Gen Tang (葛根湯)** variant with its cool acrid exterior resolution actions combined with other medicinals such as Di Long (地龍) that free the orifices. However, the typical protocol is as follows: **Paralysis Formula #1 (Di Long San Variant) (截癱一號方) (地龍散加方)** – acute stage (approximately ≤ 1 week following onset of symptoms unless corticosteroids have already been administered) with static blood and metabolic waste (e.g., hyaline degeneration, inflammatory factors) congesting the vasculature, channels, and network vessels that can be identified as collection of static blood pattern; **Paralysis Formula #2 (Shi Quan Da Bu Tang Variant) (截癱二號方) (十全大補湯加方)** – post-acute and chronic stage (approximately ≥ 1 week) with enduring symptoms that can be identified as dual qi and blood vacuity pattern, and specifically for cases involving cervical and thoracic spine injuries; and **Paralysis Formula #3 (You Gui Yin**

Variant) **(截癱三號方) (右歸飲加方)** – post-acute and chronic stages (approximately ≥ 1 week) with enduring symptoms that can be identified as kidney yang vacuity pattern, and specifically for cases involving lumbar spine injuries.

Paralysis Formula #1 (Di Long San Variant)
(截癱一號方) (地龍散加方)

Ma Huang (麻黃), Hong Hua (紅花) 1.5 qian each

Tao Ren (桃仁), Gan Cao (甘草), Gan Jiang (乾薑), Yu Gui (玉桂), Di Long (地龍), Dang Gui (當歸), Huang Bo (黃柏) 3 qian each,

Du Zhong (杜仲) 4 qian, Wei Ling Xian (威靈仙), Niu Xi (牛膝), Fu Zi (附子) 5 qian each

The Yu Sheng version is composed of the original formula's essential medicinals – Di Long (地龍), Tao Ren (桃仁), Yu Gui (玉桂), Huang Bo (黃柏), Gan Cao (甘草), Ma Huang (麻黃), and Dang Gui (當歸) – along with the addition of Hong Hua (紅花), Niu Xi (牛膝), Wei Ling Xian (威靈仙), Gan Jiang (乾薑), and Fu Zi (附子), and Du Zhong (杜仲). Hong Hua, Niu Xi, and Wei Ling Xian enhance the formula's blood-quickening, blood-breaking, blood-supplementing, stasis-dispelling, and channel-freeing actions. Wei Ling Xian is also a Urinary Bladder channel medicinal that perfuses the twelve channels and network vessels; and Du Zhong and Niu Xi are channel conductors directing medicinals into the lumbus (spine) and lower limbs. Fu Zi and Gan Jiang combine with Yu Gui to form one of the pillars of Dr. Lee's treatment approaches – "the Three Great Yang-Supplementers" – that boosts the metabolism by innervating the central nervous system (CNS) and peripheral nervous system (PNS), repairs damaged cells and rejuvenating weakened cells, and promotes tissue regeneration. Ma Huang "opens up" and transports other medicinals across all membranes of the body down to the cellular level, thus making it an effective "channel-conductor," and its action of "opening the nine orifices" innervates the nervous system (i.e., CNS, PNS, ANS). Di Long is a Urinary Bladder Tai Yang channel medicinal that clears heat, extinguishes wind, frees the channels, quickens the network vessels, and disinhibits urine; Huang Bo clears heat, dries dampness, drains fire, resolves toxin, abates heat, elminates steam in the lower burner, and counteracts the heat of "the Three Great Yang-Supplementers"; and Gan Cao supplements the center and harmonizes the nature of medicinals. The original formula is traditionally prescribed for the treatment of knocks and falls; pain in the cervical, thoracic, and lumbar spine; pain in the arms; accumulations and gatherings in the abdomen; and blood stasis and static blood pain. As mentioned in the **Paralysis Formula (截癱方)** series introduction, Dr. Lee typically administers this formula during the acute stage (approximately ≤ 1 week following onset of symptoms unless corticosteroids have already been administered) with static blood and metabolic waste (e.g., hyaline degeneration, inflammatory factors) congesting the vasculature, channels, and network vessels that can be identified as collection of static blood pattern.

Paralysis Formula #2 (Shi Quan Da Bu Tang Variant) (截癱二號方) (十全大補湯加方)

Da Huang (大黃) 5 fen, Ma Huang (麻黃) 1.5 qian

Dan Shen (丹參), Chao Bai Zhu (炒白朮), Fu Ling (茯苓), Gan Cao (甘草), Dang Gui (當歸), Chuan Qiong (川芎), Chi Shao (赤芍), Gan Di (乾地黃), Huang Qi (黃耆), Yu Gui (玉桂), Di Long (地龍), Niu Xi (牛膝), Huang Qin (黃芩), Gan Jiang (乾薑) 3 qian each, Fu Zi (附子) 5 qian

This formula is composed of **(Yu Sheng) Shi Quan Da Bu Tang (十全大補湯)** with Chao Bai Zhu (炒白朮) replacing Cang

Zhu (蒼朮) for its emphasis on supplementing qi and fortifying the spleen, along with the addition of Da Huang (大黃), Ma Huang (麻黃), Di Long (地龍), and Niu Xi (牛膝). Da Huang drains precipitation (laxative) and damp heat, disperses accumulation, quickens the blood, and transforms stasis to lower intracranial pressure, relieves tension in the diaphragm, and promotes lysis of hyaline degeneration and the removal of metabolic waste that obstructs neurotransmitters. Ma Huang "opens up" and transports other medicinals across all membranes of the body down to the cellular level, thus making it an effective "channel-conductor," and its action of "opening the nine orifices" innervates the nervous system (i.e., CNS, PNS, ANS). Di Long is a Urinary Bladder Tai Yang channel medicinal that clears heat, extinguishes wind, frees the channels, quickens the network vessels, and disinhibits urine. Niu Xi quickens the blood, frees the channels, supplements the liver and kidney, strengthens the sinews and bones, disinhibits water, and serves as a channel conductor directing medicinals into the lumbus (spine) and lower limbs. This formula provides the enhanced qi and blood warming and supplementing, yin-enriching and yang-upbearing, and kidney yang-supplementing actions of Shi Quan Da Bu Tang along with the precipitation-draining (laxative), accumulation-dispersing, blood-quickening, stasis-transforming, water-disinhibiting actions (e.g., lower intracranial pressure), wind-extinguishing, channel-freeing, and network vessel-quickening actions of the additional medicinals. As mentioned in the **Paralysis Formula (截癱方)** series introduction, Dr. Lee typically administers this formula during the post-acute and chronic stage (approximately ≥ 1 week) with enduring symptoms that can be identified as dual qi and blood vacuity pattern, and specifically for cases involving cervical and thoracic spine injuries.

Paralysis Formula #3 (You Gui Yin Variant)
(截癱三號方) (右歸飲加方)

Da Huang (大黃) 5 fen, Ma Huang (麻黃) 1.5 qian

Fu Ling (茯苓), Dang Gui (當歸) 2 qian each

Gou Qi Zi (枸杞子), Niu Xi (牛膝), Du Zhong (杜仲), Huang Bo (黃柏), Di Long (地龍), Gan Jiang (乾薑), Yu Gui (玉桂) 3 qian each, Gan Di Huang (乾地黃), Shan Zhu Yu (山茱萸), Shan Yao (山藥), Tu Si Zi (菟絲子) 4 qian each, Fu Zi (附子) 5 qian

This formula is derived from **(Yu Sheng) You Gui Yin (右歸飲)** subtracting Cang Zhu (蒼朮) and adding Di Long (地龍), Da Huang (大黃), and Ma Huang (麻黃) just as in the **Paralysis #2 Formula (Shi Quan Da Bu Tang Variant)** above. Ma Huang "opens up" and transports other medicinals across all membranes of the body down to the cellular level, thus making it an effective "channel-conductor," and its action of "opening the nine orifices" innervates the nervous system (i.e., CNS, PNS, ANS). Di Long is a Urinary Bladder Tai Yang channel medicinal that clears heat, extinguishes wind, frees the channels, quickens the network vessels, and disinhibits urine. Da Huang drains precipitation (laxative) and damp heat, disperses accumulation, quickens the blood, and transforms stasis to lower intracranial pressure, relieves tension in the diaphragm, and promotes lysis of hyaline degeneration and the removal of metabolic waste that obstructs neurotransmitters. These additions complement and enhance the overall kidney yang-warming and supplementing, blood-quickening, sinew and bone-strengthening, and liver and kidney-supplementing actions of this formula. As mentioned in the **Paralysis Formula (截癱方)** series introduction, Dr. Lee typically administers this formula during the post-acute and chronic stage (approximately ≥ 1 week) with enduring symptoms that can be identified as kidney yang vacuity pattern, and specifically for cases involving lumbar spine injuries.

Po Xiao Dang Bao Tang (朴硝盪胞湯)

Da Huang (大黃), Mang Xiao (芒硝) 1 qian, Yu Gui (玉桂), Fu Ling (茯苓), Mu Dan Pi (牡丹皮), Chi Shao (赤芍), Tao Ren (桃仁),

Dang Shen (黨參), Gan Cao (甘草), Niu Xi (牛膝), Dang Gui (當歸), Hou Po (厚朴), Xi Xin (細辛), Jie Geng (桔梗), Huang Qin (黃芩), Qing Pi (青皮) 3 qian, Cang Zhu (蒼朮) 4 qian, Gan Jiang (乾薑), Fu Zi (附子) 5 qian, Meng Chong (䗪蟲) 20 pieces, Shui Zhi (水蛭) 3 qian

The Yu Sheng version is virtually identical to the original formula with the exception of Dang Shen (黨參) replacing Ren Shen (人參) and the addition of Huang Qin (黃芩), Cang Zhu (蒼朮), and Gan Jiang (乾薑). Meng Chong (䗪蟲), Shui Zhi (水蛭), Hou Po (厚朴), Da Huang (大黃), and Mang Xiao (芒硝) are among the essential medicinals combining to provide an effective formula for treating female infertility with its stasis-dispeling, accumulation-breaking, accumulation-dispersing, qi-moving downward, channel-freeing, phlegm-transforming, and draining-precipitation actions. As its name indicates – Dang Bao (盪胞) means to "flush the uterus" – this formula functions to "flush away" the residual metabolic waste (e.g., pus, cellular matter, blood clots) that may stagnate on the uterine lining and fallopian tube junctions (i.e, uterotubal junction) as a result of inflammation, adhesions, polyps, endometrial hyperplasia, endometriosis, and leiomyomas. This formula also elicits uterine contractions which sends a definitive feedback signal to the hypothalamus and pituitary gland so that the body clearly recognizes it should recalibrate normal hormone regulation and continue the regeneration process once again (e.g., a pathophysiological phenomenon occurring in some women whom have already given birth or have had a spontaneous abortion, either knowingly or unknowingly). Dr. Lee administers this formula specifically as a first-line treatment for female infertility (i.e., defined as absence of a live birth despite ≥ 1 years of efforts with a male partner (primary infertility) during which they have not used contraceptives or in women whom have consummated a live birth previously but are subsequently unable to despite ≥ 1 years of efforts (secondary infertility) during which they have not used contraceptives). The treatment regimen involves administration of this formula for 1 week starting a few days before menstruation with the couple subsequently proceeding in attempts at natural insemination over a 6-month period. In approximately 70% of these cases this approach will lead to pregnancy within that 6-month period. If this treatment does not result in pregancy, then Dr. Lee will advise the couple to undergo further evaluation (e.g., ultrasound to determine the thickness of the endometrial lining, scrotal ultrasound) and testing (e.g., postcoital test (PCT), semen analysis) to determine the presence of anti-sperm antibodies) prior to conducting further pattern identification and proceeding with other treatment approaches.

Qi Chuan Fang (氣喘方)
(aka Asthma Formula)

Ma Huang (麻黃) 1.5 qian, Dan Shen (丹參), Cang Zhu (蒼朮), Fu Ling (茯苓), Gan Cao (甘草), Mu Xiang (木香), 砂仁 (Sha Ren), Wu Wei Zi (五味子) 3 qian each, Chen Pi (陳皮), Ban Xia (半夏), Xing Ren (杏仁), Bai Guo (百果) 4 qian each, Shan Yao (山藥), Yu Gui (玉桂) 5 qian each

This original Yu Sheng formula contains the qi-boosting and spleen-fortifying and qi-moving and phlegm-transforming actions of **Xiang Sha Liu Jun Zi Tang (香砂六君子湯)** adding Ma Huang (麻黃), Wu Wei Zi (五味子), Xing Ren (杏仁), Bai Guo (白果), Shan Yao (山藥), and Yu Gui (玉桂). Ma Huang promotes sweating and resolves the exterior; Wu Wei Zi constrains the lung and stabilizes panting; Xing Ren suppresses cough and calms panting; Bai Guo constrains the lung and dispels phlegm; Shan Yao supplements the spleen, lung, and kidneys and nourishes yin; and Yu Gui supplments fire and aides yang for vacuity asthma debilitation of the life gate fire. Dr. Lee will also add Ren Shen (powder) (人參粉), which enters the lung and spleen channels, greatly supplements original qi, and supplements the spleen and boosts the lung. As its name indicates, this formula is designed for the treatment of asthma, and specifically for the spleen yang vacuity pattern type that presents with panting (asthma) and shortness of breath (dyspnea).

Spleen yang vacuity pattern presents in the early stages of this pathocondition and can often be either cured or at least well controlled so that it does not progress to the more severe chronic stage of kidney yang vacuity pattern for which Dr. Lee typically prescribes **You Gui Yin (右歸飲)** variants. For acute flare-ups, heat-clearing and toxin resolving, lung-depurating and phlegm-transforming, and cough-suppressing and panting calming medicinals will be added to the main formula; or the original formula will be substituted with a heat-clearing, cough-suppressing, and panting calming formula until the flare-up subsides.

Ru Mo Si Wu Tang (乳沒四物湯)

Dang Gui (當歸), Chuan Qiong (川芎), Chi Shao (赤芍), Gan Di Huang (乾地黃), Ru Xiang (乳香), Mo Yao (沒藥), Cang Zhu (蒼朮), Gan Cao (甘草), Tao Ren (桃仁) 3 qian each, Hong Hua (紅花) 1.5 qian

This Yu Sheng formula is a variant of **Si Wu Tang (四物湯)** with Gan Di Huang (乾地黃) replacing Shu Di Huang (熟地黃) and Chi Shao (赤芍) replacing Bai Shao (白芍), and adding Tao Ren (桃仁) and Hong Hua (紅花). Gan Di Huang supplements yin and cools the blood; Chi Shao cools the blood and expels stasis; Tao Ren quickens the blood and dispels stasis; and Hong Hua quickens the blood, dispels stasis, and frees the channels (menstruation). These additions complement Si Wu Tang's blood-supplementing, blood-quickening, and qi-moving actions with enhanced stasis-dispeling and channel-freeing actions. Dr. Lee prescribes this formula for treating a broad spectrum of pathoconditions involving blockage of the flow of blood both inside the vessels (e.g., thrombus, embolus) and outside in the interstitium (e.g., hemorrhage) where it is capable of promoting absorption of blood and stanching bleeding. It is a commonly prescribed formula for gynecological pathoconditions involving blood stasis and concretions, conglomerations, accumulations, and gatherings such as uterine fibroids (leiomyomas), endometrial hyperplasia, ovarian cysts, and menstrual irregularities. And it is also one of the main formulas prescribed in Dr. Lee's cancer treatment protocol, specifically administered for malignant (or benign) tumors of the smooth muscle (soft tissue) such as carcinomas, fibromas, leiomyosarcomas, and hamartomas involving the breast, urinary bladder, uterus, gastrointestinal tract, and respiratory tract.

Sai Ji (塞劑) (aka Vaginal Suppository)

She Chuang Zi (蛇床子) 1g, Xiong Huang (powder) (雄黃粉) 0.3g, Liu Huang (powder) 0.3g, Da Huang (大黃) 0.3g

The **(Yu Sheng) Sai Ji (塞劑) (aka Vaginal Suppository)** is a vaginal suppository prescribed for various types of vaginal infections including yeast (e.g., candidiasis), bacterial (e.g., gonorrhea), trichomoniasis, and genital herpes that present with itching, irritation, and watery or viscous vaginal discharge that occur inside the vaginal cavity. This formula is typically prescribed as part of a therapeutic regimen that includes decocted formulas taken orally such as **Long Dan Xie Gan Tang (龍膽瀉肝湯)**, **Jin Suo Gu Jing Wan (金鎖固經丸)**, or **Bu Zhong Yi Qi Tang (補中益氣湯)**.

Seborrheic Dermatitis Formula (脂漏方)

Ma Huang (麻黃) 1.5 qian, Huang Qin (黃芩) 3 qian Cang Zhu (蒼朮) 4 qian, Gan Cao (甘草) Jin Yin Hua (金銀花) 5 qian each, Lu Lu Tong (路路通) 10 pieces, Shi Gao (石膏), Yi Yi

Ren (薏苡仁) 1 liang

This Yu Sheng original formula is composed of **(Yu Sheng) Ma Xing Yi Gan Tang (麻杏薏甘湯)** adding Huang Qin (黃芩), Jin Yin Hua (金銀花), and Lu Lu Tong (路路通). Huang Qin clears heat and dries dampness, drains fire and resolves toxin; Jin Yin Hua clears heat and resolves toxin and courses wind, dissipates heat dissipates well-abscess and disperses swelling, and is an essential medicinal for the treatment of all types of yang pattern swollen welling-abscess and clove sores (carbuncles, faruncles, boils); and Lu Lu Tong dispels wind, eliminates dampness, and resolves toxin for the treatment of wind-damp streaming sores, welling-abscesses, scab, and lichen. As the name indicates, this Yu Sheng formula is specifically designed for the treatment of seborrheic dermatitis, which correlates with "wandering wind of the face" and "white scaling wind" described in classical TCM texts.

Sheng Yu Tang (聖愈湯)

Dang Gui (當歸), Chuan Qiong (川芎), Chi Shao (赤芍), Gan Di Huang (乾地黃), Cang Zhu (蒼朮) 3 qian each, Dan Shen (丹參) 5 qian, Huang Qi (黃耆) 1.5 liang

The Yu Sheng version is similar to the original formula except that Gan Di Huang (乾地黃) replaces Shou Di Huang (熟地黃) and Dan Shen (丹參) replaces Ren Shen (人參), and Chi Shao (赤芍) and Cang Zhu (蒼朮) have been added. Due to the time-consuming and costly method of traditional processing, Shou Di Huang (熟地黃) on the market today is either very expensive or uses modern processing methods resulting in inferior quality; thus, Dr. Lee typically substitutes it with Gan Di Huang (乾地黃), which also has yin-supplementing and blood-cooling actions. Depending on the presenting symptoms, signs, and pattern, Dr. Lee may prescribe Ren Shen (powder) (人參粉) (or Ren Shen (powder) and Chuan Qi (powder) paired). Chi Shao cools the blood and expels stasis; Dan Shen engenders blood, dispels stasis, cools the blood, regulates menses, and calms the fetus; and Cang Zhu fortifies the spleen and dries dampness, thus counteracting the potential for digestion impairment and loose stools induced by the blood-nourishing and yin-enriching medicinals. These additions complement and enhance this formula's overall blood-supplementing, yin-nourishing, blood-regulating, stasis-dispeling, blood-cooling, and qi-supplementing actions. Dr. Lee utilizes this formula's actions of dispelling stasis and cooling the blood for the treatment of vascular wall pathologies such as chemotherapy-induced nephrototoxicity (e.g., interstitial nephritis), chemotherapy-induced hepatotoxicity (e.g., hepatitis), aneurysm, and retinopathy (e.g., diabetic). For the treatment of chemotherapy side effects manifesting as vascular wall pathoconditions Dr. Lee will typically prescribe **Xiao Chai Hu Tang (小柴胡湯)** combined with **Sheng Yu Tang**. **Sheng Yu Tang** is an excellent formula for providing stable and lasting effects in the promotion of blood perfusion, but it neither controls blood as effectively as **Xue Ku Fang (血枯方)** (aka **Blood Desiccation Formula**), nor does it promote blood perfusion as rapidly as **Bu Yang Huan Wu Tang (補陽還五湯)**.

Shi Quan Da Bu Tang Tang (十全大補湯)

Qin Huang (黃芩) 2 qian, Dan Shen (丹參), Cang Zhu (蒼朮), Fu Ling (茯苓), Gan Cao (甘草), Dang Gui (當歸), Chuan Qiong (川芎), Chi Shao (赤芍), Gan Di Huang (乾地黃), Gan Jiang (乾薑), Fu Zi (附子) 3 qian each, Yu Gui (玉桂) 5 qian, Huang Qi (黃耆) 1 liang

This formula combines the blood-quickening and blood-supplementing actions of **(Yu Sheng) Si Wu Tang (四物湯)**

(Dang Gui (當歸), Chuan Qiong (川芎), Chi Shao (赤芍), Gan Di Huang (乾地黃)) and the qi-boosting and spleen-fortifying actions of **(Yu Sheng) Si Jun Zi Tang (四君子湯)** (Dan Shen (丹參), Cang Zhu (蒼朮), Fu Ling (茯苓), Gan Cao (甘草)); replaces Sheng Jiang (生薑) with Gan Jiang (乾薑) instead of adding Fu Zi (附子), Huang Qin (黃芩), large doses of Huang Qi (黃耆) and Yu Gui (玉桂), and includes. Huang Qin (黃芩) is added to counteract the great heat medicinals. The Yu Sheng version of this formula provides enhanced qi and blood warming and supplementing, yin-enriching and yang-upbearing, and kidney yang-supplementing actions making this dual blood-quickening and blood-supplementing actions and qi-boosting and spleen-fortifying formula applicable for the treatment of a broad range of pathoconditions and complications. In addition to other applications, Dr. Lee commonly uses this formula for pediatric patients with delayed growth (e.g., height and weight), cerebral palsy (congenital or acquired), and congenital developmental delay (e.g., physical, cognitive, emotional, speech and language).

Tong Jing Fang (通經方)

Cang Zhu (蒼朮) 4 qian, Gan Cao (甘草) 5 qian

Niu Xi (牛膝), Xu Duan (續斷), Gu Sui Bu (骨碎), Qian Cao (茜草) 8 qian each

The Yu Sheng version is designed with similar therapeutic actions as the original, but Dr. Lee has overhauled the composition and increased the dose of its essential medicinals. Niu Xi (牛膝) dissipates stasis, quickens the blood, frees the channels (menstruation), supplements the liver and kidney, and relieves pain; Xu Duan (續斷) quickens the blood, joins sinew and bones, quiets the fetus, and supplements the liver and kidney; Gu Sui Bu (骨碎補) quickens the blood, strengthens the sinew, supplements the kidney, and settles pain; and Qian Cao (茜草) cools blood and moves blood.

Cang Zhu (蒼朮) has the action of drying dampness and fortifying the spleen to counteract the potential of digestion impairment and loose stools resulting from blood-nourishing and yin-enriching medicinals; and Gan Cao supplements the center and harmonizes the nature of medicinals. The addition of liver and kidney-supplmenting and sinew and bone-strengthening medicinals complement the original formula's blood-breaking, channel-freeing, and pain-relieving actions. Dr. Lee typically prescribes this formula for fractures and trauma injuries; osteoporosis; and as adjuvant therapy for the side efforts of chemotherapy in bone and uterine cancer patients. It is also one of the commonly prescribed formulas in Dr. Lee's cancer treatment protocol specifically administered for malignant (or benign) tumors of the striated muscle and marrow (e.g., rhabdomyosarcoma, osteosarcoma) with its capacity to inhibit tumor-cell mediated angiogenesis and neovascularization and the proliferation of cancer stem cells.

Wan Ling Dan (萬靈丹) (aka Unlimited Efficacy Elixir) – refer to Bao An Wan Ling Dan (保安萬靈丹) (aka Safeguard Unlimited Efficacy Elixir)

Wen Dan Tang (溫膽湯)

Huang Qin (黃芩), Zhi Shi (枳實) 3 qian each

Chen Pi (陳皮), Ban Xia (半夏), Fu Ling (茯苓), GanCao (甘草) 4 qian each, Zhu Ru (竹茹) 3 pieces

Hong Zao (紅棗) 4 pieces

The Yu Sheng version is virtually the same as the original formula except for the addition of Huang Qin (黃芩) and the subtraction of Sheng Jiang (生薑). The heat-clearing and dampness-drying actions of Huang Qin complement this formula's overall qi-moving, phlegm-transforming, and harmonizing the gallbladder and stomach actions making it suitable for the treatment of pathoconditions involving heat phlegm with repletion heat or residual heat patterns. Dr. Lee prescribes variants of this formula for a broad scope of ailments such as external contraction (common colds), insomnia, rhinitis, otitis, glaucoma, infertility (both male and female), and myasthenia gravis (damp-heat pattern type).

Wu Ling San (Calculi Formula)
(五苓散) (結石方)

Yu Gui (玉桂) 2 qian, Yan Hu Suo (延胡索), Mu Xiang (木香), Huang Bo (黃柏), Gan Cao (甘草) 3 qian each, Cang Zhu (蒼朮), Zhu Ling (豬苓), Fu Ling (茯苓) 5 qian each, Dang Gui (當歸) 8 qian, Ze Xie (澤瀉) 1 liang

This Yu Sheng version contains the essential components of the original formula except for Yu Gui (玉桂) replacing Gui Zhi (桂枝) and Cang Zhu (蒼朮) replacing Bai Zhu (白朮), and adding Dang Gui (當歸), Yan Hu Suo (延胡索), Mu Xiang (木香), Huang Bo (黃柏), and Gan Cao (甘草). This formula includes large doses of Ze Xie (澤瀉) for its water-inhibiting, dampness-percolating, and heat-draining actions and large doses of Dang Gui (當歸) for its blood-supplementing and blood-quickening actions – a medicinal pair that promotes smooth muscle contractions of the bile ducts, kidneys, and urinary tract thus resulting in dislogdement and evacuation of calculi. Mu Xiang moves qi, relieves pain, and relaxes smooth muscle; and Yan Hu Suo quickens the blood, moves qi, and functions as a strong analgesic to promote evacuation of calculi and provide relief for pain. Huang Bo drains lower burner fire, dries dampness, resolves toxin, and disinhibits the gallbladder to treat inflammation. As its name infers, Dr. Lee has specifically designed this formula for the treatment of calculi in the bile ducts (gallstones (choledocholithiasis)), pancreatic duct, kidneys (nephrolithiasis), and urethra.

Wu Ling San (Nephritis Formula)
(五苓散) (腎炎方)

Dang Gui (當歸) 2 qian, Gan Jiang (乾薑), Fu Zi (附子), Huang Bo (黃柏) 3 qian each, Zhu Ling (豬苓), Fu Ling (茯苓), Cang Zhu (蒼朮), Ze Xie (澤瀉), Yu Gui (玉桂) 5 qian each, Huang Qi (黃耆) 1 liang

This Yu Sheng version contains the essential components of the original formula except for Yu Gui (玉桂) replacing Gui Zhi (桂枝) and Cang Zhu (蒼朮) replacing Bai Zhu (白朮), and adding Dang Gui (當歸), Huang Qi (黃耆), Gan Jiang (乾薑), Fu Zi (附子), and Huang Bo (黃柏). Huang Qi supplements qi, disinhibits water and disperses swelling, increases myocardial contractility, promotes passage across membranes, and functions as a broad spectrum antimicrobial, which complements Dang Gui's actions of supplementing and quickening blood as these medicinals combine to improve renal blood flow and filtration through the glomeruli. Yu Gui reinforces yang, greatly supplements life gate fire, promotes blood circulation, and conducts medicinals throughout the entire body. Fu Zi supplements kidney yang and strengthens cardiac contractility. Together they function to increase stroke volume and reduce heart rate. This formula warms kidney yang, transforms qi, disinhibits water, and percolates dampness for the treatment of water-damp collecting internally, edema, and inhibited urination. Dr. Lee commonly prescribes this formula for the treatment of post-acute and chronic pathoconditions involving intrinsic renal disease which result in proteinuria, edema, uremia, and hypoalbuminemia (e.g., nephrotic syndrome, glomeronephritis, chronic kidney failure); pulmonary edema (e.g., intrinsic lung disease, congestive heart failure, kidney failure); and increased intracranial pressure (ICP).

Xi Ji (洗劑) (aka Vaginal Wash/Douche)

Long Dan Cao (龍膽草), She Chuang Zi (蛇床子), Xiong Huang (powder) (雄黃粉), Liu Huang (powder) (硫磺粉), Lu Gan Shi (powder) (爐甘石)

This formula composition is similar to **(Yu Sheng) Sai Ji (塞劑) (aka Vaginal Suppository)** except for the substraction of Da Huang (大黃) and the addition of Long Dan Cao (龍膽草) and Lu Gan Shi (powder) (爐甘石). It is prescribed for various types of vaginal infections presenting externally at the vulva including yeast (e.g., candidiasis), bacterial (e.g., gonorrhea), trichomoniasis, and genital herpes that present with itching, irritation, and watery or viscous vaginal discharge that occur inside the vaginal cavity. This formula is typically prescribed as part of a therapeutic regimen that includes decocted formulas taken orally such as **Long Dan Xie Gan Tang (龍膽瀉肝湯)**, **Jin Suo Gu Jing Wan (金鎖固經丸)**, or **Bu Zhong Yi Qi Tang (補中益氣湯)**.

Xian Fang Huo Ming Yin (仙方活命飲)

Chen Pi (陳皮), Tian Hua (天花), Jin Yin Hua (金銀花), Ru Xiang (乳香), Mo Yao (沒藥), Fang Feng (防風), Zao Jiao Ci (皂角刺), Dang Gui (當歸), Niu Bang Zi (牛蒡子), Chi Shao (赤芍), Bai Zhi (白芷), Gan Cao (甘草) 3 qian each, Cang Zhu (蒼朮) 4 qian Sheng Shi Gao (生石膏) 1 liang

The Yu Sheng version is similar to the original formula except for the exclusion of Bei Mu (貝母) and Chuan Shan Jia (穿山甲), which is an endangered animal species now prohibited. Instead, Dr. Lee includes Niu Bang Zi (牛蒡子) with its wind-coursing, heat-dissipating, papule-outthrusting, toxin-resolving, and swelling-dispersing actions; Sheng Shi Gao (生石膏) with its heat-clearing and fire-draining actions; and Cang Zhu (蒼朮) with its drying dampness and fortifying the spleen actions. These additions complement the blood-quickening, swelling-dispersing, pus-expelling, and channel passage-freeing actions of Zao Jiao Ci (皂角刺) and provide an effective alternative for the absence of Chuan Shan Jia. In TCM classical texts this formula is classified as a "sore sage formula" with its heat-clearing and toxin-resolving, swelling-dispersing and hardness-breaking, and blood-quickening and pain-relieving actions traditionally prescribed for the treatment of acute and post-acute stage swelling and toxin of welling-abscess (carbuncle, faruncle, boils) and sores in which there is localized redness, heat, swelling, and pain or generalized heat with mild aversion to cold. In addition to these types of external medicine pathoconditions, Dr. Lee prescribes this formula for pathoconditions such as innominate toxin swelling (both benign and malignant), cellulitis, appendicitis, postherpetic neuralgia, and pulmonary abscesses.

Xiang Sha Liu Jun Zi Tang (香砂六君子湯)

Dan Shen (丹參), Cang Zhu (蒼朮), Fu Ling (茯苓), Gan Cao (甘草), Mu Xiang (木香), Sha Ren (砂人) 3 qian each, Chen Pi (陳皮), Ban Xia (半夏) 4 qian each

The Yu Sheng version is similar to the original formula except that Dan Shen (丹參) replaces Ren Shen (人參) and Cang Zhu (蒼朮) replaces Bai Zhu (白朮), and Sheng Jiang (生薑) and Da Zao (大棗) are subtracted. Dan Shen engenders blood and dispels stasis; and Cang Zhu fortifies the spleen and dries dampness, which is ideal for northern Taiwan's humid climate. Depending on the presenting symptoms, signs, and pattern, Dr. Lee may prescribe Ren Shen (powder) (人參粉) (or Ren Shen (powder) and Chuan Qi (powder) paired). Also, for Sheng Jiang may be included as in the original formula for the treatment of morning sickness during first trimester of pregnancy. This formula's qi-boosting and spleen-fortifying and qi-moving and phlegm-transforming actions are traditionally administered for pathoconditions involving spleen and stomach vacuity, dampness obstructing and qi stagnation, abdominal distention after food intake, acid reflux, and poor appetite. Some specific pathoconditions Dr. Lee typically prescribes this formula for are gastrointestinal reflux disease (GERD), gastritis, autoimmune diseases (e.g., SLE), ascites (e.g., hepatic disorders), renal disease (e.g., azotemia), and poor appetite and malnutrition during the late stages of cancer.

The qi-boosting and spleen-fortifying and qi-moving and phlegm-transforming actions of **Xiang Sha Liu Jun Zi Tang (香砂六君子湯)** forms the foundation of the three formulas that treat the "allergic triad" manifestions of atopy – **Qi Chuan Fang (氣喘方) (aka Asthma Formula)** (i.e., lung), **Yi Wei Xing Pi Fu Yan Fang (異位性皮膚炎方) (aka Atopic Dermatitis Formula)** (i.e., skin), and **Ying Feng Luo Lei Fang (迎風落淚方) (aka Tearing on Exposure to Wind Formula)** (i.e., sinuses). These hyperallergic reactions may present as inflammatory responses in the lungs. In TCM theory, the spleen belongs to earth and engenders metal, governs movement and transformation of the essence of grain and water, and also governs the flesh. The lung belongs to metal, governs qi, skin and hair, opens at the nose, and has an upward and outward diffusing movement, which is responsible for carrying moisture and nourishment to the skin. These descriptions of physiological mechanisms correlate with the lymphatics, immune system, metabolism, ANS, and CNS in modern biomedicine and provide the foundations for pattern identification as the basis of treatment.

Xiao Chai Hu Tang (小柴胡湯)

Huang Qin (黃芩) 3 qian, Dan Shen (丹參), Ban Xia (半夏), Gan Cao (甘草), Sheng Jiang (生薑) 5 qian each Hong Zao (紅棗) 5 pieces, Chai Hu (柴胡) 6 qian

The Yu Sheng version is nearly identical to the original formula except for Dan Shen (丹參) replacing Ren Shen (人參). However, depending on the presenting symptoms, signs, and pattern identification, Ren Shen (powder) (人參粉) (or Ren Shen (powder) and Chuan Qi (powder) paired) may also be included. Traditionally, this is a commonly prescribed formula for the treatment of lesser yang (Shao Yang)-harmonizing pathoconditions (e.g., alternating heat and cold, fullness in the chest and rib-side, no desire for food and drink), general discomfort or pain in the hypochondriac region, heat entering the blood chamber, and pathoconditions of the liver, gallbladder, and spleen (e.g., hepatitis, cholecystitis, splenitis). Dr. Lee's application of this formula can be classified into three broad categories: 1) Depressed heat (i.e., persisten low-grade fever) following external contraction (common colds) in pediatric patients and in tuberculosis (TB) patients whom have been administered antibiotic treatment; 2) Microbial infections, toxins (e.g., noxious chemicals), or autoimmune reaction leading to metabolic waste buildup that disrupts the capacity of the nervous system (specifically, the coordianted interactions of the CNS, ANS, and PNS) to regulate bodily functions and maintain homeostasis, thus resulting in dyscrasias (e.g. leukemia, hemophilia, multiple myeloma); and 3) For complex pattern pathoconditions that are difficult to diagnose and pathoconditions in a transitional state this half-interior half exterior (midstage penetration) formula is prescribed until definitive pattern identification can be ascertained (e.g., whether a pathocondition is passing from the exterior into the interior or from the interior into the exterior).

Xue Ku Fang
(血枯方) (aka Blood Desiccation Formula)

Cang Zhu (蒼朮), Ci Ji Li (刺蒺藜) 4 qian each

Dang Gui (當歸), He Shou Wu (何首烏), Tu Si Zi (菟絲子), Sha Yuan Ji Li (沙苑蒺藜) 8 qian each

The term blood dessication first appears in the *The Yellow Emperor's Inner Cannon* and refers to this pathocondition as blood vacuity following hemorrhage. Indeed, Dr. Lee's adaptation of this term covers a much broader scope of applications. This Yu Sheng original formula has similar actions and clinical applications as **Dang Gui Yin Zi (當歸飲子)** containing the essential medicinals Dang Gui (當歸), He Shou Wu (何首烏), and Ci Ji Li (刺蒺藜). However, it replaces Shao Yao (芍藥), Chuan Qiong (川芎), and Sheng Di Huang (生地黃) with large doses of Dang Gui and He Shou Wu; subtracts Fang Feng (放風), Jing Jie (荊芥), and Huang Qi (黃耆); and adds Sha Yuan Ji Li (沙苑蒺藜), Tu Si Zi (菟絲子), and Cang Zhu (蒼朮). Sha Yuan Ji Li and Tu Si Zi both supplement the kidney, secure essence, and nourish the liver; and Cang Zhu dispels wind-damp and dries dampness and fortifies the spleen to counteract the potential of digestion impairment and loose stools resulting from blood-nourishing and yin-enriching medicinals. These additions complement this formula's overall actions of nourishing the blood, moistening dryness, dispeling wind, and relieving itching for the treatment of yin vacuity, blood vacuity, and blood desiccation patterns. For the treatment of skin pathoconditions the relatively hardier Ma Huang (麻黃) is added in place of Fang Feng and Jing Jie whose volatile oils and exterior-resolving actions easily vaporize upon decoction requiring large doses to achieve efficacy; and if itchiness presents, then Lu Lu Tong (路路通) will also be added. Dr. Lee typically prescribes this formula for wind-dryness presenting as dry, itchy skin, and possibly mild redness (e.g., pruritis, erythema, urticaria, eczema, atopic dermatitis), liver blood vacuity (e.g., hepatic cirrhosis during late stages with darkened skin and compromised hematopoiesis), and endometrial hypoperfusion (e.g., causing infertility and miscarriage).

Yi Wei Xing Pi Fu Yan Fang
(異位性皮膚炎方) (aka Atopic Dermatitis Formula)

Ma Huang (麻黃) 1.5 qian, Dan Shen (丹參), Cang Zhu (蒼朮), Fu Ling (茯苓), Gan Cao (甘草), Chen Pi (陳皮), Ban Xia (半夏), Mu Xiang (木香), Sha Ren (砂仁), Xing Ren (杏仁), Bai Guo (百果), Wu Wei Zi (五味子), Shan Yao (山藥) 3 qian each, Dang Gui (當歸), He Shou Wu (何首烏), Tu Si Zi (菟絲子), Sha Yuan Zi (沙苑子) 5 qian each

This is an Yu Sheng original compound formula derived from **Qi Chuan Fang (氣喘方) (aka Asthma Formula)** (subtracting Yu Gui (玉桂)) and **Xue Ku Fang (血枯方) (aka Blood Desiccation Formula)** (subtracting Ci Ji Li (刺蒺藜)). **Qi Chuan Fang (氣喘方) (aka Asthma Formula)** supplements the spleen, lung, and kidneys, nourishes yin, resolves the exterior, opens the pores, and dispels phlegm; and **Xue Ku Fang (血枯方) (aka Blood Desiccation Formula)** nourishes blood, enriches yin, and dispels wind. As its name indicates, Dr. Lee administers this formula for the treatment of atopic dermatitis, and specifically spleen yang vacuity patttern type.

Depending on the patient's presenting symptoms and pattern, the following medicinals are commonly added: Shi Gao (石膏), Lu Lu Tong (路路通), and Hua Shi (滑石) for severe pruritis; Bai Xian Pi (白鮮皮), Huang Qin (黃芩), Yi Yi Ren (薏苡仁) for flare-ups with excessive suppuration; and for chronic persistent cases with erythematous lesions in body creases (or generalized), cracking, suppuration, pruritis, and agitation the dose of **Xue Ku Fang (血枯方) (aka Blood Desiccation Formula)** will be increased and small doses of Gan Jiang (乾薑), Fu Zi (附子), and Yu Gui (玉桂) added to supplement kidney and spleen vacuity and return and reinforce yang.

Ying Feng Luo Lei Fang (迎風落淚方) (aka Tearing on Exposure to Wind Formula)

Ma huang (麻黃) 1.5 qian, Dan Shen (丹參), Cang Zhu (蒼朮), Fu Ling (茯苓), Gan Cao (甘草) Chen Pi (陳皮), Ban Xia (半夏), Mu Xiang (木香), Sha Ren (砂仁), Xi Xin (細辛), Wu Wei Zi (五味子) 3 qian each, Bai Guo (白果) 4 qian, Yu Gui (玉桂) 5 qian

This original Yu Sheng formula is similar to **Qi Chuan Fang (氣喘方) (aka Asthma Formula)** above except for the substractions of Shan Yao (山藥) and Xing Ren (杏仁) and the addition of Xi Xin (細辛). Xi Xin dispels wind and dissipates cold, frees the orifices, relieves pain, and warms the lung and transforms rheum; Ma Huang (麻黃) promotes sweating, resolves the exterior, and frees the nasal orifices; Wu Wei Zi (五味子) constrains the lung and stabilizes panting; Bai Guo (白果) constrains the lung and dispels phlegm; and Yu Gui warms and supplements qi and aides spleen and kidney yang for vacuity asthma. Depending on the presenting signs and symptoms, Dr. Lee may also add Gan Jiang (乾薑) and Fu Zi (附子) to further enhance this formula's spleen and kidney yang-supplementing actions. Together, these medicinals complement the qi-boosting and spleen-fortifying and qi-moving and phlegm-transforming actions of **Xiang Sha Liu Jun Zi Tang (香砂六君子湯)**.

As its name indicates, this formula is specifically designed for the treatment of "tearing on exposure to wind," the classical TCM pathological term that directly correlates with allergic rhinitis and other pathoconditions of the sinuses in modern biomedicine. The underlying pathomechanism of "tearing on exposure to wind" is spleen yang vacuity pattern, which inhibits the spleen's capacity to absorb and diffuse nutrients throughout the entire body resulting in a compromised immune system and the inability to govern flesh. Dr. Lee explains this pathocondition as follows: "Persistent and prolonged sneezing, nasal discharge, and post-nasal drip further irritates the lacrimal gland causing slackening of the lacrimal gland at the inner canthus of the eye and the exacerbation of profuse eye tearing."

You Gui Yin (右歸飲)

Dang Gui (當歸), Fu Ling (茯苓) 2 qian each

Gou Qi Zi (枸杞子), Huang Bo (黃柏), Gan Jiang (乾薑) 3 qian each, Gan Di Huang (乾地黃), Shan Zhu Yu (山茱萸), Shan Yao (山藥), Cang Zhu (蒼朮), Du Zhong (杜仲), Tu Si Zi (菟絲子) 4 qian each

Fu Zi (附子), Niu Xi (牛膝), Yu Gui (玉桂) 5 qian each

The Yu Sheng version combines medicinals from **(Yu Sheng) Shen Qi Wan (腎氣丸)** and the original version of **You Gui Wan (右歸丸)**, but adds medicinals to enhance its kidney yang-warming and supplementing actions. Gan Di Huang (乾地黃) is included instead of Shou Di Huang (熟地黃), and Huang Bo (黃柏), Gan Jiang (乾薑), Cang Zhu (蒼朮), and Niu Xi (牛膝) are added. Along with providing blood-quickening, sinew and bone-strengthening, and liver and kidney-supplementing actions, Niu Xi (牛膝) and Du Zhong (杜仲) serve as channel conductors directing medicinals to the lower limbs. Huang Bo counteracts the heat of the great yang supplementing medicinals and Cang Zhu dries dampness and fortifies the spleen to counteract the potential of digestion impairment and loose stools resulting from large doses of blood-nourishing and yin-enriching and yang-supplementing medicinals. Dr. Lee commonly prescribes this formula for a wide range of yang vacuity and depletion pattern pathoconditions such as lumbar and back pain (e.g., radiculopathy (sciatica) from herniated intervertebral disc, spondylolisthesis, spinal stenosis), limp knees and weak legs (e.g., various post-acute articular cartilage, ligament, and tendon injuries), congenital development disorders, and atopy (especially in male patients) (i.e., chronic stage asthma, tearing on exposure to wind, atopic dermatitis).

Yu Sheng Wan (育生丸)

Man Tuo Luo Hua (曼陀羅花) 0.04g/pill

Shan Yao (山藥) 0.6g/pill

This is a commonly prescribed pill that Dr. Lee includes in the treatment regimen for a broad spectrum of pathoconditions. The principal medicinal in this pill is Man Tuo Luo Hua (曼陀羅花) (white flower of the datura plant, *Datura metel L.*) whose bioactive compounds are the anticholinergics scopolamine and hyoscyamine. Dr. Lee believes that the pharmacodynamics involve this pill's capacity to stimulate cerebral collateral circulation and rejuvenate the brain's self-regulating (autoregulation) function. Cerebral circulation fluctuates in response to the physical and mental activities and metabolic processes and normally the brain is able to self-regulate (autoregulation) in oder to maintain homeostasis. However, certain pathoconditions as well as the process of aging may lead to microvascular changes, decreased vascular density, and pericyte degeneration that cause the brain to "misinterpret" the internal environment it holds dominion over, becoming "fooled" into a compromised state of errantly perceived homeostasis in the midst of actual imbalance. Dr. Lee utilizes the actions of these properties to supplement the brain, remedy insomnia and depression, eliminate anxiety and stress, slow the degenerative process of aging and disease (e.g., dementia, Alzheimer's disease, Parkinson's disease), relieve all types of pain, check spasm, and stabilize panting (asthma). Its capacity to relax smooth muscle makes it effective for treating overactive bladder (females) and enlarged prostate (males) and promoting the passage of urinary tract stones (urolithiasis) and gallstones (cholelithiasis) (i.e., large 1x dose of 4~6 pills (males) and 4~8 pills (females) accompanied by acupuncture). It is also prescribed as a part of Dr. Lee's cancer treatment protocol. The efficacy of this pill is very much dose-related with large doses potentially causing side effects such as dry mouth, drowsiness, blurry vision, and confusion; thus, it is essential to limit the standard dosage to 1~3 pills per day.

Zhi Bo Di Huang Tang (知柏地黃湯)

Gan Cao (甘草), Huang Bo (黃柏) 3 qian, Zhi Mu (知母), Shan Zhu Yu (山茱萸), Shan Yao (山藥), Fu Ling (茯苓), Mu Dan Pi (牡丹皮) Ze Xie (澤瀉), Niu Xi (牛膝), Cang Zhu (蒼朮) 4 each qian, Gan Di Huang (乾地黃) 8 qian

The Yu Sheng version is similar to the original formula except for Gan Di Huang (乾地黃) replacing Shu Di Huang (熟地黃) and the addition of Niu Xi (牛膝), Cang Zhu (蒼朮), and Gan Cao (甘草). Niu Xi (牛膝) quickens the blood, strengthens the sinews and bones, and is a channel conductor leading other medicinals downward; Cang Zhu supplements the spleen and dries dampness; and Gan Cao supplements the center and harmonizes the nature of medicinals. The combination of Huang Bo (黃柏), Niu Xi, and Cang Zhu forms **San Miao San (三妙散)**, a commonly prescribed heat-clearing and dampness-drying formula used for pathoconditions in the lower burner and lower limbs such as genitourinary (damp-heat pouring downward) and arthritic ailments. Dr. Lee typically prescribes this yin-enriching and fire-downbearing formula for effulgent yin vacuity fire and steaming bone pathoconditions such as osteoarthritis, pulling of the sinews (e.g., sprains, strains osteomyelitis), bone fractures, heel pain syndrome, tuberculosis, "yin vacuity cough" (aka dryness cough) in the kidney channel, epilepsy, diabetes, genitourinary tract disorders, seminal emission, and menopausal symptoms. This is an essential formula for acute and sub-acute muskuloskeletal injuries (e.g., arthritic, traumatic, autoimmune) manifesting in swelling and inflammation because of its capacity to promote self-repair and prevent the potential development of further degeneration (e.g., fibrosis, enthesopathy) that may arise as complications following aspiration, bleeding, and administration of anti-inflammatory agents.

Zuo Gui Yin (左歸飲)

Dang Gui (當歸) 2 qian, Gou Qi Zi (枸杞子), Fu Ling (茯苓), Gan Cao (甘草) 3 qian each, Gan Di Huang (乾地黃), Shan Zhu Yu (山茱萸), Shan Yao (Shan Yao), Tu Si Zi (菟絲子), Du Zhong (杜仲), Cang Zhu (蒼朮) 4 qian each, Niu Xi (牛膝) 5 qian

The Yu Sheng version is similar to the original formula except for replacing Shou Di Huang (熟地黃) with Gan Di Huang (乾地黃) and adding Niu Xi (牛膝), Du Zhong (杜仲), and Tu Si Zi (菟絲子). Niu Xi quickens the blood, frees the channels, supplements the liver and kidney, strengthens sinews and bones, and conducts medicinals downward to the lumbus and lower limbs; Du Zhong supplements the liver and kidney, strengthens sinews and bones, and conducts medicinals downward to the lumbus and lower limbs; and Tu Si Zi supplements the kidney and secures essence. These additions enhance this formula's essence replenishing and blood-supplmenting actions and complements it with warm natured kidney yang supplementation medicinals targeting the lumbus and lower limbs. In the early years of Dr. Lee's clinical practice, he would prescribe this formula for lumbar and back pain (e.g., back muscle strains and sprains) and limp knees and weak legs (e.g., various articular cartilage, ligament, and tendon injuries) in which heat pattern (inflammation) was still presenting or for certain patients with yin vacuity constitiutions. Nowadays, Dr. Lee does not prescribe this formula, choosing instead to use **Zhi Bo Di Huang Tang (知柏地黃湯)** variants instead.

BIBLIOGRAPHY

Bensky, Dan, Steve Clavey, Erich Stoger. *Chinese Herbal Medicine: Materia Medica* (3rd Edition). Eastland Press, 2015.

Chang, Hsian-che; Tsai, Gui-hua. *Processing of Traditional Chinese Medicine Materia Medica* Second Edition. Taichung, Taiwan (R.O.C.): China Medical University, 2003.

Chen, Shi-gong. *Orthodox Manual of External Medicine.* China: Qing Dynasty (1617).

Clinical Applications of Traditional Chinese Medicinals. Taipei, Taiwan (R.O.C.): Cheers Books Co., 1988.

Harrison's Principles of Internal Medicine 19th Edition. McGraw-Hill, 2015.

Lee, Chen-yu. *Neuropathy: Traditional Chinese Herbal Treatment in a Modern Medical Environment.* tr. Daniel L. Altschuler. Taipei, Taiwan (R.O.C.): Cheers Books Co., 2005.

Lee, Chen-yu. *Traditional Chinese Medicine Treatment of Common Liver Diseases.* Taipei, Taiwan (R.O.C.): Cheers Books Co., 2001.

Neal, Anthony J., Peter J. Hoskin. Clinical Oncology Basic Principles and Practice (Third Edition). London, UK: Arnold, 2003.

Oswald, Cyril, Frank Delaigue. *Les Hommes de l'Art*. You-Feng (Librairie), 2013.

The Yellow Emperor's Inner Cannon. China: Eastern Han Dynasty.

Wang, Ang. *The Essential Herbal Foundation*. China: Qing Dynasty (1694).

Wang, Qing-ren. *Correction of Errors in Medical Classics*. China: Qing Dynasty (1830).

Wiseman, Nigel and Ye, Feng. *A Practical Dictionary of Chinese Medicine* Second Edition. Brookline, Massachusetts: Paradigm Publications, 1998.

Wu, Qian. *The Golden Mirror of Medicine*. China: Qing Dynasty (1742).

Wu, Qian. *Essential Teachings on Miscellaneous Diseases*. China: Qing Dynasty (1742).
Zhang Ji [Zhong-jing]. *On Cold Damage and Miscellaneous Diseases*. China: Eastern Han Dynasty.

https://www.cancer.org/

http://www.cancer.net/

https://www.cancerresearchuk.org/

https://my.clevelandclinic.org/

http://www.mayoclinic.org/

http://www.merckmanuals.com/professional

http://www.pathophys.org/

http://yibian.hopto.org/ (a Chinese language online TCM databank)

ABOUT THE AUTHOR

The author has spent the better part of the past 25 years in Taiwan and China immersed in Chinese culture and pursuing related studies in literature, philosophy, religion, music, martial arts, and of course traditional Chinese medicine (TCM).

From 1993 to 1996, he learned Mandarin at Normal Taiwan University Mandarin Training Center; from 2001 to 2007, he precepted under the tutelage of Dr. Lee Chen-Yu at the Yu Sheng Chinese Medicine Clinic; and from 2007 to 2012, he studied in the Post-baccalaureate Chinese Medicine program at China Medical University in Taichung, Taiwan, which included a Western medicine clerkship at Tri-Service General Hospital and TCM internships at Taipei Municipal Heping Hospital, Taipei City Hospital – Kunming TCM Branch, and Taipei City Hospital – Linsen TCM Branch.

Upon completion of his Chinese medicine degree in 2012 to the present, he has had the honor and privilege of returning to assist Dr. Lee in the clinical setting as well as compiling and translating academic papers, case study presentations, and now this three volume series of correspondences.

ABOUT THE EDITOR

Marc Wasserman studied under Dr. Lee Chen Yu from 2004 through 2014. During those years, he worked directly with patients in the clinic while also assisting Dr. Lee with research, translation, and publication projects. He and Dr. Lee often travelled together, making presentations at various international medical conferences.

Marc is a graduate of the doctoral program at Liaoning University of Traditional Chinese Medicine, a prestigious medical school in northeastern China. He is the first American of non-Asian heritage to complete the program. He holds a visiting professorship with Liaoning University of Traditional Chinese Medicine, and is an adjunct professor at Virginia University of Oriental Medicine.

Currently, Dr.Wasserman runs a small clinic in Hunt Valley, Maryland. For more information on his practice, please visit www.flowhealthclinic.com

www.ingramcontent.com/pod-product-compliance
Lightning Source LLC
Chambersburg PA
CBHW020631220526
45464CB00001B/106